Next-Generation Therapeutics Using Internet of Things and Machine Learning

Mohammed Shuaib
Jazan University, Saudi Arabia

Shadab Alam
Jazan University, Saudi Arabia

A. Rajaram
E.G.S. Pillay Engineering College, India

Kishor Kumar Reddy C.
Stanley College of Engineering and Technology for Women, India

IGI Global
Scientific Publishing
Publishing Tomorrow's Research Today

Vice President of Editorial Melissa Wagner
Director of Acquisitions Mikaela Felty
Director of Book Development Jocelynn Hessler
Production Manager Mike Brehm
Cover Design Jose Rosado

Published in the United States of America by
IGI Global Scientific Publishing
701 East Chocolate Avenue
Hershey, PA, 17033, USA
Tel: 717-533-8845
Fax: 717-533-7115
Website: https://www.igi-global.com E-mail: cust@igi-global.com

Library of Congress Cataloging-in-Publication Data

Names: Shuaib, Mohammed, 1989- editor | Alam, Shadab, 1985- editor | Ayyasamy, Rajaram, 1982- editor | Reddy, C. Kishor Kumar editor
Title: Next-generation therapeutics using Internet of Things and machine learning / edited by Mohammed Shuaib, Shadab Alam, Rajaram Ayyasamy, Kishor Kumar Reddy C.
Description: Hershey, PA : IGI Global Scientific Publishing, [2025] | Includes bibliographical references and index. | Summary: "The objective of this book is to provide a comprehensive framework for understanding and implementing IoT and ML in healthcare and environmental monitoring. By exploring practical applications, this book aims to equip researchers, practitioners, and students with insights into how these technologies are reshaping diagnostics, patient care, operational efficiencies, and environmental sustainability"-- Provided by publisher.

Identifiers: LCCN 2024060445 (print) | LCCN 2024060446 (ebook) | ISBN 9798337310220 hardcover | ISBN 9798337310237 paperback | ISBN 9798337310244 ebook
Subjects: LCSH: Artificial intelligence--Medical applications | Internet of things--Medical applications
Classification: LCC R859.7.A78 N498 2025 (print) | LCC R859.7.A78 (ebook) | DDC 610.285--dc23/eng/20250515
LC record available at https://lccn.loc.gov/2024060445
LC ebook record available at https://lccn.loc.gov/2024060446
British Cataloguing in Publication Data
A Cataloguing in Publication record for this book is available from the British Library.

Table of Contents

Detailed Table of Contents

The integration of cutting-edge technology such as artificial intelligence and the Internet of Things has altered the landscape of healthcare delivery. This study investigates current advances in digital health technology, such as electronic health records, wearable devices, and health monitoring systems, that have dramatically improved patient treatment and outcomes. As healthcare expenses grow internationally and sustainability becomes a significant problem, AI and IoT provide potential solutions to improve healthcare efficiency, lower costs, and solve difficulties such as aging population and environmental concerns. The combination of AI and IoT results in smarter systems that optimise healthcare operations by providing remote patient monitoring, predictive equipment maintenance, and improved data security. This study also discusses significant AI functions and the constraints of AI and IoT in healthcare are explored, such as data privacy, high prices, interoperability issues. Future advances in the industry to improve healthcare sustainability.

The Internet of Things (IoT) has transformed healthcare by enabling smart healthcare systems focused on real-time monitoring, data-driven insights, and improved patient outcomes. IoMT (Internet of Medical Things) and Healthcare 4.0 are evolving with technologies like AI, edge computing, and 5G, supporting efficient, connected, and mobile health services. Despite rapid progress, gaps remain in understanding implementation challenges, design complexities, and adoption barriers. This study reviews recent advancements, identifies enabling technologies, and outlines future requirements for scalable, secure, and intelligent healthcare systems. It also proposes research directions to enhance IoT-driven healthcare delivery in the post-pandemic era.

Machine learning (ML) is revolutionizing healthcare by offering innovative solutions that enhance delivery, outcomes, and efficiency. This chapter highlights ML's significance in healthcare, addressing current trends, challenges, and techniques like supervised, unsupervised, and reinforcement learning. Applications in disease diagnosis, medical imaging, drug discovery, personalized treatments, and remote monitoring are explored. It also delves into data sharing, security, and real-time monitoring through IoT and blockchain, along with NLP advancements automating clinical documentation and sentiment analysis. Real-life case studies on AI-based radiology and chronic disease prediction demonstrate its impact. Ethical and regulatory issues, such as data privacy, biases in AI models, and emerging paradigms like federated learning for secure, decentralized healthcare, are discussed. The chapter envisions a future where ML transforms healthcare to become more efficient, personalized, and accessible while addressing critical ethical considerations.

Collecting, organizing, analyzing, and managing health data is the focus of health information management. Computer Science, Data Analytics, Information Science, Medicine, Business, And Information Management are all parts of it. A new topic within healthcare, machine learning (ML) is rapidly developing. They provide faster and more accurate analysis of health data. Artificial intelligence (AI) is a crucial area within software engineering. Drawing on knowledge gained from prior experiences or lessons learned, it provides a simplified solution to these problems of the present. As a field, software engineering makes use of specialized machine learning computations. Machine learning techniques such as Recurrent Neural Networks, Decision Trees, Naive Bayes Classifier, Ensemble Vector Machine, and Linear discriminant Analysis are introduced in this chapter. The methods are all laid out in great detail, allowing the reader to come up with their solutions to the problems provided.

Improving patient risk score structures, anticipating the start of illness, and optimizing hospital operations are just a few examples of the practical insights that may be generated by applying machine learning to electronic health records (EHRs). Better patient outcomes, more efficient operations, and better decision-making are all possible thanks to predictive analytics in healthcare. Discover the ways this technology revolutionizes patient care by facilitating early intervention, cutting expenses, and enhancing overall efficiency. There is a promising gap in the literature about statistical models that take use of the diversity and depth of data obtained from HER. We review the benefits of machine learning over more conventional analytical techniques and provide an outline of its use in clinical settings in this chapter. We outline the practical and methodological difficulties when applying machine learning in both academia and industry. As a conclusion, we provide our thoughts on potential machine learning uses in the future that might have far-reaching effects on healthcare.

Real-time remote patient monitoring, enabled by the integration of biosensors and multi-hop Internet of Things (IoT) networks, marks a transformative shift in modern healthcare. Biosensors placed throughout healthcare environments transmit vital data via interconnected microcontrollers to centralized servers using secure cloud infrastructure. Emphasizing systems developed for elderly care, this study categorizes key architectures, examines deployment challenges, and identifies opportunities for further innovation. Remote health monitoring solutions enhance continuous care, support independent living, and ensure rapid medical response through real-time access to patient data. By leveraging IoT and cloud connectivity, these systems promise to overcome traditional care limitations and elevate healthcare accessibility and quality.

The healthcare industry is currently experiencing a significant and groundbreaking change as a result of the integration of fifth-generation (5G) mobile communication technologies, Artificial Intelligence (AI), Machine Learning, Deep Learning, and Internet of Things (IoT). This research paper explores the complex interaction of various technologies, with a specific focus on the crucial role of 5G in enabling and improving healthcare applications. The study examines the potential of 5G-enabled IoT technologies in the field of smart healthcare, focusing on their ability to bring about significant changes in terms of network performance, device density, energy efficiency, and security. The paper addresses necessary prerequisites for the effective implementation of 5G scenarios in healthcare settings as it evolves. The technical requirements, analyzed key performance indicators (KPIs), and deployment circumstances together provide a roadmap for the future development and integration of advanced healthcare solutions that utilize the latest technology breakthroughs.

Automated healthcare systems, powered by artificial intelligence are revolutionizing medical diagnosis, treatment, and patient care by offering enhanced precision, efficiency, and scalability. However, their deployment raises critical ethical considerations. Issues such as patient privacy, data security, and informed consent are paramount, given the sensitive nature of healthcare data. Bias in algorithms can lead to unequal treatment and exacerbate healthcare disparities, while the lack of transparency and explainability in AI decision-making challenges trust and accountability. Furthermore, determining liability in cases of errors or harm caused by autonomous systems complicates legal and ethical responsibility. The balance between AI autonomy and human oversight is crucial to ensure safety and fairness. As automated healthcare continues to evolve, fostering ethical frameworks that prioritize equity, inclusivity, and patient rights is essential for building systems that enhance health outcomes while maintaining public trust and adherence to societal values.

Preface

The convergence of advanced technologies such as Artificial Intelligence (AI), the Internet of Things (IoT), Machine Learning (ML), and blockchain is redefining the healthcare ecosystem on a global scale. Next-Generation Therapeutics Using Internet of Things and Machine Learning presents a curated collection of scholarly contributions that explore the dynamic intersections of technology and healthcare innovation. As global healthcare systems grapple with increasing demands for accessibility, personalization, and sustainability, this volume aims to provide a multidisciplinary blueprint for the future of digital health interventions.

This edited volume gathers contributions from leading researchers and practitioners across academia and industry. The chapters collectively offer a unique blend of theoretical frameworks, empirical studies, practical implementations, and future outlooks. Topics range from intelligent diagnostics and remote health monitoring to ethical considerations in automated healthcare, all framed within the evolving technological, regulatory, and societal landscapes.

The primary audience for this volume includes academic researchers, graduate students, healthcare professionals, technologists, hospital administrators, and policymakers interested in the transformative potential of AI and IoT. Additionally, it serves as a reference guide for courses in health informatics, machine learning applications, and digital transformation in healthcare.

CHAPTER OVERVIEW

Chapter 1 examines the transformative potential of integrating AI and IoT in healthcare ecosystems, emphasizing enhanced efficiency, real-time decision-making, and sustainability goals.

Chapter 2 explores the application of IoT technologies in revolutionizing healthcare delivery and patient monitoring, detailing remote sensing architectures and intelligent patient engagement strategies.

Chapter 3 investigates machine learning techniques applied to healthcare, showcasing advancements in diagnostics, predictive analytics, and treatment personalization.

Chapter 4 delves into advanced machine learning techniques driving innovations in personalized medicine and clinical decision-making frameworks.

Chapter 5 emphasizes the role of predictive analytics in proactive healthcare management, highlighting how predictive modeling can improve patient outcomes and reduce healthcare costs.

Chapter 6 presents innovative architectures for remote health monitoring systems, aiming to improve accessibility and care delivery in underserved regions through IoT and AI solutions.

Chapter 7 discusses the convergence of personalized medicine and IoT technologies, proposing models for precision healthcare that adapt dynamically to individual patient needs.

Chapter 8 focuses on operational improvements in healthcare organizations driven by AI, addressing process optimization, workflow automation, and decision-support systems.

Chapter 9 builds on operational improvements, examining how AI enhances clinical workflows, optimizes resource allocation, and transforms patient care models.

Chapter 10 examines AI's impact on transforming healthcare operations and boosting clinical efficiency, offering empirical insights into digital transformation strategies.

Chapter 11 tackles security and privacy challenges in IoT-enabled healthcare ecosystems, proposing robust frameworks for safeguarding sensitive medical data.

Chapter 12 explores blockchain technology as a transformative solution for secure and transparent medical data exchanges, ensuring data integrity and patient trust.

Chapter 13 analyzes the interoperability of health data systems, emphasizing the technical and regulatory frameworks needed for seamless digital healthcare integration.

Chapter 14 reviews advancements in remote health monitoring technologies, discussing current applications, emerging trends, and future research directions.

Chapter 15 highlights how integrating 5G and emerging technologies enables smart healthcare systems, discussing real-time data processing and low-latency remote care.

Chapter 16 concludes by critically examining ethical considerations in automated healthcare and advocating for responsible AI deployment and transparent governance models.

This compilation captures the transformative technological trends shaping modern healthcare and reflects the urgent need for interdisciplinary, secure, and ethically grounded solutions. Through bridging engineering innovations with medical practice, Next-Generation Therapeutics Using Internet of Things and Machine Learning aspires to inspire researchers, practitioners, and decision-makers to collaboratively navigate and accelerate the future of healthcare innovation.

Mohammed Shuaib, Shadab Alam, Kishor Kumar Reddy C, Rajaram Ayyasamy

Chapter 1
Transforming Healthcare With AI and IoT:
A Path Towards to Efficiency and Sustainability

Shivani Bhardwaj
Shoolini University, India

Gaurav Gupta
https://orcid.org/0000-0002-5192-4428
Shoolini University, India

Sultan Ahmad
https://orcid.org/0000-0002-3198-7974
Prince Sattam Bin Abdulaziz University, Alkharj, Saudi Arabia & Chandigarh University, Mohali, India

Md. Alimul Haque
https://orcid.org/0000-0002-0744-0784
Veer Kunwar Singh University, India

ABSTRACT

The integration of cutting-edge technology such as artificial intelligence and the Internet of Things has altered the landscape of healthcare delivery. This study investigates current advances in digital health technology, such as electronic health records, wearable devices, and health monitoring systems, that have dramatically improved patient treatment and outcomes. As healthcare expenses grow internationally and sustainability becomes a significant problem, AI and IoT provide potential solutions to improve healthcare efficiency, lower costs, and solve difficulties such as aging population and environmental concerns. The combination of AI and IoT results in smarter systems that optimise healthcare operations by providing remote patient monitoring, predictive equipment maintenance, and improved data security. This study also discusses significant AI functions and the constraints of AI and IoT in healthcare are explored, such as data privacy, high prices, interoperability issues. Future advances in the industry to improve healthcare sustainability.

DOI: 10.4018/979-8-3373-1022-0.ch001

INTRODUCTION

Globally, there has been a surge of interest in engineering approaches to healthcare delivery. Because of fast advancements in medical equipment, clinical procedures, data analytics and information technology. Recent advances in digital health technology, such as electronic health records, health monitoring systems, and wearable devices, alter care delivery and improve outcomes such as treatment quality and patient safety. These developments have important socioeconomic ramifications, as healthcare expenses contribute to approximately 20% of US GDP(Li and Carayon 2021).The healthcare sector has several sustainability issues, including rising prices, ageing populations, and growing environmental concerns. The convergence of Internet of Things (IoT) with Artificial Intelligence (AI) technology shows promises in addressing these difficulties. Internet of things enabled devices offers remote patient monitoring, predictive medical equipment maintenance, and energy efficiency optimization in healthcare facilities and systems(Akhter 2023). Modern healthcare has several issues, including handling massive volumes of patient data, assuring correct diagnoses, providing efficient remote patient monitoring, and protecting data. Integrating Artificial Intelligence with the internet of Things provides answers to these issues by enabling smarter, more efficient systems. AI and IoT work together to improve healthcare efficiency, patient outcomes, and data security, solving crucial concerns in today's healthcare landscape.

Figure 1. Number of Publication per year on AI and IoT in healthcare.

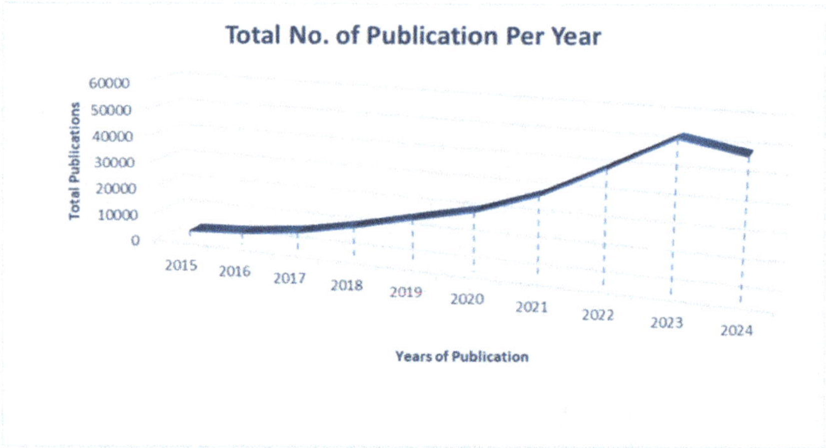

Figure 1 shows the publication per year in artificial intelligence and Internet of things in healthcare. Sustainable health care is an important part of connected life. Smart health care is expected to generate billions of dollars in income, fulfilling a fundamental human need. Smart health care involves various components, including IoT, IoMT, medical sensors, AI, edge computing, cloud computing, and next-generation wireless communication technologies. Several studies in the literature focus on smart health care or healthcare in general(Alshehri and Muhammad 2021). Renewable health care is a vital part of linked living. Smart health care is predicted to earn billions of dollars in revenue while meeting a basic human need. Smart health care consists of several components, including IoT, IoMT, medical sensors, AI, edge computing, cloud computing, and next-generation wireless communication technologies. Several studies in the literature examine smart health care or healthcare in general(Saraswat et al. 2022). Life sciences and pharmaceutical industries have a substantial potential and difficulty in accessing large-scale real-world data (RWD) to assist basic and translational science in clinical research and accepted manuscript development. Randomized, controlled trials provide high-quality data on limited patient populations, while high-volume, routinely collected data can provide insights into the health situation and treatment effectiveness in a more diverse patient population. This also allows for hypothesis generation regarding rare conditions, effects, and biomarkers. Using RWD in population health data analysis is not a novel approach, since it has been used for decades to acquire knowledge(Singh et al. 2018).

Role of AI in healthcare These days AI plays a vital role in healthcare, AI transformed healthcare and focuses on important areas such as medical research and drug discovery, patient engagement and adherence, administrative duties. AI's impact can be seen in improving diagnostic accuracy through medical imaging, controlling the speed of COVID-19 through early detection, providing virtual patient care through AI-tools, managing and improving health records, accelerating drug and vaccine discovery, minimizing prescription errors, and enabling technology-assisted rehabilitation(Al Kuwaiti et al. 2023).

Figure 2. Role of Artificial Intelligent in Healthcare

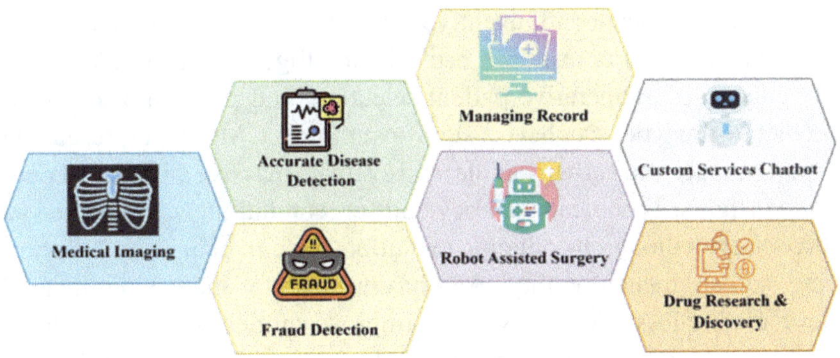

Figure 1 highlights the key roles of artificial intelligence in healthcare, which will be discussed in detail in the following section.

- Medical Imaging
- Healthcare Assistant
- Accurate Diagnosis of Disease
- Robot-Assisted Surgery
- Managing Records
- Custom Services Chatbots
- Combating Services

Medical Imaging: AI is becoming a useful tool for radiology specialists, assisting in the early detection of many diseases and reducing diagnostic mistakes, particularly in preventative treatment. Similarly, AI plays an important role in evaluating ECG and echocardiogram charts, allowing cardiologists to make better decisions. For example the ultromics platform, utilized at an Oxford hospital, uses artificial intelligence to analyze echocardiogram images, detect heartbeat patterns, and identify ischemic heart disease(Gosh 2018). Machine learning, a subset of AI, has been employed in diagnostic imaging since the 1980s. Users first specify certain image attributes and features using their expert's knowledge in this method. They may extract characteristics likes shapes, areas, or pixel distributions in regions of interest, such as tumor areas(Panayides et al. 2020).

Healthcare Assistant: AI has revolutionized patient care by changing how medical practitioners identify illnesses an create treatment strategies, leading to substantial improvements in the field. Among the most noteworthy developments is the emergence of virtual health aides. The accessibility of health-care services has been greatly enhanced by these AI-driven solutions, especially for the elderly and those with mobility impairments who frequently find it difficult to get in-person care(Chavali, Dhiman, and Katari 2024). Healthcare Cognitive Assistants (HCAs) are set to play a transformational role soon, enabling evidence-based, accurate, sustainable, and efficient healthcare delivery on a large scale. This article will investigate the technological capabilities of existing HCAs, highlight essential characteristics and developing trends, and identify critical research problems and application gaps. These findings will serve as the foundation for furthering cognitive assistant technology in healthcare, allowing future advancements and meeting unmet requirements(Preum et al. 2021).

Robot-Assisted Surgery: Robotic surgery is one of the medical fields where artificial intelligence is seeing some of the most significant and inventive developments. AI is changing almost every area of modern life(Knudsen et al. 2024). For example, artificial intelligence can significantly transform whole spine treatment. By enhanced preoperative patient selection, and personalized postoperative care, its evidence-based, predictive analytics can have a significant impact. Moreover, research can benefit from the use of AI's computer capacity to gather, handle, and evaluate massive amounts of patient data to derive important therapeutic insights. Technical accuracy and surgeon fatigue are expected to be improved by robotic-assisted surgery, even though its ongoing evolution(Rasouli et al. 2021). Robot-assisted surgery is quickly advancing, and augmented reality (AR) has promise for increasing doctors' visual insights. This paper proposes a marker less AR framework to improve surgical safety by reducing intraoperative bleeding caused by tool collisions with sensitive blood arteries. The framework uses powerful stereo reconstruction and segmentation networks to generate 3D models of intraoperative blood arteries and link them with preoperative data. A collision detection device keeps track of the minimal distance between instruments and boats to avoid mishaps. The framework was tested in a simulated lymphadenectomy with the da Vinci Research Kit and proved its capacity to prevent vascular collisions without putting the operator under pressure. This adaptable AR integration improves safety and efficiency in robot-assisted procedures(Chen et al. 2024).

Accurate Diagnosis of Disease: Artificial Intelligence (AI) has a lot to offer when it comes to disease diagnosis. Medical experts work in an ever-changing environment in the healthcare system, where they face new tasks, responsibilities that change often, and disruptions. Because of this dynamic nature, diagnosing disease frequently falls to the back of healthcare workers' minds(Mirbabaie, Stieglitz, and Frick 2021). AI-powered surgical robotics provide accuracy and minimally invasive solutions, which improve recovery times and results. AI accelerates drug discovery by refining prediction models and clinical trials, lowering costs and shortening development times. Despite these developments, issues like as data quality, algorithmic bias, privacy problems, and ethical application remain crucial. Addressing these concerns is critical for ensuring fair access and confidence in AI-powered healthcare(Zeb et al. 2024).

Managing Records: the privacy and security of sensitive patient data are becoming more and more important as healthcare records become more digitally connected. Healthcare companies may improve records and security and lower the risk of data breaches or unauthorized access with the use of artificial intelligence (AI) technology like machine learning and natural language processing. Large amounts of patient data may be evaluated to find trends and abnormalities using AI-based algorithms, which makes it easier to identify any security issues realy on. Healthcare practitioners may react swiftly and reduce hazards before they worsen thanks to these preventive strategies. AI can help to create strong authentication systems that improve access restrictions and lessen dependency on easily cracked passwords, including biometric recognition and behavioral analysis(Nitsa J. Herzog n.d.).

Custom Services Chatbot: AI-driven communication is demonstrated by chatbots, a kind of conversational software agent driven by natural language processing. It is a program that enabled users to busy in conversations with machines. Utilizing Artificial Intelligence technology, chatbots may be created for a range of platforms, such as messaging online and mobile apps. Chatbots may provide human-like interactions by using natural language processing to comprehend and reply to user inquiries. Chatbots have a revolutionary impact on the healthcare industry by providing a productive means of interacting with members of affiliations. By handling one-on-one patient conservations and answering particular patient questions, chatbots with a health emphasis can improve patient support and care(Bulla et al. 2020).

Combating Frauds: Corruption poses a severe danger to global health outcomes, including financial waste and negative health repercussions. However, kinds of corruption that have an influence on global health are widespread in both the public and commercial sectors, as well as in rich and resource-poor countries. Allegations of money mismanagement and fraud in global health efforts can jeopardize future funding. Domestic and sectoral solutions are now fragmented and condemned for being inefficient. To address this issue, we propose a global health governance structure that includes international acknowledgment of "global health corruption" and the creation of a treaty convention to tackle this critical issue(MacKey and Liang 2012). With the growing adoption of online payment systems and electronic health records by healthcare institutions, effective fraud detection models are now critical. The use of advanced AI-driven technology is becoming crucial for identifying and categorizing fraudulent activity. Organizations are strengthening their security frameworks with cutting-edge solutions made to project their networks and data to successfully battle digital crime and fraud. A thorough grasp of fraud dynamics and the most recent techniques for preventing cybercrime are necessary for successful fraud detection, and this knowledge lays the groundwork for more reliable and efficient AI-based learning models(Iqbal, Abd-Alrazaq, and Househ 2022).

Drug Research and Drug Discovery: Artificial Intelligence is a technique that replicates human intellect through sophisticated computing processes and has transformed research and drug development. For instance, the use of machine learning to early-stage drug discovery expedites the screening of candidate therapeutic molecules and forecasts success rate by taking biological factors include instruments that greatly increase the efficiency of research and development operations, including next-generation protein sequencing(Subasi 2024). The healthcare system always demands new medications to fulfill unmet medical needs in a variety of therapeutic areas. Pharmaceutical firms play an important role in satisfying these demands by navigating the complex procedures of medication research and development. Drug discovery entails numerous essential processes, including target selection and validation, hit identification, lead creation and optimization, and finally choosing a candidate for future development. In contrast, the development phase focuses on improving the drug's chemical production and formulation, performing animal toxicity studies, executing clinical trials, and obtaining regulatory approval. These methods are both time consuming and expensive. Furthermore, the pharmaceutical business is facing new obstacles, such as severe regulatory requirements, environmental concerns, and decreased profitability due to patent expirations(Sinha and Vohora 2017).

Web-based Application used in healthcare

Table 1. Web-based application of healthcare using AI and IoT

Year	References	Web Application/ Models	Services Provided	Methodology	Outcomes
2021	(Computational et al. 2023)	Web system for E-Mental Health	Provide E-mental care along with the cities and outside the city as well	NLP, LSTM	Recognizing facial expressions and conducting online meeting
2022	(Xu et al. 2022)	Risk Assessment Tool	Predicting HIV infection using risk assessment tool	Machine Learning Models (Gradient Boosting Machine and Random Forest)	Used to improve the rate of prediction and reduce the future risk.
2022	(Ashfaq et al. 2022)	AI-based diggi Healthcare	Remote patient monitoring system for cardiovascular patients	Linear Regression, Logistic Regression, Naïve Bayes, KNN, SVM and NN	User friendly interface to record the patients as well as doctor meetings.
2022	(Silvestri et al. 2023)	NLP-based Cyber threat analysis in healthcare	To analyze threat and vulnerabilities in healthcare	Logistic Regression and XGBoost	Detection of threat using existing dataset from CVE
2021	(Khan et al. 2021)	Personal Healthcare system	Proposed system is deployed using RFID and steganography for better health analyses	NodeMCU, Arduino and RFID sensors	Successfully deployed Wi-Fi based Arduino with MATLAB using different GUI to provide safe and secure
2021	(Vijayasarveswari et al. 2021)	E-Healthcare Management system	Offering doctor appointment online	CSS, PHP, JavaScript and CSS	Online appointments and doctors can arrange their time according to their free slots.

Table 1 lists the several web-based healthcare applications. A variety of healthcare requirements are met by these apps, including the provision of E-mental health services, HIV risk assessments, and remote patient monitoring for cardiovascular patients. Recent advances in healthcare technology have resulted in novel online apps and models that considerably improve patient care and system efficiency. In 2021, a web-based E-Mental Health system was created combining NLP and LSTM to provide remote mental healthcare services and improve facial expression identification during online consultations. Similarly, in 2022, a risk assessment tool that used machine learning algorithms such as Gradient Boosting and Random Forest increased the accuracy of HIV infection forecasts while decreasing future risks. Diggi Healthcare, an AI-based company, launched a remote monitoring solution for cardiovascular patients that incorporates machine learning algorithms to give a user-friendly interface for patient-doctor interaction. In cybersecurity, an NLP-driven application used Logistic Regression and XGBoost to analyse risks and vulnerabilities in healthcare systems, utilizing existing datasets for better identification.

Role of Internet of Things in Healthcare

Despite enormous expenditures in information technology, the healthcare sector confronts significant worldwide difficulties. Unfortunately, no good security solution has been identified, and many medical facilities continue to use paper-based record-keeping, making it impossible to maintain the confidentiality of patient information. Addressing these difficulties, the internet of things emerges as a viable alternative for improving data security and healthcare record management(Saif et al. 2024) (Herrera Perez, Fajes Alfonso, and Alvarez 1989). The Internet of things is a fast-expanding sector to revolutionize healthcare delivery. Healthcare has benefited greatly from IoT's advancements, which also present enormous development potential. Notable inventions like the IoT-enabled AliveCor cardiac monitor illustrate the importance of this technology to saving lives. IoT devices are being used in the healthcare industry for a variety of purposes. One prominent use is remote health monitoring, which enables patients to be seen at home rather than in hospitals. In doing so, fewer hospital visits occur and patient care is improved(Chataut, Phoummalayvane, and Akl 2023). The internet has grown rapidly, allowing people all over the world to access an unprecedented number of services via smartphones and other World Internet Web-connected technology. The Internet of Things (IoT) extends this connectedness by integrating the internet into common things, allowing them to interact and share data via sensors and smart technology. IoT-enabled gadgets are intended to link numerous things to a system, either wirelessly or via cable connections, altering the way we communicate with the world around us(Indrakumari et al. 2019). Extensive study has explored how information technology (IT) might enhance and strengthen healthcare services. The Internet of Things (IoT) has been widely used to connect medical resources and deliver dependable, effective, and smart healthcare services for the elderly and those with chronic illnesses. This study aims to describe IoT applications in healthcare, highlight intelligentization trends, and outline future research prospects(YIN et al. 2016). Advancements in communication and embedded systems enable low-power, high-performance mobile communication systems. These properties are critical for developing mobile health monitoring systems(Rajagopal et al. 2023). As the population ages and chronic diseases become more common, there is a growing demand for at-home health care. However, hiring medical workers can lead to higher medical expenditures. Remote monitoring, also known as telemonitoring, allows clinicians to watch patient progress and determine if a medical assistant or doctor should be present or relocate the patient to another hospital. This approach ensures patients receive high-quality medical treatments(Chiuchisan, Costin, and Geman 2014). The Internet of Things (IoT) is crucial for today's healthcare system. IoT in healthcare entails using embedded sensors and actuators to treat patients. IoT-based invasive monitoring devices provide comprehensive monitoring and tracking of patients' physiological condition. RFID technology was employed at a top Ohio hospital to monitor medical practitioners' hand washing habits. The implementation of such IoT-based technologies helped to avert infection-related deaths and also decreased financial loss for the companies(Ajazmoharkan et al. 2017). Internet-based healthcare services, particularly IoT technologies, can help public health institutions improve their efficacy. To build e-loyalty towards public internet-based healthcare services, users must perceive the advantage and comfort of using the internet over traditional face-to-face options. To prevent wasting resources, patient e-loyalty is crucial for implementing these services, which demand significant expenditure(Martínez-Caro et al. 2018). Figure 3 depicts the role of Internet of things in healthcare sector for managing different tasks individually by modern technology. This may leads to the advancement in the medical field for achieving the sustainability in healthcare.

Figure 3. Role of IoT in Healthcare

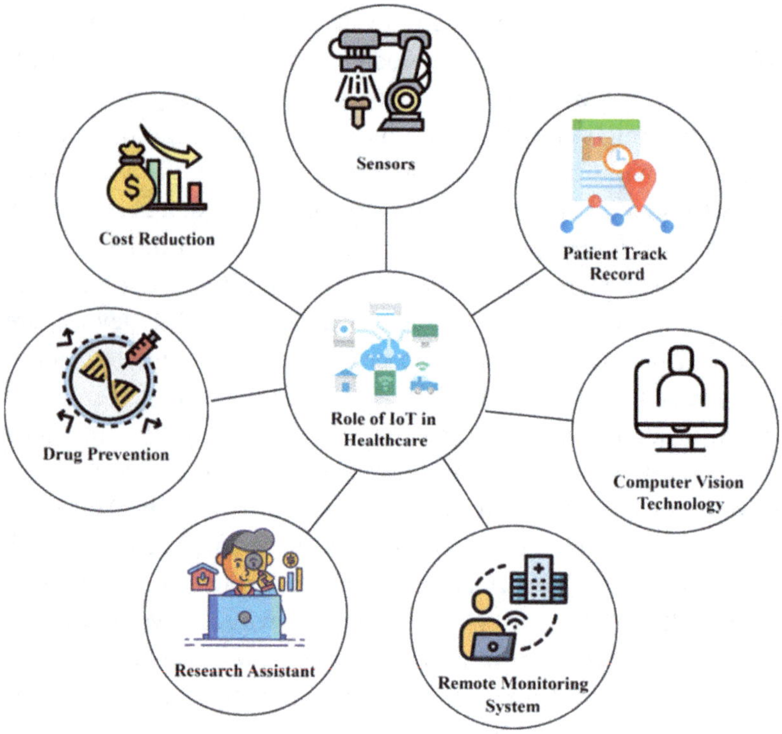

- IoT devices are used in many different contexts, such as educational institutions, smart homes, and security management. IoT devices are having a big influence in a lot of fields, one of which is healthcare. They are being used a lot there to improve patients outcomes and lower risk factors(Huifeng, Kadry, and Raj 2020).
- Medical sensors can be put as motion detectors in homes or combined with other wearable electronics like watches, clothes, shoes, and beds. Physiological and environmental sensors are the two main categories. Wearable physiological sensors monitor blood pressure, heart rate, blood oxygen, saturation, and body temperature. Environmental sensors, track exterior factors such as lighting, sound, and temperature in the space and are employed to identify events like falls(Parihar et al. 2024).
- Healthcare is the major concern, as India is one of the populous nations, a sizeable section of the populace lives in rural regions with little access to real-time healthcare services. The demand for a smart health monitoring system that facilitates smooth communication between network devices and applications is pressing as technology becomes more and more commonplace. A system like this would make it easier for physicians and patients to keep record of confidential medical information(Badiganti et al. 2022).
- The use of computer vision in healthcare applications, particularly for medical imaging, is growing worldwide. For the advancement of such applications machine learning approaches used in medical imaging(Gao et al. 2018).

Artificial Intelligence and Internet of Things combined to work together for the evolution of healthcare.

AI-powered intelligent internet of things devices has the potential to make decisions on their own, which has the potential to completely change the healthcare industry. Small wearable, and implanted sensors have been made possible by recent developments in wireless communication and sensor technology(Pandimurugan et al. 2024). These developments open the door to individualized healthcare plans and real-time monitoring, which improves the effectiveness and responsiveness of the healthcare system(Zahid et al. 2022). AI has the capability to derive precise and significant insights from sensor data when it is combined with Internet of Things-based healthcare monitoring systems. It is possible to bring processing capacity closer to the data source and facilitate quicker and more effective decision-making by utilizing the edge computing paradigm. Large-scale data management made possible by big data computing also improves internet of things healthcare system by facilitating the analysis of massive volumes of health data for more accurate monitoring and predictive therapy(Khan et al. 2022) (Abdul-malek et al. 2022). AI has progressed beyond emulating human thought to encompass a wider range of functions due to increased processing power in computer systems. AI encompasses data collecting, modelling, and processing (e.g., machine learning, deep learning, natural language processing), as well as analytics and visualization. AI approaches will be integrated into the IoT Stack, leading to the development of AIoT applications for the future(Serrano, Dang, and Nguyen 2018). AI has advanced beyond replicating human mind to embrace a broader variety of functions as computer processing power has risen. AI includes data collection, modelling, and processing (such as machine learning, deep learning, and natural language processing), as well as analytics and visualization. AI techniques will be incorporated into the IoT Stack, enabling future AIoT applications(Ud Din et al. 2019). New technology and fast-paced lifestyles necessitate personalized smart healthcare for patients. Edge computing, together with 5G and IoT sensors, enables real-time healthcare solutions that meet energy and latency requirements. Prior research on smart healthcare systems focused on cloud and fog computing architectures, security and authentication, and edge computing frameworks with various sensors and devices(Amin and Hossain 2021).

Figure 4. AI and IoT worked together for healthcare system

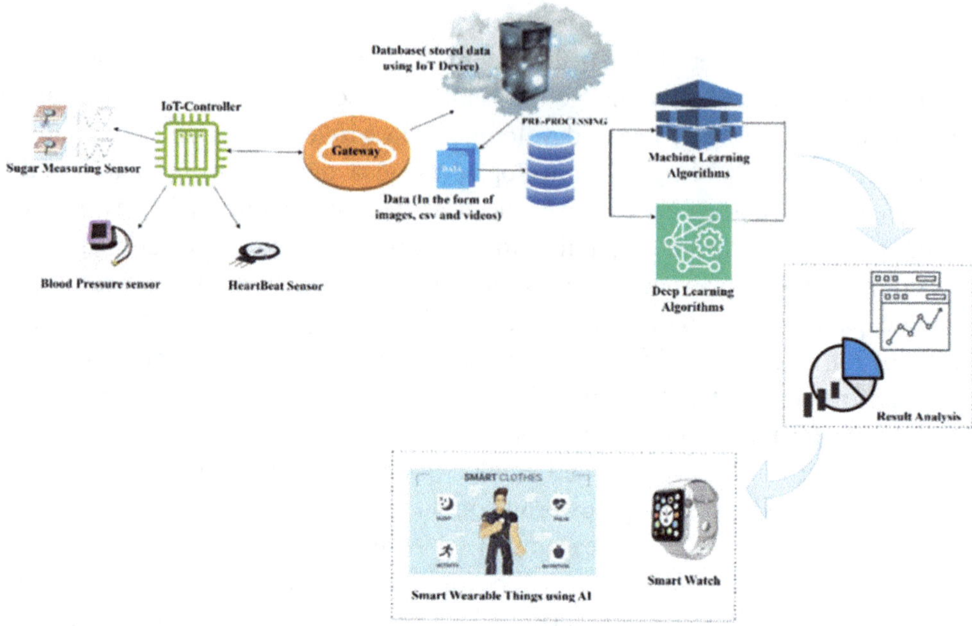

Above figure 4 uses IoT devices such as sensors, smartwatches, sensors to track a patient's health in real-time. These devices are used to collect data including heart rate or blood sugar levels, which AI examines to analyze possible issues and spot patterns. This will lead to early detection, personalized treatments, and manage care more efficiently, all leads to reducing hospital visits and improving overall patient outcomes.

IoT Devices and Sensors: Role in collecting Healthcare Data

Sensor technologies, cloud computing, wireless sensor networks (WSNs), and big data have transformed healthcare by enabling the building of linked systems. These systems maximize the use of medical equipment and provide tailored patient care(Whig et al. 2022). Connected healthcare systems save money and time by remotely monitoring medical devices, healthcare staff, and patients(Haque et al. 2023). Among the several problems discussed in this chapter, privacy and security emerge as major concerns due to the sensitive nature of healthcare data and the large volume processed(Mathew, Pillai, and Palade 2018). Integrating cloud computing with WSNs can improve network stability and availability. However, it is critical to have strong security measures during this integration process. Cloud-based sensor frameworks can also improve interoperability, scalability, and effective exploitation of WSNs in healthcare. This chapter delves into numerous facets of the HIoT system, providing a thorough overview of its architecture, components, and communication procedures amongst them. It also showcases contemporary healthcare services that use IoT-based technology. Using these technologies, IoT has enabled healthcare practitioners to monitor and diagnose a wide range of health disorders, measure various health indices, and provide diagnostic services in remote places. This transition has shifted the healthcare sector away from a hospital-centric strategy.

The chapter also looks at several uses of the HIoT system and current trends in the sector. Furthermore, it examines the problems and concerns involved in the design, development, and implementation of HIoT systems, laying the groundwork for future developments and research initiatives(Pradhan, Bhattacharyya, and Pal 2021). The Internet of Things (IoT) is a pioneering technology that incorporates billions of sensors into a variety of applications. Sensors play an important part in the IoT ecosystem by gathering data required for focused analytics. IoT and sensors are critical to progress in smart cities, smart agriculture, smart education, healthcare systems, and a variety of other industries(Vaiyapuri et al. 2023). In healthcare, the Internet of Things solves global health concerns, with the COVID-19 pandemic serving as a noteworthy example. During this time, the demand for remote and digital healthcare services increased, allowing patients to get care from home. Healthcare systems may deliver better treatments, boost computational skills, and make IoT solutions more prevalent, cost-effective, and available at any time(Al-kahtani, Khan, and Taekeun 2022).

Table 2. Overview of sensors and IoT devices used in healthcare

Sensor Name	Description	Applications
Wearable Devices	These are portable devices that use embedded sensors to track vital indicators such as heart rate, blood pressure,	Continuous surveillance of health, early detection of cardiac arrhythmias, exercise and sleep tracking, and chronic illness management, including hypertension and diabetes.
Teeth Sensor	Small sensors embedded in the mouth to monitor oral health by detecting changes in saliva composition, pH levels, and chemical markers.	Monitoring oral hygiene, detecting disease like diabetes through saliva markers, and tracking nutritional intake.
Microneedle Patches	Microneedle patches that pierce the skin to detect glucose levels, administer medications, and analyze biomarkers in interstitial fluid.	Non-invasive glucose monitoring in diabetics, transdermal medicine administration, and biomarker analysis for early illness identification.
Smart Lenses	Contact lenses have built-in sensors to track eye health concerns, measure intraocular pressure, or identify glucose levels in tears.	Glaucoma management, noninvasively glucose monitoring, and surveillance of dry eye or other ocular diseases.
Smart Textile	Fabrics integrated with sensors that can detect heart rate, respiration rate, posture, and activity levels.	Monitoring athletes performance rehabilitation for patients with mobility issues, and remote monitoring of elderly patients.
Electronic Tattoos	Brittle and malleable digital patches that adhere to the skin and track health parameters including heart rate, hydration, and muscular activity.	Real-time health vitals tracking during exercise, dehydration monitoring, and stroke or accident rehabilitation.
Face Mask Sensors	Face masks with sensors that monitor respiratory metrics, air quality, and humidity levels.	Monitoring respiratory problems like asthma, identifying pollutants or allergens in the environment, and tracking the development of airborne infections such as COVID-19.
Smart Shoes	Shoes equipped with pressure and motion sensors to monitor gait, balance, and physical activity.	Early neurological problem detection, injury rehabilitation, and workout metric tracking.
Implantable Sensors	Miniaturized sensors are implanted in the body to monitor internal physiological factors like blood pressure, glucose levels, and oxygen levels.	Managing chronic diseases, monitoring patients after surgery, and tracking internal health issues in real time.
Environmental Sensors	Sensors are put in the atmosphere to measure variables such as air quality, temperature, and humidity.	Creating a healthier indoor environment, managing allergies, and providing early warnings for asthma triggers.

continued on following page

Table 2. Continued

Sensor Name	Description	Applications
Pulse Oximeters	Devices that use light sensors to measure oxygen saturation levels in the blood and pulse rate.	Monitoring respiratory diseases, managing chronic obstructive pulmonary disease, and ensuring oxygen levels during critical conditions like COVID-19.
Body Temperature Sensors	Sensors that measure and monitor body temperature in real-time.	Early detection of fever or infections, monitoring temperature changes during physical exertion or illness, and remote monitoring of patients during pandemics.

The Table 2 describes several forms of sensor technology used in medical treatment, such as wearable devices, tooth sensors, microneedle patches, and smart lenses, which monitor vital signs, glucose levels, and health issues. Several sensors, including smart fabrics, electronic tattoos, face masks, smart shoes, implanted sensors, environmental sensors, pulse oximeters, and body temperature sensors, aid in illness management, recovery, and real-time tracking of health.

BLOCKCHAIN TECHNOLOGY'S ROLE IN SECURING DATA SHARED BY IOT DEVICES

Blockchain is a continually increasing chain of blocks that keeps user records in a distributed manner while protecting them with cryptographic procedures. Each block is linked to the next, resulting in an interconnected structure that shares information across the network. Stuart Haber and W. Scott Stornetta established the notion of blockchain for the first time in 1991. Later, in 2009, a developer or group of developers under the pseudonym Satoshi Nakamoto created the first functional Blockchain, which allowed transactions using the electronic currency Bitcoin. These transactions were recorded in a public ledger, which is now commonly known as the Blockchain(Kumar and Sharma 2022). Blockchain is an application of distributed ledger technology. The ledger records all transactions in the order they occur. In blockchain, transactions are recorded in blocks. Blocks are linked by including the preceding block's cryptographic hash value in the following block. This chaining approach uses linked hash values to avoid tampering without detection. Smart contracts are computer programs that execute agreed-upon business logic among network users. They utilize blockchain technology and offer a user-friendly platform for data interaction. This code is exposed to all members of the network(Truong et al. 2019).

These modern innovations provide enhanced security and usefulness, making them vital in healthcare settings. They serve several objectives, such as identity verification, biometric data rectification, data collecting and analysis, and security reinforcement. These small monitoring devices can measure various physiological parameters, including blood pressure, oxygen saturation, body temperature, heart rate, respiratory rate, weariness, weight, height, and sleep duration, while individuals are being observed. This vast amount of data gives crucial insights into patient health and well-being(Ghadi et al. 2024).

Blockchain is a cutting-edge technology with promising applications in healthcare.

Efficient data sharing and distribution among network members and healthcare professionals leads to the development of cost-effective and advanced medicines for various ailments.

This will hasten growth in healthcare in the future years. Blockchain technology has recently been found to provide prospects in the logistics business, which can also benefit the healthcare sector. Digital transformation has a direct impact on living quality, making it a priority area for improvement and innovation(Haleem et al. 2021).

ALGORITHMS USED IN SMART HEALTHCARE

As it addresses mathematics or engineering challenges, optimization algorithms are significant because people want to choose the best (usually better) answer from many options based on certain criteria. The difficulty of the optimization task is determined by its type and complexity. Convex optimization issues are often easier to solve than non-convex problems because the local minimum must be a global solution, which means that first-order conditions are ideally adequate. Mult objective optimization issues (which frequently involve numerous competing objectives) are more complicated than single-objective optimization problems. When the global optimal solution is unknown or takes a significant amount of computational effort, a compromise or near optimal solution is sometimes chosen(Chui et al. 2017). AI algorithms involved for the innovation of the smart healthcare to improve the sustainability in healthcare.

Machine Learning Algorithms

- **Supervised Learning:** Supervised machine learning trains techniques using a labeled dataset, with every point of data assigned to a preset category. The algorithm is designed to learn patterns and discriminate between categories, such as detecting malignant tumors from non-cancerous ones. Supervised learning is particularly useful for classification and regression issues. During development, the system generates predictions, compares them to labeled data, and tweaks its strategy to enhance accuracy. This method continues until the forecasts nearly match the actual results. The quality and variety of the training dataset are critical to supervised learning's effectiveness in ensuring accurate and generalized results. While supervised learning gives exact control over the training process and generates predictable outcomes, it takes significant work to create massive, labeled datasets(Godewatte Arachchige, Branch, and But 2023).
- **Unsupervised Learning:** The unsupervised algorithms employed throughout the implementation phase are explained. The study employs three unsupervised methods: IF, K-Means, and LOF. The fundamental difficulty with this unsupervised model is that a subjective threshold must be established. There is limited knowledge about fraud situations, yet a suitable threshold was chosen for a fraudulent event. As a result, when a forest of random trees produces shorter path lengths for specific samples, they are very always aberrations. Isolated forest detects abnormalities by randomly partitioning the domain space. It primarily acts as a Decision Tree Algorithm, with a root node at the beginning and partitioning the space following. We arbitrarily divide in isolation, similar to how decision trees partition based on knowledge gain(Kanksha et al. 2021).
- **Reinforcement Learning:** Reinforcement Learning (RL), a subset of Machine Learning (ML), is gaining popularity in the medical profession due to its capacity to offer individualized therapies in accordance with precision medicine. Unlike older approaches, RL learns dynamically by interacting with its surroundings and improving tactics based on the results. Its versatility makes it perfect for improving complicated healthcare scenarios including treatment protocols, chronic

illness management, and personalised medication regimens. By integrating real-time data and patient-specific input, RL systems improve treatment efficacy and customisation, supporting the ideal of individualized, patient-centered healthcare(Coronato et al. 2020).

Deep learning Algorithms

- **Convolutional Neural Networks:** The CNN model successfully detects disease-related knowledge from unstructured medical records. CNN requires a significant amount of memory when using a fully linked network topology. Adding more layers to a model might raise its complexity analysis(Ismail et al. 2020). One of the most common types of neural networks is CNN. CNN image classifications take input photographs, process them, and assign them to certain categories, such as cat and dog. CNN's function is to reduce a picture to a form that is easier to comprehend while retaining any acute elements that are required for a successful prediction. CNN has a great capacity to process photos and learn features. CNN plays a crucial role in several deep neural network applications(Arabahmadi and Farahbakhsh 2022).
- **Recurrent Neural Networks and Long Short-Term Memory:** A Convolutional Neural Network (CNN) is combined with an LSTM recurrent network. CNNs are meant to identify spatial correlation patterns in pictures. Our network will recognize spatial patterns connected to skeletal joint positions in 3D space. The LSTM recurrent network captures spatiotemporal patterns of the skeletal joint's 3D coordinates across time. However, we first train the CNN independently of the LSTM. This is performed by linking the CNN to a fully connected multilayer perceptron (MLP) with two hidden layers. To complete the training process, we link the pre-trained CNN output to the LSTM(Núñez et al. 2018).
- **Autoencoders**: Autoencoder is a neural network used for unsupervised learning that recreates input rather than classifying it. The input layer has the same number of neurons as the output layer does. Hidden layers in neural networks have fewer neurons than input/output layers due to the usage of autoencoders to encode lower-dimensional data and extract discriminative features(Al-Marridi, Mohamed, and Erbad 2018).

Natural Language Processing Algorithms: A natural language processing (NLP) technique is critical to enable continuous remote monitoring in digital health. This technology uses powerful deep learning (DL) algorithms to evaluate data from wearable devices and other remote monitoring technologies, resulting in a holistic perspective of patient health. NLP is primarily focused on reading patient comments and extracting insights from electronic medical records (EMRs), which improves knowledge of individual health issues.A variety of deep learning techniques are used to assist this. For example, convolutional neural networks (CNNs) are used to assess medical pictures, whereas recurrent neural networks (RNNs) manage time-series data from wearable devices such as heart rate and glucose levels. Furthermore, unsupervised learning approaches, such as autoencoders, are used for feature extraction, allowing the discovery of significant patterns and abnormalities in healthcare(Shastry and Shastry 2023).

Optimization Algorithms: The optimization technique is included into the healthcare monitoring system to improve predicted accuracy and computational efficiency. The Centered Convolutional Restricted Boltzmann Machines-based Whale Optimization (CCRBM-WO) algorithm is the foundation of this optimization strategy. The CCRBM-WO algorithm combines the structural strengths of CCRBMs and the Whale Optimization Algorithm (WOA). The CCRBM reduces concerns such as approximation and structural instability, enhancing the model's capacity to handle complex, nonlinear healthcare data. WOA improves CCRBM initialization and parameter adjustment by emulating whales' bubble-net hunting behavior, resulting in faster convergence and higher prediction accuracy(Irshad et al. 2023). This hybrid optimization strategy successfully refines critical parameters like network weights and thresholds, resulting in strong classification and prediction performance. It minimizes noise, stabilizes gradients during training, and dramatically improves the model's ability to detect and categorize illnesses using patient data. The optimization approach assures that the algorithm achieves superior outcomes while being computationally efficient, making it ideal for real-time healthcare applications.

Predictive Analytics Algorithms: Machine learning is used in healthcare to diagnose and forecast tumors. Dealing with heterogeneous, remote, diversified, and highly dynamic data sets, as well as unstructured and non-standardized information related to various cancer kinds, poses significant hurdles. Developing novel tools for integrating, analyzing, and interpreting complex biomedical data is crucial in clinical practice and biomedical research. This allows for the identification of testable hypotheses and the creation of accurate models for cancer diagnosis and prediction(Nithya and Ilango 2017). Redictive analytics are essential in the healthcare business. Accurate and timely illness prediction can save patients' lives, while inaccurate predictions can put them at risk. Diseases must be precisely anticipated and estimated. Therefore, accurate and efficient approaches for healthcare predictive analysis are necessary(Badawy, Ramadan, and Hefny 2023).

Data Fusion and Integration Algorithms: In clinical decision-making, relying solely on one source of information may lead to inaccurate results. Fusing heterogeneous data allows for more accurate analysis and better knowledge of a specific condition. Integrating data from many sources, including clinical archives, sensory equipment, and historical/textual data, is crucial for both patients and healthcare practitioners. As the number of sensory devices increases, data fusion becomes more complicated. Several difficulties have been observed, including sophisticated distributed processing, unstable data connectivity, ambiguity in data interpretation, and varying data transmission speeds. Further research is needed in areas such as data privacy and security, inconsistent variable definitions, heterogeneous data collection, decision fusion, patient identification, data management, computationally efficient in-depth learning development, and multimodal data fusion for context-aware detection(Kalamkar and Mary 2020).

Edge AI algorithms: Edge AI is the deployment of algorithms for AI directly on edge devices such as smartphones, IoT devices, and embedded systems rather than depending on cloud servers for computing. This strategy has various benefits, including speedier decision-making with low latency, improved data privacy, and decreased reliance on internet access(Haq et al. 2021). Edge AI algorithms are meant to be lightweight and efficient, allowing devices with minimal processing resources to do tasks in real time. Common algorithms used in Edge AI include Convolutional Neural Networks (CNNs) for image and video analysis, Recurrent Neural Networks (RNNs) for time-series prediction, and decision trees or Random Forests for categorization(Greco et al. 2020).

Image Processing Algorithms: Computerized clinical images are crucial for illness detection and treatment in modern hospitals, which are integrated with the internet of things.

Medical photos can contain sensitive and personal patient information. Unauthorized access and usage of private photographs might lead to disastrous consequences(Khan et al. 2019). Smart healthcare systems capture pictures, including X-rays and Magnetic Resonance Imaging. The security and integrity of pictures are vital for databases used in knowledge-based learning systems, fostering organized decision-making and improving AI learning skills. Furthermore, in knowledge-driven systems, the storing and transmission of HD medical pictures imposes a stress on the restricted bandwidth of the communication channel, causing data transmission delays(Rehman et al. 2024).

Rule-Based Systems: Rule-based systems play a crucial role in these applications, replicating logical reasoning procedures and explaining their conclusions. Rule-based systems, particularly on mobile devices with limited resources, lose efficiency as the volume of data fulfilling the criteria and the complexity of the rule base increase. This paper proposes an optimization approach to improve the structure of ontologies and rules in a rule-based system. The goal is to reduce the cost of evaluating all rules by operating directly at the knowledge level(Minutolo, Esposito, and De Pietro 2017). This study proposes a rule-based information extraction (IE) system designed for Polish medical texts. It provides two programs for extracting data from Polish medical documentation: mammography reports and diabetic hospital records. A customized ontology was initially developed, and its ideas were then translated into two different models, expressed as typed feature structure (TFS) hierarchies that followed the syntax specified by the selected IE platform. Dedicated IE grammars were used to parse the documents and generate templates depending on the models(Mykowiecka, Marciniak, and Kupść 2009).

THE LIMITATION OF AI AND IOT IN HEALTHCARE

The given Table 3 describes the limitation of artificial intelligence and Internet of Things in healthcare field on different factors.

Table 3. Limitation depending on different factors of AI and IoT in healthcare.

Factors	Artificial Intelligence in Healthcare	Internet of Things in Healthcare
Data Privacy and Security Risk	Challenges with efficient data anonymization, inadequate security precautions, threats posed by third parties and weakness in the integration of new technologies.	Ensuring data security, privacy, and accuracy is crucial for IoT-based healthcare. Access should be limited to authorized individuals, and auditability should be preserved for transparency.
High Cost of Implementation	Making advancements in technology, skilled professionals, making costly for small organizations. In addition, the updating and maintenance leads high expenses	Requires skilled workers, secure networks, and robust infrastructure. Ongoing monitoring, maintenance, and upgrades add to the financial challenges, limited widespread adoption.
Data Quality and Integrity	Due to the poor quality of algorithms, less accurate predictions can affect patient outcomes.	Quality of data collected from IoT devices may be affected from environmental conditions, device inaccuracies which leads of incomplete data.
Limited Interoperability	Leads to restricts their ability to effectively communicate and share data with existing technologies	Inconsistent data formats and communication protocols hinder seamless integration and data sharing.
Ethical Concern	The ethical consideration around data usage and AI systems must be addressed with consideration for informed permission, safety and transparency, and algorithmic fairness and discrimination.	Privacy breaches, informed consent challenges, accountability issues, unequal access, and the impact on the doctor-patient relationship.

Table 3 explores the limitation in Artificial intelligence (AI) and the Internet of Things (IoT) are transforming healthcare, but both confront enormous difficulties that must be overcome before their full promise can be realized. Data privacy and security remain significant concerns, as AI systems face risks from insufficient security measures and integration flaws, but IoT-based healthcare stresses-controlled access and auditability to maintain transparency. The high cost of implementation, which includes the requirement for qualified specialists, secure infrastructure, and continuous maintenance, creates financial barriers that limit access, particularly for smaller enterprises. Furthermore, data quality and integrity are jeopardized, with AI forecasts hampered by algorithmic flaws and IoT devices vulnerable to incomplete or erroneous data owing to environmental conditions. Limited interoperability further impedes smooth integration and data sharing, since conflicting standards and protocols impede effective communication between technology. Ethical considerations for AI and IoT include securing informed consent, maintaining data openness, and addressing issues of responsibility and justice. Overcoming these obstacles is critical to offering safe, efficient, and fair healthcare solutions using these disruptive technologies.

DISCUSSION

The combination of artificial intelligence (AI) and the Internet of Things (IoT) is altering the healthcare industry by improving patient care, diagnostics, and overall healthcare administration. This study demonstrates how merging these sophisticated technologies results in a smarter, more efficient healthcare ecosystem that emphasizes improved patient outcomes and operational excellence. One of AI and IoT's most significant contributions to healthcare is its capacity to enable real-time monitoring and early identification of health concerns. IoT allows for continuous data collecting using wearable devices and smart sensors, such as monitoring blood pressure, glucose levels, heart rate, and other vital indications. This massive amount of data is then analyzed using AI algorithms to provide predictive insights, individualized treatment plans, and early detection of potential health issues. By changing from reactive to proactive.

Beyond monitoring, AI has transformed medical diagnosis. AI-powered systems can scan medical pictures, identify trends, and help healthcare practitioners diagnose complicated disorders more accurately. For example, in radiology and cardiology, AI systems may detect illnesses like cancer and cardiovascular abnormalities more sooner than traditional approaches, allowing for early therapies. This not only improves diagnosis accuracy, but it also reduces the workload of healthcare personnel, allowing them to concentrate on more complicated and vital responsibilities.

The combination of AI and IoT also improves the sustainability of healthcare systems. AI-driven optimization has the potential to expedite operations, minimize waste, and enhance energy efficiency in healthcare facilities. For example, IoT devices can forecast when equipment requires maintenance, reducing downtime and ensuring that resources are spent efficiently. The combination of AI and IoT also improves the sustainability of healthcare systems. AI-driven optimization has the potential to expedite operations, minimize waste, and enhance energy efficiency in healthcare facilities. For example, IoT devices can forecast when equipment requires maintenance, reducing downtime and ensuring that resources are spent efficiently. AI also plays an important role in expediting drug development and clinical trials, making research procedures faster and less expensive, resulting in more economical and efficient healthcare solutions. The ongoing progress of AI and IoT in healthcare bodes well for the future. These technologies open the path for more intelligent systems that provide customized, predictive, and sustainable treatment. By improving patient experiences and operational efficiency, the marriage of AI and IoT has the potential to totally redefine how healthcare is provided.

FUTURE TRENDS OF AI (ARTIFICIAL INTELLIGENCE) AND IOT (INTERNET OF THINGS)

By Integrating new framework like those used in mysignals like sensor networks, serverless computing, device-less edge computing, and data analytics, healthcare system can be improved by putting computation closer to sensors and wearable through mobile computation nodes. This strategy will help respond times even more, which is very helpful in emergency medical situations(Tuli et al. 2020).

Robotic nurses and other AI-embedded technologies are integrated into the healthcare modelling framework to improve patient care through automation and efficiency. Smart IoT devices are also used for individualized healthcare solutions and real-time.

Recent research rely heavily on clinical and laboratory factors, which might be a limitation. These technologies may be useful for hospitalized patients but are not accessible to those with limited healthcare access or in telemedicine applications. As a result, they have little usefulness outside of clinical settings. Future AIoMT studies should focus on developing systems that monitor and diagnose using data from wearables and ambient sensors, rather than relying on clinical factors(Baker and Xiang 2023).

The role of AI in smart cities is to efficiently manage and analyze the vast amounts of data generated by IoT devices, ensuring accurate and precise decision-making. For instance, data from public transportation systems, traffic lights, and citizens' daily activities can be harnessed by AI to derive actionable insights, improving the efficiency and productivity of municipal operations while reducing costs. Additionally, AI minimizes human errors, enables automated data-driven decision-making, streamlines urban management, and unlocks new commercial opportunities. By integrating AI with 5G technology, energy providers can optimize renewable energy sources such as solar and wind power. AI can predict weather patterns, such as sunlight availability or wind conditions, while 5G ensures instant communication of this information to energy providers, enabling real-time adjustments to energy supply. Furthermore, in the transportation sector, AI and 5G work together to alleviate traffic congestion and reduce emissions by optimizing traffic flow and determining the most efficient vehicle routes(Alahi et al. 2023).

Future research will focus on cutting edge technologies including blockchain, cloud computing, artificial intelligence, and wireless body sensor networks. Along with providing the collection of substantial physiological data from patients, the confluence of these breakthroughs with IoT offers the promise of delivering more accurate diagnosis and treatment suggestions and resulting in considerable cost savings in healthcare. Smart hybrid technologies improve decision-making in a business, education, such as business, education, security, and healthcare(Aldahiri, Alrashed, and Hussain 2021).

CONCLUSION

The integrated use of artificial intelligence and the internet of things is transforming healthcare by tackling many of the most significant issues in industry. These technologies improve patient care, resources management, and diagnostic accuracy, resulting in better healthcare outcomes and lower costs. Despite the potential, issues like data privacy, security threats, high implementation costs, and restricted compatibility must be addressed. As AI and IoT technologies advance, they provide enormous opportunities for tailored, real-time healthcare systems that can adapt more rapidly and efficiently to patient demands. Future Breakthroughs in blockchain, cloud computing, and wireless sensor networks will allow healthcare systems to gather and analyze massive volumes of patient data, giving more accurate diagnosis and treatments while contributing to more accurate diagnosis and treatments while also adding to the general sustainability of healthcare. By overcoming existing limits, AI and IoT have the potential to significantly enhance the healthcare industry, changing it into a more efficient, responsive, and patient-centered model.

REFERENCES

Abdulmalek, S., Nasir, A., Jabbar, W. A., Almuhaya, M. A. M., Bairagi, A. K., Md, A. M. K., & Kee, S. H. (2022). IoT-Based Healthcare-Monitoring System towards Improving Quality of Life: A Review. *Healthcare (Basel)*, *10*(10), 1993. Advance online publication. DOI: 10.3390/healthcare10101993 PMID: 36292441

Ajazmoharkan, Z., Choudhury, T., Gupta, S. C., & Raj, G. 2017. "Internet of Things and Its Applications in E-Learning." *3rd IEEE International Conference On* 10(1):447–52. DOI: 10.1109/CIACT.2017.7977333

Akhter, N. (2023).. . *Harnessing IOT and Artificial Intelligence for Sustainable Healthcare.*, (March). Advance online publication. DOI: 10.25215/138757678X.35

Al-kahtani, M. S., Khan, F., & Taekeun, W. (2022). Application of Internet of Things and Sensors in Healthcare. *Sensors (Basel)*, *22*(15), 5738. Advance online publication. DOI: 10.3390/s22155738 PMID: 35957294

Al Kuwaiti, A., Nazer, K., Al-Reedy, A., Al-Shehri, S., Al-Muhanna, A., Subbarayalu, A. V., Al Muhanna, D., & Al-Muhanna, F. A. (2023). A Review of the Role of Artificial Intelligence in Healthcare. *Journal of Personalized Medicine*, *13*(6), 1–22. DOI: 10.3390/jpm13060951 PMID: 37373940

Al-Marridi, A. Z., Mohamed, A., & Erbad, A. 2018. "Convolutional Autoencoder Approach for EEG Compression and Reconstruction in M-Health Systems." *2018 14th International Wireless Communications and Mobile Computing Conference, IWCMC 2018* 370–75. DOI: 10.1109/IWCMC.2018.8450511

Alahi, E. E., Sukkuea, A., Tina, F. W., Nag, A., Kurdthongmee, W., Suwannarat, K., & Mukhopadhyay, S. C. 2023. "Integration of IoT-Enabled Technologies and Artificial Advancements and Future Trends." *Sensors (Switzerland)* 23(5206).

Aldahiri, A., Alrashed, B., & Hussain, W. (2021). Trends in Using IoT with Machine Learning in Health Prediction System. *Forecasting*, *3*(1), 181–206. DOI: 10.3390/forecast3010012

Alshehri, F., & Muhammad, G. (2021). A Comprehensive Survey of the Internet of Things (IoT) and AI-Based Smart Healthcare. *IEEE Access : Practical Innovations, Open Solutions*, *9*, 3660–3678. DOI: 10.1109/ACCESS.2020.3047960

Amin, S. U., & Shamim Hossain, M. (2021). Edge Intelligence and Internet of Things in Healthcare: A Survey. *IEEE Access : Practical Innovations, Open Solutions*, *9*, 45–59. DOI: 10.1109/ACCESS.2020.3045115

Arabahmadi, M., & Farahbakhsh, R. (2022). Deep Learning for Smart Healthcare: A Survey on Brain Tumor. *Sensors (Basel)*, *22*, 1–27. DOI: 10.3390/s22051960 PMID: 35271115

Arachchige, G., Kithmini, P. B., & But, J. (2023). Evaluation of Blockchain Networks' Scalability Limitations in Low-Powered Internet of Things (IoT) Sensor Networks. *Future Internet*, *15*(9), 317. Advance online publication. DOI: 10.3390/fi15090317

Ashfaq, Z., Mumtaz, R., Rafay, A., Mohammad, S., Zaidi, H., Saleem, H., Mumtaz, S., Shahid, A., De Poorter, E., & Moerman, I. (2022). Applied Sciences Embedded AI-Based Digi-Healthcare. *Applied Sciences (Basel, Switzerland)*, *12*(519), 1–17.

Badawy, M., Ramadan, N., & Hefny, H. A. (2023). Healthcare Predictive Analytics Using Machine Learning and Deep Learning Techniques: A Survey. *Journal of Electrical Systems and Information Technology*, *10*(1), 40. Advance online publication. DOI: 10.1186/s43067-023-00108-y

Badiganti, P. K., Peddirsi, S., Alla, T. J. R., & Tripathi, S. L. (2022). Design and Implementation of Smart Healthcare Monitoring System Using FPGA. *Lecture Notes in Networks and Systems*, *329*, 205–213. DOI: 10.1007/978-981-16-6246-1_18

Baker, S., & Xiang, W. (2023). Artificial Intelligence of Things for Smarter Healthcare: A Survey of Advancements, Challenges, and Opportunities. *IEEE Communications Surveys and Tutorials*, *25*(2), 1261–1293. DOI: 10.1109/COMST.2023.3256323

Bulla, C., Parushetti, C., Teli, A., Aski, S., & Koppad, S. (2020). A Review of AI Based Medical Assistant Chatbot. *HBRP Publication*, *3*(2), 1–14. DOI: 10.5281/zenodo.3902215

Chataut, R., Phoummalayvane, A., & Akl, R. (2023). Unleashing the Power of IoT: A Comprehensive Review of IoT Applications and Future Prospects in Healthcare, Agriculture, Smart Homes, Smart Cities, and Industry 4.0. *Sensors (Basel)*, *23*(16), 7194. Advance online publication. DOI: 10.3390/s23167194 PMID: 37631731

Chavali, D., Dhiman, V. K., & Katari, S. C. (2024). AI-Powered Virtual Health Assistants. *Transforming Patient Engagement Through Virtual Nursing.*, *2*(2), 613–624. DOI: 10.5281/zenodo.10691495

Chen, Z., Cruciani, L., Fan, K., Fontana, M., Lievore, E., De Cobelli, O., Musi, G., Ferrigno, G., & De Momi, E. (2024). Towards Safer Robot-Assisted Surgery: A Markerless Augmented Reality Framework. *Neural Networks*, *178*(March), 106469. DOI: 10.1016/j.neunet.2024.106469 PMID: 38925030

Chiuchisan, I., Costin, H. N., & Geman, O. 2014. "Adopting the Internet of Things Technologies in Health Care Systems." *EPE 2014 - Proceedings of the 2014 International Conference and Exposition on Electrical and Power Engineering* (Epe 2014):532–35. DOI: 10.1109/ICEPE.2014.6969965

Chui, K. T., Alhalabi, W., Sally, S. H. P., Ordóñez de Pablos, P., Liu, R. W., & Zhao, M. (2017). Disease Diagnosis in Smart Healthcare: Innovation, Technologies and Applications. *Sustainability (Basel)*, *9*(12), 1–23. DOI: 10.3390/su9122309

Coronato, A., Naeem, M., De Pietro, G., & Paragliola, G. (2020). Reinforcement Learning for Intelligent Healthcare Applications: A Survey. *Artificial Intelligence in Medicine*, *109*, 101964. DOI: 10.1016/j.artmed.2020.101964 PMID: 34756216

Din, U., Ikram, A. A., Guizani, M., & Zuair, M. (2019). A Decade of Internet of Things: Analysis in the Light of Healthcare Applications. *IEEE Access : Practical Innovations, Open Solutions*, *7*, 89967–89979. DOI: 10.1109/ACCESS.2019.2927082

Gao, J., Yang, Y., Lin, P., & Park, D. S. (2018). Editorial: Computer Vision in Healthcare Applications. *Journal of Healthcare Engineering*, *2018*, 1–4. Advance online publication. DOI: 10.1155/2018/5157020 PMID: 29686826

Ghadi, Y. Y., Mazhar, T., & Shahzad, T. Muhammad Amir khan, Alaa Abd-Alrazaq, Arfan Ahmed, and Habib Hamam. 2024. *The Role of Blockchain to Secure Internet of Medical Things*. Vol. 14. Nature Publishing Group UK.

Gosh, P. (2018). *AI Early Diagnosis Could Save Heart and Cancer Patients*. BBC.

Greco, L., Percannella, G., Ritrovato, P., Tortorella, F., & Vento, M. (2020). Trends in IoT Based Solutions for Health Care: Moving AI to the Edge. *Pattern Recognition Letters*, *135*, 346–353. DOI: 10.1016/j.patrec.2020.05.016 PMID: 32406416

Haleem, A., Javaid, M., Singh, R. P., Suman, R., & Rab, S. (2021). Blockchain Technology Applications in Healthcare: An Overview. *International Journal of Intelligent Networks*, *2*(May), 130–139. DOI: 10.1016/j.ijin.2021.09.005

Haq, A. U., Jian, P. L., Ahmad, S., Khan, S., Alshara, M. A., & Alotaibi, R. M. (2021). Diagnostic Approach for Accurate Diagnosis of COVID-19 Employing Deep Learning and Transfer Learning Techniques through Chest X-Ray Images Clinical Data in E-Healthcare. *Sensors (Basel)*, *21*(24), 8219. DOI: 10.3390/s21248219 PMID: 34960313

Haque, M. A., Ahmad, S., Sonal, D., Haque, S., Kumar, K., & Rahman, M. (2023). Analytical Studies on the Effectiveness of IoMT for Healthcare Systems. *Iraqi Journal of Science*, •••, 4719–4728. DOI: 10.24996/ijs.2023.64.9.34

Herrera Perez, J. L., Fajes Alfonso, A., & Alvarez, D. (1989). Retinopatia Diabetica E Hiperlipoproteinemia. *Revista Cubana de Medicina*, *28*(4), 333–340.

Herzog, N. J. (n.d.). *Dilek Celik &. Rejwan Bin Sulaiman*. Artificial Intelligence in Healthcare and Medical Records Security.

Huifeng, W., Kadry, S. N., & Raj, E. D. (2020). Continuous Health Monitoring of Sportsperson Using IoT Devices Based Wearable Technology. *Computer Communications*, *160*, 588–595. DOI: 10.1016/j.comcom.2020.04.025

Indrakumari, R., Poongodi, T., Suresh, P., & Balamurugan, B. (2019). *The Growing Role of Internet of Things in Healthcare Wearables*. Elsevier Inc.

Iqbal, M. S., Abd-Alrazaq, A., & Househ, M. (2022). Artificial Intelligence Solutions to Detect Fraud in Healthcare Settings: A Scoping Review. *Studies in Health Technology and Informatics*, *295*(July), 20–23. DOI: 10.3233/SHTI220649 PMID: 35773795

Irshad, R. R., Alattab, A. A., Omar, A. S. A., Sohail, S. S., Aziz, A., Madsen, D. Ø., & Alalayah, K. M. (2023). An Optimization-Linked Intelligent Security Algorithm for Smart Healthcare Organizations. *Healthcare (Basel)*, *11*(4), 580. Advance online publication. DOI: 10.3390/healthcare11040580 PMID: 36833114

Ismail, W. N., Hassan, M. M., Alsalamah, H. A., & Fortino, G. (2020). CNN-Based Health Model for Regular Health Factors Analysis in Internet-of-Medical Things Environment. *IEEE Access : Practical Innovations, Open Solutions*, *8*, 52541–52549. DOI: 10.1109/ACCESS.2020.2980938

Kalamkar, S., & Mary, G. A. 2020. “Clinical Data Fusion and Machine Learning Techniques for Smart Healthcare.” *2020 International Conference on Industry 4.0 Technology, I4Tech 2020* 211–16. DOI: 10.1109/I4Tech48345.2020.9102706

Kanksha, A. B., Pande, S., Malik, R., & Khamparia, A. (2021). An Intelligent Unsupervised Technique for Fraud Detection in Health Care Systems. *Intelligent Decision Technologies*, *15*(1), 127–139. DOI: 10.3233/IDT-200052

Khan, H. A., Abdulla, R., Selvaperumal, S. K., & Bathich, A. (2021). IoT Based on Secure Personal Healthcare Using RFID Technology and Steganography. *International Journal of Electrical and Computer Engineering*, *11*(4), 3300–3309. DOI: 10.11591/ijece.v11i4.pp3300-3309

Khan, J., Khan, G. A., Jian, P. L., Alajmi, M. F., Haq, A. U., Khan, S., Ahmad, N., Parveen, S., Shahid, M., Ahmad, S., Raji, M., Ahamad, B., Alghamdi, A. A., & Ali, A. (2022). Secure Smart Healthcare Monitoring in Industrial Internet of Things (IIoT) Ecosystem with Cosine Function Hybrid Chaotic Map Encryption. *Scientific Programming*, *2022*, 1–22. Advance online publication. DOI: 10.1155/2022/8853448

Khan, J., Li, J., Haq, A. U., Parveen, S., Khan, G. A., Shahid, M., Monday, H. N., Ullah, S., & Sun, R. 2019. “Medical Image Encryption into Smart Healthcare IOT System.” *2019 16th International Computer Conference on Wavelet Active Media Technology and Information Processing, ICCWAMTIP 2019* 378–82. DOI: 10.1109/ICCWAMTIP47768.2019.9067592

Knudsen, J. E., Ghaffar, U., Ma, R., & Hung, A. J. (2024). Clinical Applications of Artificial Intelligence in Robotic Surgery. *Journal of Robotic Surgery*, *18*(1), 1–10. DOI: 10.1007/s11701-024-01867-0 PMID: 38427094

Kumar, R., & Sharma, R. (2022). Leveraging Blockchain for Ensuring Trust in IoT: A Survey. *Journal of King Saud University. Computer and Information Sciences*, *34*(10), 8599–8622. DOI: 10.1016/j.jksuci.2021.09.004

Li, J., & Carayon, P. (2021). Health Care 4.0: A Vision for Smart and Connected Health Care. *IISE Transactions on Healthcare Systems Engineering*, *11*(3), 171–180. DOI: 10.1080/24725579.2021.1884627 PMID: 34497970

MacKey, T. K., & Liang, B. A. (2012). Combating Healthcare Corruption and Fraud with Improved Global Health Governance. *BMC International Health and Human Rights*, *12*(1), 23. Advance online publication. DOI: 10.1186/1472-698X-12-23 PMID: 23088820

Martínez-Caro, E., Cegarra-Navarro, J. G., García-Pérez, A., & Fait, M. (2017, July). 2018. “Healthcare Service Evolution towards the Internet of Things: An End-User Perspective.”. *Technological Forecasting and Social Change*, *136*, 268–276. DOI: 10.1016/j.techfore.2018.03.025

Mathew, P. S., Pillai, A. S., & Palade, V. (2018). Applications of Iot in Healthcare. *Lecture Notes on Data Engineering and Communications Technologies*, *14*, 263–288. DOI: 10.1007/978-3-319-70688-7_11

Minutolo, A., Esposito, M., & De Pietro, G. (2016, December). 2017. “Optimization of Rule-Based Systems in MHealth Applications.”. *Engineering Applications of Artificial Intelligence*, *59*, 103–121. DOI: 10.1016/j.engappai.2016.12.007

Mirbabaie, M., Stieglitz, S., & Frick, N. R. J. (2021). *Artificial Intelligence in Disease Diagnostics: A Critical Review and Classification on the Current State of Research Guiding Future Direction* (Vol. 11). Springer Berlin Heidelberg.

Mykowiecka, A., Marciniak, M., & Kupść, A. (2009). Rule-Based Information Extraction from Patients' Clinical Data. *Journal of Biomedical Informatics*, *42*(5), 923–936. DOI: 10.1016/j.jbi.2009.07.007 PMID: 19646551

Nithya, B., & Ilango, V. 2017. "Predictive Analytics in Health Care Using Machine Learning Tools and Techniques." *Proceedings of the 2017 International Conference on Intelligent Computing and Control Systems, ICICCS 2017* 2018-January:492–99. DOI: 10.1109/ICCONS.2017.8250771

Núñez, J. C., Cabido, R., Pantrigo, J. J., Montemayor, A. S., & Vélez, J. F. (2018). Convolutional Neural Networks and Long Short-Term Memory for Skeleton-Based Human Activity and Hand Gesture Recognition. *Pattern Recognition*, *76*, 80–94. DOI: 10.1016/j.patcog.2017.10.033

Panayides, A. S., Amini, A., Filipovic, N. D., Sharma, A., Tsaftaris, S. A., Young, A., Foran, D., Do, N., Golemati, S., Kurc, T., Huang, K., Nikita, K. S., Veasey, B. P., Zervakis, M., Saltz, J. H., & Pattichis, C. S. (2020). AI in Medical Imaging Informatics: Current Challenges and Future Directions. *IEEE Journal of Biomedical and Health Informatics*, *24*(7), 1837–1857. DOI: 10.1109/JBHI.2020.2991043 PMID: 32609615

Pandimurugan, V., & Sultan Ahmad, A. (2024). CNN-Based Deep Learning Model for Early Identification and Categorization of Melanoma Skin Cancer Using Medical Imaging. *SN Computer Science*, *5*(7), 1–20. DOI: 10.1007/s42979-024-03270-w

Parihar, Akshay, Jigna B. Prajapati, Bhupendra G. Prajapati, Binti Trambadiya, Arti Thakkar, and Pinalkumar Engineer. 2024. "Role of IOT in Healthcare: Applications, Security & Privacy Concerns." *Intelligent Pharmacy* (December 2023). .DOI: 10.1016/j.ipha.2024.01.003

Pradhan, B., Bhattacharyya, S., & Pal, K. (2021). IoT-Based Applications in Healthcare Devices. *Journal of Healthcare Engineering*, *2021*, 1–18. Advance online publication. DOI: 10.1155/2021/6632599 PMID: 33791084

Preum, S. M., Munir, S., Ma, M., Yasar, M. S., Stone, D. J., Williams, R., Alemzadeh, H., & Stankovic, J. A. (2021). A Review of Cognitive Assistants for Healthcare: Trends, Prospects, and Future Directions. *ACM Computing Surveys*, *53*(6), 1–37. Advance online publication. DOI: 10.1145/3419368

Rajagopal, A., Ahmad, S., Jha, S., Alagarsamy, R., Alharbi, A., & Alouffi, B. (2023). A Robust Automated Framework for Classification of CT Covid-19 Images Using MSI-ResNet. *Computer Systems Science and Engineering*, *45*(3), 3215–3229. DOI: 10.32604/csse.2023.025705

Rasouli, J. J., Shao, J., Neifert, S., Gibbs, W. N., Habboub, G., Steinmetz, M. P., Benzel, E., & Mroz, T. E. (2021). Artificial Intelligence and Robotics in Spine Surgery. *Global Spine Journal*, *11*(4), 556–564. DOI: 10.1177/2192568220915718 PMID: 32875928

Rehman, M. U., Shafique, A., Khan, M. S., Driss, M., Boulila, W., Ghadi, Y. Y., Changalasetty, S. B., Alhaisoni, M., & Ahmad, J. (2024). A Novel Medical Image Data Protection Scheme for Smart Healthcare System. *CAAI Transactions on Intelligence Technology*, *9*(4), 821–836. DOI: 10.1049/cit2.12292

Saif, S., Das, P., Biswas, S., Khan, S., Haq, M. A., & Kovtun, V. (2024). A Secure Data Transmission Framework for IoT Enabled Healthcare. *Heliyon, 10*(16), e36269. DOI: 10.1016/j.heliyon.2024.e36269 PMID: 39224301

Saraswat, D., Bhattacharya, P., Verma, A., Prasad, V. K., Tanwar, S., Sharma, G., Bokoro, P. N., & Sharma, R. (2022). Explainable AI for Healthcare 5.0: Opportunities and Challenges. *IEEE Access : Practical Innovations, Open Solutions*, *10*(July), 84486–84517. DOI: 10.1109/ACCESS.2022.3197671

Serrano, M., Dang, H. N., & Hoan, M. Q. N. 2018. "Recent Advances on Artificial Intelligence and Internet of Things Convergence for Human-Centric Applications." *ACM International Conference Proceeding Series*. DOI: 10.1145/3277593.3277638

Shastry, K. A., & Shastry, A. (2023). An Integrated Deep Learning and Natural Language Processing Approach for Continuous Remote Monitoring in Digital Health. *Decision Analytics Journal*, *8*(August), 100301. DOI: 10.1016/j.dajour.2023.100301

Silvestri, S., Islam, S., Papastergiou, S., Tzagkarakis, C., & Ciampi, M. (2023). A Machine Learning Approach for the NLP-Based Analysis of Cyber Threats and Vulnerabilities of the Healthcare Ecosystem †. *Sensors (Basel)*, *23*(2), 1–26. DOI: 10.3390/s23020651 PMID: 36679446

Singh, G., Schulthess, D., Hughes, N., Vannieuwenhuyse, B., & Kalra, D. (2018). Real World Big Data for Clinical Research and Drug Development. *Drug Discovery Today*, *23*(3), 652–660. DOI: 10.1016/j.drudis.2017.12.002 PMID: 29294362

Sinha, S., & Vohora, D. (2017). *Drug Discovery and Development: An Overview*. Elsevier Inc.

Subasi, A. (2021, August). 2024. "Artificial Intelligence in Drug Discovery and Development.". *Applications of Artificial Intelligence in Healthcare and Biomedicine*, *23*, 417–454. DOI: 10.1016/B978-0-443-22308-2.00018-4

Truong, H. T. T., Almeida, M., Karame, G., & Soriente, C. 2019. "Towards Secure and Decentralized Sharing of IoT Data." *Proceedings - 2019 2nd IEEE International Conference on Blockchain, Blockchain 2019* 176–83. DOI: 10.1109/Blockchain.2019.00031

Tuli, S., Tuli, S., Wander, G., Wander, P., Gill, S. S., Dustdar, S., Sakellariou, R., & Rana, O. (2020). Next Generation Technologies for Smart Healthcare: Challenges, Vision, Model, Trends and Future Directions. *Internet Technology Letters*, *3*(2), 1–6. DOI: 10.1002/itl2.145

Vaiyapuri, T., Mahalingam, J., Ahmad, S., Abdeljaber, H. A. M., Yang, E., & Jeong, S.-Y. (2023). Ensemble Learning Driven Computer-Aided Diagnosis Model for Brain Tumor Classification on Magnetic Resonance Imaging. *IEEE Access : Practical Innovations, Open Solutions*, *11*, 91398–91406. DOI: 10.1109/ACCESS.2023.3306961

Vijayasarveswari, V., & Lim Jia Chyin, N. M. (1962). Wafi, and I. Iszaidy. 2021. "Development of E-Healthcare Management System Using PHP, Javascript and Cascading Style Sheets.". *Journal of Physics: Conference Series*, (1). Advance online publication. DOI: 10.1088/1742-6596/1962/1/012030

Whig, V., Othman, B., Gehlot, A., Haque, M. A., Qamar, S., & Singh, J. 2022. "An Empirical Analysis of Artificial Intelligence (AI) as a Growth Engine for the Healthcare Sector." Pp. 2454–57 in *2022 2nd International Conference on Advance Computing and Innovative Technologies in Engineering (ICACITE)*. IEEE. DOI: 10.1109/ICACITE53722.2022.9823607

Xu, X., Ge, Z., Chow, E. P., Yu, Z., Lee, D., Wu, J., & Zhang, L. (2022). A machine-learning-based risk-prediction tool for HIV and sexually transmitted infections acquisition over the next 12 months. *Journal of Clinical Medicine*, *11*(7), 1818.

Yin, Y., Zeng, Y., Chen, X., & Fan, Y. (2016). The Internet of Things in Healthcare: An Overview. *Journal of Industrial Information Integration*, *1*, 3–13. DOI: 10.1016/j.jii.2016.03.004

Zahid, N., Sodhro, A. H., Kamboh, U. R., Alkhayyat, A., & Wang, L. (2022). AI-Driven Adaptive Reliable and Sustainable Approach for Internet of Things Enabled Healthcare System. *Mathematical Biosciences and Engineering*, *19*(4), 3953–3971. DOI: 10.3934/mbe.2022182 PMID: 35341282

Zeb, S., Fnu, N., Abbasi, N., & Fahad, M. (2024). AI in Healthcare: Revolutionizing Diagnosis and Therapy. *International Journal of Multidisciplinary Sciences and Arts*, *3*(3), 118–128. DOI: 10.47709/ijmdsa.v3i3.4546

Chapter 2
The Role of Internet of Things Technologies in Revolutionizing Healthcare Delivery and Patient Monitoring

D. Prabakar
https://orcid.org/0009-0002-1558-5251
SRM Institute of Science and Technology, India

Nirmalkumar S. Benni
RNS Institute of Technology, India

B. Arunsundar
SRM Institute of Science and Technology, India

Satyajeet Sahoo
Vignan's Foundation for Science, Technology and Research, India

N. Keerthy
Global Academy of Technology, India

K. Suganthi
SRM Institute of Science and Technology, India

Khaja Raoufuddin Ahmed
Infosol IT Solutions, UK

ABSTRACT

The Internet of Things (IoT) has transformed healthcare by enabling smart healthcare systems focused on real-time monitoring, data-driven insights, and improved patient outcomes. IoMT (Internet of Medical Things) and Healthcare 4.0 are evolving with technologies like AI, edge computing, and 5G, supporting efficient, connected, and mobile health services. Despite rapid progress, gaps remain in understanding implementation challenges, design complexities, and adoption barriers. This study reviews recent advancements, identifies enabling technologies, and outlines future requirements for scalable, secure, and intelligent healthcare systems. It also proposes research directions to enhance IoT-driven healthcare delivery in the post-pandemic era.

DOI: 10.4018/979-8-3373-1022-0.ch002

1. INTRODUCTION

The phrase "Internet of Things" (IoT), first used by Kevin Ashton in 1999, describes information stored online and linked to a dynamic global service architecture. Advanced studies in information and communication technologies have resulted in the IoT. The quality of life for city dwellers may be improved. There is a rising need to develop efficient health systems that can manage and deliver a variety of medical treatments while lowering overall costs, as the world's population is expanding at an unprecedented rate and chronic diseases are becoming more common (Alam et al., 2023). When it comes to improving healthcare monitoring systems, the IoT has lately emerged as a crucial area for growth. The goal of the IoT healthcare monitoring system is to precisely monitor individuals while also linking different services and objects throughout the globe via the Internet in order to gather, exchange, keep tabs on, store, and evaluate the data produced by these things. However, the IoT is a new paradigm that allows for the remote control and management of any intelligent application's linked physical items (Chinthala et al., 2022). This includes smart cities, smart homes, and smart healthcare. Medical treatment relies on accurate diagnosis and close patient monitoring; integrating sensor networks into the human body would greatly facilitate these tasks (Alqahtani et al., 2023). Also, you can get the data whenever you want, no matter where you are on the globe. When it comes to healthcare, the IoT is all about a mix of hardware and software that can talk to one another and the healthcare IT infrastructure over the Internet. The IoT paves the way for a system of seamless data exchange and analysis by allowing machine-to-machine connections via Wi-Fi-enabled medical equipment. In the 1990s, the IoT in healthcare made its debut with the introduction of simple telemedicine and RPM systems (Hasan et al., 2024). Miniaturization with data analytics breakthroughs in the early 2000s led to intelligent medical equipment and wearable health gadgets. The IoT is now transforming the healthcare business by enabling personalized therapy and real-time data-driven decision-making with remote patient monitoring.

Figure 1. IoT Healthcare

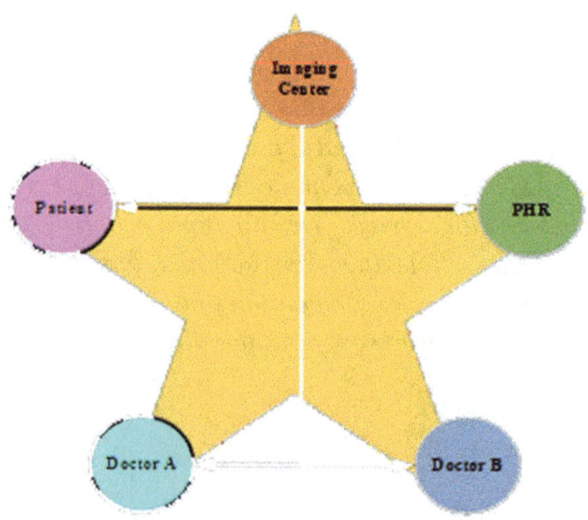

The hospital may be out of reach for patients from certain locations or those with very serious injuries. As a result, individuals may save time and money by communicating with their physicians via video conferencing, which can enhance their health (Kumar et al., 2023). Using this technology, patients may document their health issues directly on their phones. Improved patient outcomes and reduced healthcare administration expenses are two expected results of the IoT's personalized treatment capabilities. IoT solutions enable doctors to monitor their patients and make appointment scheduling more streamlined remotely. Additionally, patients have the power to enhance their home healthcare in order to lessen the frequency of doctor's appointments and the possibility of obtaining unneeded or improper medical treatments at healthcare facilities. Costs associated with medical treatment may go down, while patient safety and care quality may go up for this reason. The Internet of Things has enormous promise in the medical field. It won't be long before we can expedite hospital operations with a health-monitoring device that we can utilize from the convenience of our own homes. The extensive deployment of IoT sensors may achieve continuous monitoring of the body and surroundings (Kishor Kumar Reddy et al., 2025). As a result of these efforts, rehabilitation, and chronic illness management may be monitored. The IoT has the potential to revolutionize remote medical consultations by facilitating efficient data connections across many locales. Research and implementation of the IoT are still in their early stages, with a primary emphasis on testing and implementing technologies in different environments. But these methods aren't employed much these days. Thus, the purpose of this study is to assess relevant studies that have focused on the development and implementation of healthcare monitoring systems that make use of the IoT to provide a better quality of life. IoT gadgets and sensors play a crucial role in these systems, which aim to match patients with the most appropriate healthcare providers. This paper's primary contribution is an in-depth analysis of healthcare monitoring systems that make use of the IoT. This will help academics, researchers, and scientists of the future better understand these systems as they stand, which will allow them to develop better solutions for these vital applications. In this study, we systematically outline healthcare monitoring systems that rely on the IoT, discussing its advantages and importance while also reviewing the relevant literature. From an IoT vantage point, we also go over the ideas of wearable objects in healthcare systems. Additionally, the article discusses protocols and security for healthcare monitoring systems that rely on the IoT, and it lays out the obstacles and unanswered questions in this field. In addition, we provide recommendations on how to address these problems and obstacles in the future.

Figure 2. IoT Model for Healthcare

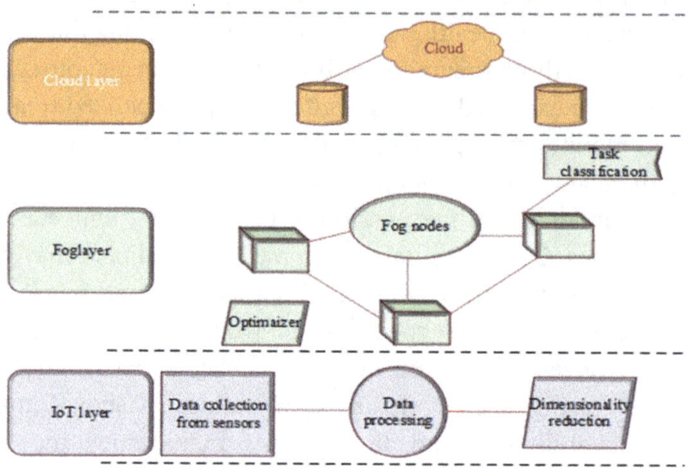

This research seeks to fill a gap in existing scholarship by expanding on these topics in order to provide a thorough knowledge of the importance and possible contributions of the IoT to the healthcare industry. We want to show how the IoT might enhance patient outcomes by analyzing and studying healthcare delivery in depth (Roy et al., 2021). The structure is made up of three separate levels, namely:

- **Device Layer:** This layer incorporates environmental or wearable smart sensors, robotic agents, and agents used for user engagement, including smartphones, virtual assistants, and gesture control devices. It covers everything that can interact with the physical environment and people.
- **IoT Fog Layer:** Decentralized devices that store and process data. They take the information collected at the device layer, preprocess it, and then transfer it to the cloud. Fog devices are often located on the user's local area network.
- **Cloud Layer:** A gathering place for analytics and storage of huge datasets. With its help, increasing the system's processing along with prediction model capacities is a breeze.

2. IOT HEALTHCARE MONITORING DEVICES

Thanks to IoT devices, healthcare providers and patients have many new possibilities for monitoring each other and themselves. The proliferation of wearable IoT devices has many implications for healthcare practitioners and patients.

IoT Medical Sensors

- **Pulse oximeters**

One medical tool for determining a patient's SpO2 level is a pulse oximeter. It is a tiny, portable gadget that commonly clips onto an index finger, toe, or earlobe. After being attached to a body part, the pulse oximeter releases two light wavelengths—usually red and infrared—into that area. The instrument then measures the light absorbed through the blood's oxygen-carrying hemoglobin. The percentage of oxygen saturation is determined from this measurement. Although pulse oximeters are more often seen in healthcare facilities, they may also be found in many homes. In particular, they help keep tabs on people who have heart or respiratory issues, as well as those who are active or at high altitudes, and to assess their overall health status. A blood oximeter may identify pneumonia, anemia, asthma, lung problems, and other medical issues. It is safe, easy, noninvasive, and inexpensive to measure peripheral SpO2 with a blood oximeter, even though it isn't always equivalent to the preferred arterial SpO2. One useful way to measure oxygen saturation in the clinic is with the use of pulse oximetry (Pradhan et al., 2021).

The underlying concept of spectrophotometry is what makes pulse oximeters function. They transmit two beams of light, commonly red and infrared, via the body area where it is connected. The absorption of infrared light is enhanced by oxygenated hemoglobin, while red light is enhanced by deoxygenated hemoglobin. The pulse oximeter analyzes how much light the blood absorbs and calculates the saturation level of oxygen by contrasting the absorbed infrared to red light ratio. The device's screen then shows the pulse rate and oxygen saturation percentage (SpO2). The results of a pulse oximeter show how well oxygen is carried to different parts of the body. Saturation levels of oxygen typically fall between 95% and 100%. Values under this range may indicate hypoxemia, which is defined as low blood oxygen levels. A typical application case of pulse oximeters is their application in airplanes. Low cabin pressure, oxygen levels, and humidity pose a threat to passengers having chronic obstructive pulmonary disease (COPD). Thus, this system is essential for airplanes. Therefore, it is crucial to track their health and notice any deviations early so that they may get proper treatment.

- **Pulse Rate Sensors**

(1) An optical sensor can measure variations in blood volume by seeing light. A light-emitting diode (LED) measures the light that is reflected, while a photodetector measures the light that is reflected. The sensor can determine the pulse rate by measuring the change in the quantity of light reflected during each heartbeat, which is caused by the increase in blood flow.
(2) The second kind of sensor is the piezoelectric, which employs materials that produce voltage in response to mechanical stress or vibration. The mechanical vibrations produced by each heartbeat may be transformed into an electrical signal by placing a piezoelectric sensor on the skin or a blood vessel, allowing for the determination of the pulse rate.
(3) A capacitive sensor can detect electrocardiogram-induced variations in capacitance among two electrodes. Because the capacitance changes with each heartbeat in response to fluctuating blood flow, these sensors usually involve putting the electrodes on the skin or blood vessels.
(4) Fourthly, an electrocardiogram (ECG) sensor can reveal details regarding the electrical activity of the heart. The electrical impulses produced by the heart's contractions and relaxations may be detected using an electrocardiogram (ECG) monitor. It is possible to extract several metrics, such as heart rate, from these signals.

- **PPG sensors**

Devices that assess modifications to peripheral blood vessel blood volume are known as photoplethysmography (PPG) sensors. Utilizing light sensors, it is able to identify fluctuations in light absorption or reflection induced by blood flow. Fitness trackers, smartwatches, and other wearables often use PPG sensors to measure heart rates and estimate blood oxygen levels. The sensor transmits light onto the epidermis and detects the strength of the light that is reflected, generating a photoplethysmography waveform. This waveform is often used in healthcare and wellness applications since it may give information about several health factors. PPG is a popular optical tracking method employed to track heart rates at a low cost. No incisions are needed for PPG. By affixing a light source along with a photodetector to the skin's surface, a PPG sensor can measure variations in blood flow. The PPG signal is currently attracting the attention of several researchers interested in extracting additional information from it. The PPG signal's second derivative wave offers critical diagnostic information. In light of this, waveform analysis is helpful for the diagnosis of numerous cardiovascular issues. Placement of the PPG sensors on the earlobe, individual's finger, or forehead is the norm. The search for more accessible measuring points has researchers investigating a number of different anatomical zones.

- **Temperature sensors**

When it comes to safe and accurate measurement of body temperature, a temperature sensor is a typical medical sensor. It is designed particularly for medical applications that track patients' temperature in clinics, hospitals, and other healthcare settings. Sensors like these use infrared, thermocouples, or thermistors to pick up body heat and transform it into an electrical signal that doctors can analyze. Medical temperature sensors exist in numerous forms, such as oral, rectal, ear, and forehead, as well as wearable patches or bands. Each variety has its benefits and limits, and its utilization relies on the individual's age and condition, along with the healthcare provider's choice. The ability to detect fever, a symptom of numerous diseases, relies heavily on these sensors. Healthcare providers can better diagnose and track the progression of illnesses and infections with accurate monitoring of body temperature. It enables prompt action as well as suitable treatment, improving the overall health of patients.

- **Blood pressure sensors**

By sensing the force that blood pressure exerts on the arteries, blood pressure monitors and measures blood pressure levels. An oscillometer, which detects variations in pressure due to the pulsating blood flow, is a common component of modern blood pressure monitors. The sensor raises the cuff to restrict blood flow temporarily before logging gradually deflates it while analyzing the pressure changes. These readings allow the sensor to calculate blood pressure in systole and diastole. There are a wide variety of blood pressure monitors on the market, including those made specifically for use in homes, hospitals, and even on wearable technology. In order to save and analyze data, certain sensors may be able to link to smartphones and other devices. It is always an excellent choice to contact a healthcare expert for assistance in choosing and utilizing blood pressure monitors since precise readings and the right technique are vital for monitoring and controlling blood pressure successfully. Instead of using a cuff, some techniques assess blood pressure using biological sensors like electrocardiogram (ECG) and photoplethysmography (PPG) sensors.

- **EEG sensors**

Electroencephalography (EEG) sensors are gadgets used to detect and record electrical activity in the brain. EEG is a non-invasive neuroimaging method that evaluates the voltage variations resulting from the ionic current flowing within the neurons of the brain. These devices have a wide variety of uses, including detecting epilepsy, sleep problems, brain traumas, and neurological illnesses. Cognitive research, neurofeedback, and brain-computer interfaces (BCI) are some of their other applications. Electroencephalogram (EEG) sensors often include a number of electrodes that are fastened to the scalp. These electrodes are tiny metal discs or sensors that rise into contact through the scalp to gather up the electrical signals generated by the brain. Wet or dry electrodes are available. For wet electrodes to work properly, a conductive gel must be placed to the area connecting the electrode along with the scalp. Impedance and interference are both mitigated by the gel. In contrast, dry electrodes may be placed straight to the scalp without the need for extra gel. Most consumer-grade EEG devices use them because they are easier to use. Depending on the degree of spatial resolution required, the total amount of electrodes utilized in an EEG system can vary from a few channels to many hundred. In order to reliably record particular patterns of brain activity, the placement of electrodes used for EEG is crucial. In addition, EEG sensors are coupled to amplifiers that enhance the feeble electrical signals picked through the electrodes. Amplifiers play an essential part in preserving a ratio of signal to noise, which is critical for getting high-quality EEG data. The following step is to use analog-to-digital converters (ADCs) to transform the amplified analog signals into digital signals. Digital signals are simpler to analyze, store, and send for future analysis. An integral part of the EEG setup is a signal processor that normalizes, amplifies, and digitizes the unprocessed EEG signals. Signal processing procedures are employed to eliminate artifacts as well as noise from the signals. Data interfaces, such as Bluetooth, are common in modern EEG systems and enable the storage of data in real-time, as well as integration with various devices and software programs.

- **EMG sensors**

Sensors that use electromyography (EMG) can pick up on the electrical signals that muscles generate. These devices are widely used in the medical and scientific communities for the purpose of monitoring muscle activity, diagnosing neuromuscular illnesses, and regulating prosthetic limbs. Surface electrodes applied to the skin just above the target muscles make up an electromyography (EMG) sensor. When you contract your muscles, they send electrical impulses that these electrodes can detect. To contract a muscle, your brain sends electrical impulses via your nervous system to its specific fibers. These electrical impulses are picked up by the EMG sensor, which then turns them into quantifiable data. Surface EMG and intramuscular EMG are the two main categories of electromyography (EMG) sensors. In contrast to intramuscular EMG sensors, which require the insertion of tiny needle electrodes into the muscle, surface EMG sensors employ adhesive electrodes applied to the skin. Among the many useful uses for electromyography (EMG) sensors are in the fields of medicine, sports science, rehabilitation, as well as HCI. They let scientists and doctors evaluate muscle function, track treatment efficacy, and create novel body-interface technologies.

Actuators of IoT for Healthcare

These environment-centric actuators engage with elements of the outside world, such as facilities, medical equipment, and technologies, rather than the human body itself. One way to characterize them is as follows:

- Linear actuators: These are widely used in healthcare and include features like movable hospital beds, patient lifts, and wheelchair lifts. They make linear motion easy and accurate, which helps with patient placement and mobility aids.
- Rotating actuators: Diagnostic tools and robotic surgical systems both use rotary actuators. Their rotary motion allows imaging components and medical devices to be precisely positioned.
- Pneumatic actuators use compressed air to provide force and motion. Medical devices that use them include compression sleeves with pneumatic components that help prevent deep vein thrombosis and assistive devices with pneumatic components that aid in patient transfers and mobility.
- Magnetic resonance imaging (MRI) and computed tomography (CT) scanners, among other medical imaging devices, rely on electrical actuators. They allow for exact regulation of these devices' moving components, which improves diagnostic precision and high-resolution imaging.
- When it comes to microscale positioning and manipulation, medical gadgets often make use of piezoelectric actuators. Surgical micromanipulation, medication delivery via microfluidics, and cellular manipulation via nanotechnology are just a few of the fields that make use of them.
- One kind of actuator is the hydraulic actuator, which produces force and motion by use of pressurized fluid. Some examples of medical equipment that make use of them include hydraulic patient lifts, operating tables, and physical therapy and rehabilitation assistive devices.

Table 1. Common sensors

Sensor Type	Measurement	Clinical Application (s)
Electrocardiogram	The heart's electrical activity	Identifying cardiac irregularities
Pulse Oximeter	Blood oxygen levels and pulse rate	Tracking oxygen levels in patients with asthma, chronic obstructive pulmonary disease, or surgery
Blood Pressure	Concentrations of glucose in the blood and interstitial fluid Blood pressure	Maintaining a close eye on blood pressure levels
Glucose	Core temperature	Tracking diabetes
Temperature	Rhythm and rate of respiration	Recognizing signs of heat illness
Respiratory	The heart's electrical activity	Keep an eye on conditions related to breathing, such as sleep apnea

Table 2. Sensors and Values

Parameter	Range measurement	Measurement precision	Sampling frequency (Hz)	Response time (s)
Heart rate	0~350/min	±2% full	100	<2
ECG	N/A	N/A	512	<2
Smart cushion	0.1~10Kg/cm^2	0.5% full	300	<1
Falling	0~350Hz, ±6g	200mV/g	300	<1
Temperature	-20~+80	±0.2	300	<1
Humidity	0~100%RH	±2%RH	300	<1
Household smart device	N/A	N/A	N/A	<1

Figure 3. IoT Dataset Model

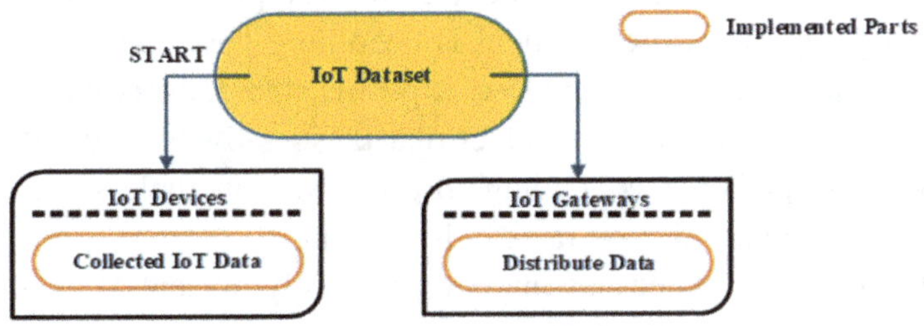

2.1 Applications

- **Parkinson's disease monitoring:** Healthcare practitioners treating Parkinson's patients should be able to track the symptom intensity throughout the day for optimal treatment. By constantly gathering data regarding Parkinson's symptoms, IoT devices claim to make this chore much simpler. Also, patients are able to go through their daily lives in the comfort of their own homes with the use of these gadgets, rather than being confined to a hospital for long periods of time for observation.
- **Glucose monitoring:** Glucose monitoring has always been challenging for the over 30 million Americans who suffer from diabetes. Manually recording findings from glucose checks is not only an inconvenience, but it also only gives a patient's glucose levels at the exact moment the test is given. The inadequacy of periodic testing to identify an issue may arise if levels exhibit large fluctuations. The IoT offers a solution to these problems by automatically monitoring patients' glucose levels in real-time. Patients may be alerted when their glucose levels become troublesome, and glucose monitoring devices eliminate the need to maintain records manually. IoT glucose monitor design is one of the obstacles that:
    - o Its little size allows for constant monitoring without disturbing patients.

- o While these may seem like insurmountable obstacles, they really hold great potential for technologies that solve them to transform the way patients manage their glucose monitoring completely.

- **Remote patient monitoring:** One of the most prevalent uses of Internet of Things devices in healthcare is remote patient monitoring. Patients who aren't physically present at a healthcare institution may nevertheless have their vitals monitored via IoT devices, which eliminates the need for them to either go to the hospital or manually gather the data themselves. A software program is notified whenever an IoT device gathers data on a patient, and either the patient or a healthcare provider may access this data. In order to provide therapy recommendations or alarms, algorithms may examine the data. An IoT sensor that notices a patient's dangerously low heart rate, for instance, may notify healthcare providers to take action. Ensuring the security and privacy of the highly sensitive data collected by these Internet of Things devices poses a significant problem to remote patient monitoring systems.
- **Hand hygiene monitoring:** There hasn't been an effective method for a long time to guarantee that healthcare workers and patients within a facility properly clean their hands to prevent the transmission of infection. The usage of IoT devices to prompt patients and visitors to wash their hands before touching any medical equipment is becoming commonplace in today's healthcare facilities. Depending on the patient's unique risk profile, the gadgets may even recommend the most effective sanitization procedures. The fact that these gadgets may only serve as reminders and not actually wash people's hands is a huge drawback. Nonetheless, studies have shown that these devices may cut hospital infection rates in half or more.
- **Heart-rate monitoring:** Even when patients are physically present at healthcare institutions, it might be difficult to monitor their heart rates, similar to glucose. Patients' movement is severely limited by the traditional methods of continuous cardiac monitoring, which involve continuously attaching them to wired apparatus and do not protect them from fast variations in heart rates. Small IoT devices are now accessible for heart rate tracking, allowing patients more freedom of movement while yet guaranteeing continuous heart monitoring. Even while it's still not easy to guarantee pinpoint precision, most current devices can provide data with a 90% accuracy rate or higher.
- **Depression and mood monitoring** Additional data types that have historically been challenging to gather regularly include information about depressive symptoms and patients' overall mood. Healthcare practitioners may inquire about patients' emotional well-being on occasion, but they couldn't foresee abrupt changes in their mood. Furthermore, patients often exaggerate their emotional states. Aware of one's emotional state IoT devices can handle these issues. A patient's mental state may be inferred from data collected and analyzed by equipment, such as their heart rate and blood pressure. The most cutting-edge IoT mood monitors can follow a patient's eye movements and other biometric data. Problematically, these measures cannot reliably foretell the onset of depressive symptoms or other alarming indicators. However, a conventional in-person evaluation of mental health also cannot.

2.2 Benefits of IoT in Healthcare

A growing number of healthcare organizations are embracing the IoT as a solution because of its many advantages.

Table 3. Benefits of IoT in Healthcare

Monitoring and Alerts	Through the use of interconnected smart devices, IoT enables continuous monitoring of patients' vital signs and medical indicators. Blood pressure and glucose levels are only two of the many characteristics that smart sensors can track. The system automatically alerts caregivers or medical personnel in the event of any abnormalities, allowing them to respond quickly. With this improvement in healthcare IoT, major health issues are less likely to occur, and patients' illnesses may be better managed.
Remote Assistance	The Internet of Things enables remote medical assistance by facilitating online consultations and connections with linked devices. Without physically meeting, patients and doctors may communicate and seek advice on healthcare matters. This is useful for those who have trouble moving around or who live in remote areas.
End-to-end Connectivity	The Internet of Things allows for smooth interactions in the healthcare system. Intelligent medical devices, doctor's offices, and hospitals all share patient information automatically. This advantage improves the precision and timeliness of patient monitoring, diagnosis, and therapy. Fully connected healthcare systems also benefit from improved efficiency, fewer mistakes, and no more double-entry of data.
Data Analysis	The automatic data collection capabilities of healthcare IoT devices provide valuable insights. Medical professionals may examine data to discover patterns and correlations between different health indicators. Based on these findings, they may make better-informed decisions about the condition's treatment and management. Statistical analysis advances modern healthcare plans and scientific investigations in medicine.
Preventive Healthcare	The healthcare IoT system may detect early warning signs of a disease and send out information quickly. This can help caregivers and patients take action against the onset of sickness and enhance their general quality of life.
Efficiency	The use of the IoT in healthcare has the potential to improve efficiency and make better use of available resources. Through improved inventory management, asset monitoring, and patient flow optimization, the IoT may reduce waste and save users' time.

3. CHALLENGES OF IOT IN HEALTHCARE

One major obstacle to the expansion of the Internet of Things is the several performance-related issues that arise from it. These include issues with efficiency, latency, security, and dependability. A better Internet of Things system should have low latency, great dependability, minimal power consumption, and strong security (Kaza et al., 2024). In the following part, we will discuss the difficulties encountered by many writers when working with IoT systems.

3.1. Low Latency

Low latency is an important goal in the IoT for many applications, including telemedicine, monitoring patients remotely, and emergency response systems that process and evaluate information in real time. Healthcare practitioners are able to react quickly to situations and make choices because of the low latency. Nevertheless, optimizing network infrastructure and using specific software and hardware may make achieving low latency a challenging task. One of the biggest problems with the Internet of Things is real-time data transmission and analysis; otherwise, healthcare practitioners won't be able to make well-informed recommendations. Very low latency in end-to-end transmission and data processing is required by an IoT system due to the system's time-critical characteristics. Finding more accessible and bandwidth-rich communication technologies shortens the transmission delay, which in turn shortens the overall latency. In contrast to the benefits of fog computing and edge computing frameworks, channel access and routing using ML algorithms might significantly reduce end-to-end latency. In addition, research has shown that integrating AI into these fog and edge computing frameworks greatly improves their efficiency. Although big data analytical systems that use deep learning techniques are better equipped to process enormous data sets, current problems make it impossible to extract all of the data from the given dataset reliably. Therefore, strong algorithms that might possibly use the dataset to their fullest extent are urgently needed. To fix this, processing and transmission delays are reduced, and computer resources close to the network edge are made less active. To guarantee low latency in time-critical IoT systems, the fog paradigm's distributed computing platforms might be used. IoT fog computing may reduce cloud latency's negative effect on EMS systems. However, there are still issues that need fixing, such as latency, energy usage, and reaction time. One solution to these problems is the EEIoMT framework, which stands for Energy-Efficient Internet of Medical Things to Fog Standardization of Task Scheduling. Optimizing task scheduling, this system manages energy usage and processes other jobs while prioritizing vital ones that must be done within a defined period.

3.2. Security Challenges

The sensitive nature of patient data makes security an important issue in the IoT. Security breaches, along with cyberattacks, are becoming increasingly common as the number of linked and accessible IoT gadgets and systems grows. Medical records might be a gold mine for fraudsters, identity thieves, and others who prey on cybercrime. In addition, patients may suffer serious consequences if a security breach occurs in an IoT system since sensitive medical data could be exposed or medical equipment could be tampered with. As a result, medical device safety and reliability, along with the availability, integrity, and confidentiality of patient data, rely on robust security mechanisms in IoT systems. It becomes laborious to frame lightweight methods for the IoT because of their resource constraints. In addition, maintaining energy efficiency is a major issue. Therefore, a deep learning or machine learning method that can manage lightweight cryptography and is energy efficient is necessary for the deployment of features designed to mitigate security concerns. But the system we just covered has computational complexity. Therefore, a federal system located close to the security equipment might be used in a fog paradigm (Zhang et al., 2022).

The Internet of Medical Things (IoMT) has the potential to provide efficient healthcare services, but it has security challenges due to its vulnerability to assaults by middlemen and the lack of security knowledge among novice users. To deal with these vulnerabilities, a security improvement strategy known as RECC-VC was suggested. By combining K-anonymity with optimized neural networks and blockchain technology, our strategy outperforms previous approaches in terms of accuracy and safety (Kumar et al., 2022).

3.3. Real-Time Operational Platforms

In general, the data obtained from the sensors could provide a more comprehensive understanding of the user's health state. It should be mentioned that the data created is large and can only be usefully extracted using specialist processing techniques. However, real-time data handling techniques are required since many current algorithms cannot handle whole data sets. It is critical to remove duplicate and numerous features from the dataset, even if machine learning techniques can manage enormous amounts of real-time data.

3.4. Energy Consumption

While it is possible to charge wearable Internet of Things devices after a certain amount of use, implants need a long-lasting battery to ensure trouble-free operation over the long haul. The literature offers a variety of remedies to this energy restriction. Minimal foreign interference to avoid harmful implementation side effects is one proposed approach to this issue. Improving the network lifespan also requires improved management of resources having limited processing capabilities, power, and memory in the IoT. A very low-power, short-range energy system has been proposed for use in fog and edge computing; however, in both scenarios, availability becomes an issue. Node energy collecting options offered in the literature should be user-safe, inexpensive, and fast-charging.

3.5. Scalability Challenges

It is necessary to resolve scalability issues in order to facilitate the widespread implementation of IoT systems. In addition, data transport is crucial in IoT systems. Thus, it's important to employ the right access method to prevent packet loss. Other than that, the inherent instability of most current protocols for routing data in IoT systems severely limits their usefulness. Furthermore, there are a number of significant concerns about coverage and localization. Wearable tech and implanted sensors must be standardized to provide seamless connection. There should be no introduction of extra expenses or computational delays into the processing of the produced data traffic. As a result, there are issues related to the ever-changing nodes' calibration in the network. Systems built on the Internet of Things also seem to face challenges related to mobility. The network performance is negatively affected if the user changes their current position due to sensors that are attached to a source, such as the human body. Therefore, trustworthy services should be implemented to ensure that the network remains available while an individual is on the go.

4. WORKING WITH IOT IN HEALTHCARE

4.1 Patients

Thanks to the many benefits of IoT in healthcare, patients are able to engage in a more active part in managing their health. Wearable IoT devices track a patient's vitals and activity levels in real time and make that information available to them via mobile applications for remote patient monitoring. People are now better able to monitor their own health and make educated choices about their care thanks to this innovation. Patients with diabetes or hypertension may keep tabs on their health with the aid of linked glucose monitors with blood pressure cuffs, which allows for regular treatment of chronic illnesses. The IoT and smart pill bottles help patients take their drugs as prescribed, which improves treatment results.

4.2 Physicians

IoT technology enhances healthcare delivery in several ways. With the use of remote monitoring and diagnostics, medical professionals are able to keep tabs on their patient's health status from afar. The data input from real-time IoT devices allows for early aberrant diagnosis and rapid response. Patient outcomes increase, and chronic illness care becomes more efficient.

4.3 Hospitals

Improvements in both efficiency and patient care may be achieved via the use of IoT in hospitals. With the use of IoT devices for asset monitoring and management, healthcare facilities are better able to monitor their medical equipment and maximize the use of their assets. This, in turn, reduces downtime and improves hospital operations by making sure that important equipment is always accessible when required. By optimizing patient flow with the help of IoT devices, hospitals may more effectively manage patient intakes, which in turn reduces waiting times and alleviates congestion in waiting rooms. Furthermore, by introducing cutting-edge hand hygiene monitoring systems, the IoT helps with infection management. In order to lower infection rates while keeping a clean atmosphere inside the hospital, these gadgets remind patients as well as doctors to sanitize their hands.

Figure 4. Data Collection from IoT Sensors

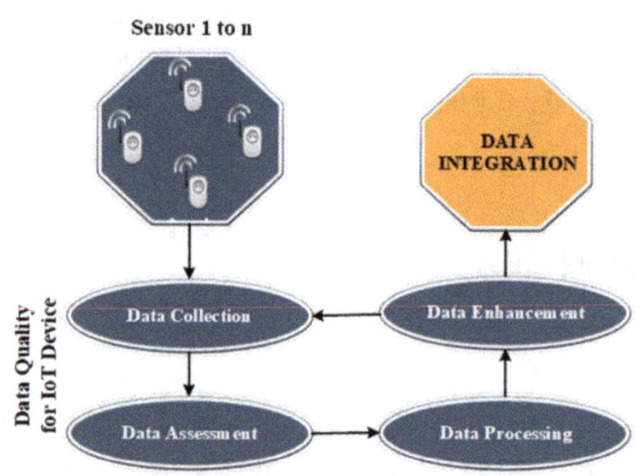

5. REVIEW OF RECENT RELATED STUDIES

By working together, they have improved healthcare workers' safety and made pandemic management more effective, which has reduced its effect on human lives as well as death rates (Rahman et al., 2023). In the field of IoMT, there have been tremendous advancements in both technology and applications. Nevertheless, it must be recognized that technical progress has brought up certain difficulties, especially regarding safety. When it comes to security and privacy, the quick and widespread deployment of IoMT throughout the globe has made things worse. Malware intrusions, remote hijacking, imitation, privileged insider threats, denial of service assaults, password guessing, and man-in-the-middle attacks are all part of that spectrum of problems. Their goal in writing that extensive research was to compare and contrast various methods now used to identify and stop malware in IoT settings.

Allowing the IoT in healthcare applications and services is the subject of a thorough systematic analysis in (Mohamad Jawad et al., 2022) that includes all publications that were assessed and published between 2015 and 2022. A systematic literature review was conducted on 106 publications that met all of the inclusion criteria. Two methods were employed to evaluate the finished papers: Study designs, published journals, and subjects/study aims, which are the primary lenses through which publications are analyzed. The second method delves into the reasons, obstacles, and suggestions for allowing the Internet of Things in healthcare systems. Research on the IoT and its applications in the smart delivery of medical care has been extensively reviewed and summarized in that article. They conclude that more studies are needed to fully use the IoT in healthcare, along with service delivery based on the papers that were examined.

The research (Tsantikidou & Sklavos, 2022) investigates well-known lightweight cryptographic primitives with their most recent architecture. The article provides information on their security, architecture, and general hardware limitations. Finally, they compare each algorithm according to how well it secures healthcare applications, the device it uses, and how efficient it is to build in general. Discusses mobile health within the framework of the Internet of Things in (Chanda et al., 2021). Healthcare system development using the Internet of Things has entered an evolutionary phase. The article explains the deployment of IoT in the medical field. That article primarily aims to highlight the rise of mobile IoT in the medical and healthcare industries. Several medical uses of M-IoT are highlighted in that chapter, including ECG monitoring, body temperature measurement, blood glucose level monitoring, and more. The Internet of Things has been permeating every facet of society, but because of the increasing importance and precision of healthcare, its impact is particularly profound. Along with the rise of mobile computing, the Internet of Things will take center stage. That expands the potential of the IoT in healthcare settings by providing substantial assistance in the realm of mobile fitness (m-fitness). These days, the healthcare business is reliant on mobile computing to aid IoT packages. IoT healthcare applications benefit from mobile computing.

The "Non-invasive monitoring and wellness assessment of older people in a smart environment (RO-SmartAgeing)" initiative was introduced in (Tudora et al., 2021). It aims to promote healthcare services that are oriented toward the elderly so that they may avoid sickness, get individualized help, and have their health monitored. Taking into account where the project is in terms of development, they lay out the essential hardware components for the RO-SmartAgeing system, show the data flow diagram, and provide a demonstration of numerical validation while filtering information from IoT devices. They also propose an architecture framework based on IoT, fog, and cloud computing.

The present research provides a current assessment of the possible healthcare applications of IoT-based technologies. From the points of view of enabling technology, healthcare providers, and applications, that article explains how Hospital IoT is being used to solve different healthcare problems. Any concerns or difficulties that may arise with the Healthcare IoT system are also handled. In conclusion, their work aims to help future scholars investigating healthcare IoT by providing a wealth of information on its many uses (Varshney, 2021).

Using the open-source IoT dataset from the Canadian Institute for Cybersecurity, the authors of (Khan & Alkhathami, 2024) simulate machine learning methods for effective anomaly identification in network traffic. The 33 distinct forms of IoT assaults included in the sample fall into 7 broad classes. That research uses pre-processed datasets to generate non-biased supervised machine learning models using a balanced representation of classes. The models include Random Forest, Adaptive Improving, Logistic Regression, Perceptron, and Deep Neural Network. Additional analysis of these models is conducted by removing characteristics with strong correlation, decreasing the number of dimensions, lowering the likelihood of overfitting, and expediting the training process. With an estimated accuracy of 99.55% under both limited and entire feature space, Random Forest was determined to perform ideally across binary along with multiclass classifications of IoT Attacks. A decrease in computing reaction time, which is critical for the detection and response to attacks in real-time, accompanied that development.

With any luck, that comprehensive overview of blockchain's IoT healthcare applications will be available in (Al-Nbhany et al., 2024). Their paper's approach is a literature review covering the years 2018–2023, with a focus on studies that combine and integrate the IoT, Blockchain technology, and healthcare applications. Types and technologies of blockchain based on the IoT, healthcare applications, sensors, application databases, coding languages, software tools, problems, open issues, and solutions—along with their pros and cons—are covered in that overview. Then, using standard measurements, they compared their findings to those of previous research. Remote patient monitoring, tracking, disease prediction, COVID-19 tracking, image retrieval, safeguarding medical information, smart telemedicine, protecting the Internet of Medical Things, large-scale data, blockchain while sensors, accurate medical choices, health surveillance, tracking soldiers, solar energy, and the blockchain IOT medical applications are all part of the research included in that paper.

That research primarily aims to propose a new model called Hybrid Ensemble Learning Enabled Sigmoid-Cosine Integrated Pigeon influenced Feature Selection Based Intrusion Detection within the context of (Rajesh et al., 2024). The model's specific purpose is to detect and mitigate threats for Tactile Internet-driven Consumer Healthcare IoT. The new Sigmoid-Cosine integrative pigeon-inspired feature selection method is part of the hybrid ensemble learning strategy that the suggested model uses. For that purpose, they ran comprehensive tests using industry-standard metric measures on four separate datasets: IoT bot, NSL-KDD, CIC2017, and KDD99. The findings show that their suggested work is better than the current methods, which shows how great an impact they might have on healthcare IoT cybersecurity.

The survey emphasizes using GAI-driven HDT in IoT healthcare (Chen et al., 2024). The history of healthcare IoT and the possibilities of GAI-driven HDT are introduced first. After that, they show the general architecture of GAI-driven HDT and get into the basic methods. Following that, they go further into the implementation of GAI-driven HDT, covering topics such as data analysis, digital modeling, communication, data administration, and GAI-enabled data gathering (Singh et al., 2025) (Ganiya et al., 2024). They also discuss several common IoT healthcare applications that might be destroyed by GAI-driven HDT, including individualized health tracking and diagnosis, medication, and rehabilitation. They wrap up their survey by outlining a few potential avenues for further study (Karthik, Aalam, et al., 2024).

5.1 Performance Evaluation of IoT Sensors

The sensors are the central nervous system of any healthcare monitoring system. Because of this, you can trust them. The ideal sensors would be those that are tiny, silent, accurate, power-efficient, and have low data transmission delays. One difficulty is that wearable sensors need to be small while yet being very accurate (Karthik, Hamatta, et al., 2024) (Karthik et al., 2025). Wearable sensors, on the other hand, prioritize outputs, which must be accurately reported for the clinician to rely on them in making judgments. Sensors designed for medical use are bulky, cumbersome, and labor-intensive to operate.

Authentication, protection, and privacy are also ongoing needs for many applications that rely on Internet of Things sensors (Poloju & Rajaram, 2024). Several protocols are easily accessible on the market to aid with security and provide certain options over a long period of time. However, the security mechanisms of these integrated and vital data-based applications are always open to attack (Maguluri et al., 2024) (Syamala et al., 2024).

5.2 Gaps in the Existing Systems

Here are the main points about the current system's shortcomings:

- The IoT offers the ability to connect with a broad range of gadgets, which is presently impossible with the majority of systems in use.
- The data that is saved may not be safeguarded by all means.
- There are a lot of loose ends between the different persons, stages, and processes in complicated systems (Chiranjeevi & Rajaram, 2024)
- Although investigations into accident causes usually find many gaps, gaps in and of themselves are seldom the culprit.
- A rise in overall safety may be achieved by comprehending and bolstering practitioners' natural capacity to bridge gaps.
- This position challenges the prevalent wisdom that systems should be protected against the unpredictable effects of people.
- Our knowledge of how experts identify newly created holes and come up with solutions to fill them during system transition is inadequate (Kalaivani et al., 2023)

6. CONCLUSION

Remote patient monitoring with data-driven decision-making is one of the many important benefits that the IoT has brought to the healthcare business. Despite concerns about data overload and security, the Internet of Things has fascinating possibilities in healthcare. In order to address issues, make the most of the benefits of the IoT, and construct a healthcare system that is data-driven, successful, and oriented on the patient, collaboration is key. Constant innovation brought about by the Internet of Things will revolutionize healthcare delivery and patient care, resulting in enhanced outcomes and a more robust health sector overall.

6.1 Future Improvements

In order to address the communication issues and constraints highlighted by prior research, it is necessary to improve and integrate wearable medical equipment in order to link it to other emerging technological developments. Scientists who want to keep their clients happy should make sure that the solutions they suggest are simple to use, flexible, and safe. New possibilities for disease management and healthcare arise when wearable sensors are integrated into healthcare systems. By linking sensors and equipment used for health monitoring to the cloud, the IoT may provide a solution that is available at all times. All patient information is safely stored on the server and may be accessed at any time.

An IoT-based healthcare system that integrates various technological approaches could one day be able to diagnose the conditions of patients with chronic diseases with COVID-19. This would allow doctors to make better decisions and optimize patients' health. The IoT, software-defined networks (SDNs), Artificial Intelligence (AI), fog computing, big data, and the Internet of Things (IoNT) are all examples of integration methodologies. By combining AI with healthcare monitoring systems built on the Internet of Things, accurate and useful findings may be extracted from sensor data. By using the fog/edge model, computing resources may be distributed closer to the point of demand. IoT healthcare monitoring systems may also benefit from Big Data computing, which enables effective management of very huge data sets. Aside from that, additional cutting-edge technologies like software-defined networks (SDNs), IoNT, and the tactile Internet (TI) might one day make IoT-based healthcare systems even more useful and increase their capabilities even further.

REFERENCES

Al-Nbhany, W. A. N. A., Zahary, A. T., & Al-Shargabi, A. A. (2024). Blockchain-IoT healthcare applications and trends: A review. *IEEE Access : Practical Innovations, Open Solutions*, *12*, 4178–4212. DOI: 10.1109/ACCESS.2023.3349187

Alam, S., Bhatia, S., Shuaib, M., Khubrani, M. M., Alfayez, F., Malibari, A. A., & Ahmad, S. (2023). An overview of blockchain and IoT integration for secure and reliable health records monitoring. *Sustainability (Basel)*, *15*(7), 5660. DOI: 10.3390/su15075660

Alqahtani, N., Alam, S., Aqeel, I., Shuaib, M., Mohsen Khormi, I., Khan, S. B., & Malibari, A. A. (2023). Deep belief networks (DBN) with IoT-based Alzheimer's disease detection and classification. *Applied Sciences (Basel, Switzerland)*, *13*(13), 7833. DOI: 10.3390/app13137833

Chanda, B., Mallick, P. K., & Chae, G.-S. (2021). An analytical study of the role of m-iot in healthcare domain. *Hybrid Artificial Intelligence and IoT in Healthcare*, 75–96.

Chen, J., Shi, Y., Yi, C., Du, H., Kang, J., & Niyato, D. (2024). Generative AI-driven human digital twin in IoT-healthcare: A comprehensive survey. *IEEE Internet of Things Journal*, *11*(21), 34749–34773. DOI: 10.1109/JIOT.2024.3421918

Chinthala, K. K. R., Thakur, M. S., Shuaib, M., & Alam, S. (2022). Prospects of Computational Intelligence in Society: Human-Centric Solutions, Challenges, and Research Areas. *Journal of Computational and Cognitive Engineering*.

Chiranjeevi, P., & Rajaram, A. (2024). A smart recommender model based on learning method for sentiment classification. *Multimedia Tools and Applications*, •••, 1–21. DOI: 10.1007/s11042-024-20347-z

Ganiya, R. K., Veeraiah, D., Thatha, V. N., Rao, K. S., Rao, J. N., Manjith, R., & Rajaram, A. (2024). Revolutionizing vascular health through the temporal convolutional transformer for drug screening and model evolution. *Biomedical Signal Processing and Control*, *95*, 106390. DOI: 10.1016/j.bspc.2024.106390

Hasan, A., Badhautiya, A., & Pandey, A. (2024). HealthNet: IoT-based healthcare monitoring and management system. *International Journal for Research in Applied Science and Engineering Technology*, *12*(3), 473–481. DOI: 10.22214/ijraset.2024.58851

Kalaivani, K., Kshirsagarr, P. R., Sirisha Devi, J., Bandela, S. R., Colak, I., Nageswara Rao, J., & Rajaram, A. (2023). Prediction of biomedical signals using deep learning techniques. *Journal of Intelligent & Fuzzy Systems*, *44*(6), 9769–9782. DOI: 10.3233/JIFS-230399

Karthik, A., Aalam, S. S., Sivakumar, M., Sundari, M. V. R., Rose, J. D., Elangovan, M., & Rajaram, A. (2024). Improving brain tumor treatment with better imaging and real-time therapy using quantum dots. *Biomedical Signal Processing and Control*, *95*, 106286. DOI: 10.1016/j.bspc.2024.106286

Karthik, A., Hamatta, H. S. A., Patthi, S., Krubakaran, C., Pradhan, A. K., Rachapudi, V., Shuaib, M., & Rajaram, A. (2024). Ensemble-based multimodal medical imaging fusion for tumor segmentation. *Biomedical Signal Processing and Control*, *96*, 106550. DOI: 10.1016/j.bspc.2024.106550

Karthik, A., Sahoo, S. K., Kumar, A., Patel, N., Chinnaraj, P., Maguluri, L. P., & Rajaram, A. (2025). Unified approach for accurate brain tumor Multi-Classification and segmentation through fusion of advanced methodologies. *Biomedical Signal Processing and Control*, *100*, 106872. DOI: 10.1016/j.bspc.2024.106872

Kaza, V. S., Alamer, A., Alam, S., Shuaib, M., Basudan, S., & Sheneamer, A. (2024). Detecting and forecasting cryptojacking attack trends in Internet of Things and wireless sensor networks devices. *PeerJ. Computer Science*, *10*, e2491. DOI: 10.7717/peerj-cs.2491 PMID: 39650421

Khan, M. M., & Alkhathami, M. (2024). Anomaly detection in IoT-based healthcare: Machine learning for enhanced security. *Scientific Reports*, *14*(1), 5872. DOI: 10.1038/s41598-024-56126-x PMID: 38467709

Kishor Kumar Reddy, C., Kaza, V. S., Madana Mohana, R., Alhameed, M., Jeribi, F., Alam, S., & Shuaib, M. (2025). Detecting anomalies in smart wearables for hypertension: A deep learning mechanism. *Frontiers in Public Health*, *12*, 1426168. DOI: 10.3389/fpubh.2024.1426168 PMID: 39850864

Kumar, M., Kumar, A., Verma, S., Bhattacharya, P., Ghimire, D., Kim, S., & Hosen, A. S. M. S. (2023). Healthcare Internet of Things (H-IoT): Current trends, future prospects, applications, challenges, and security issues. *Electronics (Basel)*, *12*(9), 2050. DOI: 10.3390/electronics12092050

Kumar, M., Verma, S., Kumar, A., Ijaz, M. F., & Rawat, D. B. (2022). ANAF-IoMT: A novel architectural framework for IoMT-enabled smart healthcare system by enhancing security based on RECC-VC. *IEEE Transactions on Industrial Informatics*, *18*(12), 8936–8943. DOI: 10.1109/TII.2022.3181614

Maguluri, L. P., Chouhan, K., Balamurali, R., Rani, R., Hashmi, A., Kiran, A., & Rajaram, A. (2024). Adversarial deep learning for improved abdominal organ segmentation in CT scans. *Multimedia Tools and Applications*, *83*(35), 82107–82129. DOI: 10.1007/s11042-024-18578-1

Mohamad Jawad, H. H., Bin Hassan, Z., Zaidan, B. B., Mohammed Jawad, F. H., Mohamed Jawad, D. H., & Alredany, W. H. D. (2022). A systematic literature review of enabling IoT in healthcare: Motivations, challenges, and recommendations. *Electronics (Basel)*, *11*(19), 3223. DOI: 10.3390/electronics11193223

Poloju, N., & Rajaram, A. (2024). Transformation with yolo tiny network architecture for multimodal fusion in lung disease classification. *Cybernetics and Systems*, •••, 1–22. DOI: 10.1080/01969722.2024.2343992

Pradhan, B., Bhattacharyya, S., & Pal, K. (2021). IoT-based applications in healthcare devices. *Journal of Healthcare Engineering*, *2021*(1), 6632599. PMID: 33791084

Rahman, S. M., Ibtisum, S., Podder, P., & Hossain, S. M. (2023). Progression and challenges of IoT in healthcare: A short review. *ArXiv Preprint ArXiv:2311.12869.*

Rajesh, R., Hemalatha, S., Nagarajan, S. M., Devarajan, G. G., Omar, M., & Bashir, A. K. (2024). Threat detection and mitigation for tactile internet driven consumer IoT-healthcare system. *IEEE Transactions on Consumer Electronics.*

Roy, C., Saha, R., Misra, S., & Niyato, D. (2021). Soft-health: Software-defined fog architecture for IoT applications in healthcare. *IEEE Internet of Things Journal*, *9*(3), 2455–2462. DOI: 10.1109/JIOT.2021.3097554

Singh, A., Nagabhooshanam, N., Kumar, R., Verma, R., Mohanasundaram, S., Manjith, R., & Rajaram, A. (2025). Deep learning based coronary artery disease detection and segmentation using ultrasound imaging with adaptive gated SCNN models. *Biomedical Signal Processing and Control, 105*, 107637. DOI: 10.1016/j.bspc.2025.107637

Syamala, M., Chandrasekaran, R., Balamurali, R., Rani, R., Hashmi, A., Kiran, A., & Rajaram, A. (2024). Evaluating generative adversarial networks for virtual contrast-enhanced kidney segmentation using Res-UNet in non-contrast CT images. *Multimedia Tools and Applications*, •••, 1–24. DOI: 10.1007/s11042-024-19626-6

Tsantikidou, K., & Sklavos, N. (2022). Hardware limitations of lightweight cryptographic designs for IoT in healthcare. *Cryptography*, *6*(3), 45. DOI: 10.3390/cryptography6030045

Tudora, E., Tîrziu, E., Nicolau, N.-D., & Gheorghe-Moisii, M. (2021). Fog and cloud computing-based IoT in healthcare monitoring system for healthy ageing. *2021 23rd International Conference on Control Systems and Computer Science (CSCS)*, 489–494.

Varshney, K. (2021).. . *Application of IoT in Healthcare*, (6), 192–196.

Zhang, L., Xu, J., Vijayakumar, P., Sharma, P. K., & Ghosh, U. (2022). Homomorphic encryption-based privacy-preserving federated learning in IoT-enabled healthcare system. *IEEE Transactions on Network Science and Engineering*, *10*(5), 2864–2880. DOI: 10.1109/TNSE.2022.3185327

Chapter 3

Machine Learning for Healthcare Applications: Transforming Patient Care, Diagnosis, and Treatment

Rithika Ango
https://orcid.org/0009-0007-3764-006X
Stanley College of Engineering and Technology for Women, India

Thakur Monika Singh
https://orcid.org/0009-0006-8534-9130
Stanley College of Engineering and Technology for Women, India

Manoj Kumar Reddy Dadireddy
Vardhman College of Engineering, India

ABSTRACT

Machine learning (ML) is revolutionizing healthcare by offering innovative solutions that enhance delivery, outcomes, and efficiency. This chapter highlights ML's significance in healthcare, addressing current trends, challenges, and techniques like supervised, unsupervised, and reinforcement learning. Applications in disease diagnosis, medical imaging, drug discovery, personalized treatments, and remote monitoring are explored. It also delves into data sharing, security, and real-time monitoring through IoT and blockchain, along with NLP advancements automating clinical documentation and sentiment analysis. Real-life case studies on AI-based radiology and chronic disease prediction demonstrate its impact. Ethical and regulatory issues, such as data privacy, biases in AI models, and emerging paradigms like federated learning for secure, decentralized healthcare, are discussed. The chapter envisions a future where ML transforms healthcare to become more efficient, personalized, and accessible while addressing critical ethical considerations.

DOI: 10.4018/979-8-3373-1022-0.ch003

1. INTRODUCTION

Machine learning (ML) has completely transformed many sectors, and its impact is the most profound in healthcare. Algorithms that learn from data empower healthcare professionals to make more accurate diagnoses, tailor treatments and predict the progression of diseases. However, encompassing machine learning in healthcare systems is, among many other challenges, increasing the efficiency of personalized medicine resource allocation and decreasing the total cost of healthcare while improving patients' outcomes (Ahmed et al., 2016; Wang & Preininger, 2019). ML disruptive capability resides in its ability to analyze large amounts of medical data in realtime, such as electronic health records (EHRs), medical imaging and genomic information. The healthcare industry is moving in the direction of intelligent, IoT connected systems by combining machine learning with cutting edge technologies, including Internet of things, natural language processing and also blockchain (Huang et al., 2018; Liu et al., 2020). This transformation raises problems such as ethical issues, data security, and the need for strong regulatory structures (Choudhury Dhar, 2023; Vayena Blasimme, 2018).

The application of machine learning to medicine has now become a tool to bring about a transformation in the style of predictive and preventive medicine, in which patient care goes way beyond the curative style, reaching a preventive one. Contemporary ML algorithms are now able to identify patterns and relationships that would otherwise be undetectable, and therefore irretrievably lost, to humankind's ability to use AI for diagnosis disease such as cancer, diabetes, and cardiovascular disease (Topol, 2019). In contrast, predictive analytics tools are also capable of processing patterns in patient data with a view to forecasting disease progression and allow clinicians the ability to intervene earlier and more accurately at an earlier stage. Furthermore, ML can also be applied to optimize operational processes such as hospital resource management, scheduling, or reduction of waiting time of patients, thus alleviating the demands of an efficient healthcare system.

Despite the promise, there is still no simple way to translate the application of machine learning into the medical context. Outcome quality depends highly on access to high quality, unbiased datasets, but those are fragmented and siloed at the level of institutions. Also, the trustworthiness and interpretability of AI models still remain an open question, because clinicians must be able to trust and understand the reason(s) behind the predictions made by the AI models in order to integrate these AI predictions into clinical workflows (Ghassemi et al., 2020). As machine learning increasingly becomes used across healthcare setups, it will be of paramount importance to address the challenges posed by these barriers, in the form of standardized data-sharing rules, robust validation structures and increased technical and clinical sharing by technologists and medical professionals, for ethical and fair adoption of these paradigm-shifting technologies.

1.1 Importance of Machine Learning in Healthcare

Machine learning offers tremendous scope in solving several of the major healthcare challenges facing us. It uses cover- from predictive analysis to real-time monitoring of patients, in order to enable early-stage interventions or more precise and advanced therapies (Kang Park, 2021; Gong Wu, 2022). Such as the utilization of ML algorithms for medical image analysis, including the detection of lesions in X-rays and MRIs, where the efficiency of the algorithm is significantly higher than that of humans, on average (Bauer et al., 2022; Esteva et al., 2017). In turn, forecasts of chronic disease management and drug discovery accelerate change, enabling the transformation of healthcare into more personalized and accessible endeavour (Kumar Sharma, 2023; Topol, 2019). Furthermore, ML enhances operational efficiency through the automation of routine administrative tasks (such as clinical documentation) and by enhancing data analysis (Naik Acharya, 2022). The use of AI-based intelligence to decision-making in healthcare has enhanced quality of life in dermatology, oncology and cardiology and has proven its immovable role in modern medicine (Dilsizian Siegel, 2014; Kelly et al., 2019).

Machine learning transformed many healthcare systems across the world. These systems show bright futures that the past has never imagined really possible. Machine learning relying on huge datasets and complex algorithms is an effective way of identifying features regarding patient data never visible to the human eye. For example, ML algorithms in genomics feature finding mutations associated with certain diseases using large-scale genetic data, which, in turn, allows early diagnosis and targeted therapy of cancers and rare genetic diseases (Huang et al ., 2020; Lee et al . 2019). Personalized medicine has much to gain in this research field, as treatments can be designed according to individual genomes, facilitating a more effective approach with fewer side effects. As a result, using better AI-driven technologies in healthcare opens up opportunities for algorithms to deliver real-time, data-driven insights to aid in clinical decision-making that attempts to improve diagnoses and at the same time offer proactive care strategies.

Figure 1. Importance of Machine Learning in Healthcare

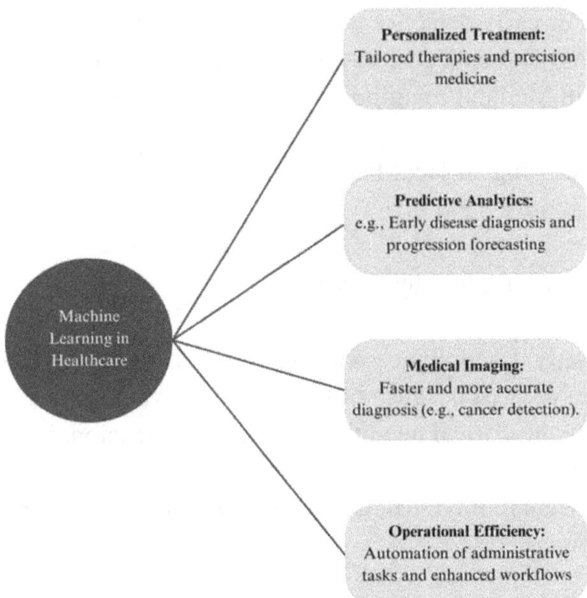

Figure 1 illustrates the importance of machine learning in its applications and impacts in healthcare. It is limited to the importance of machine learning in healthcare and delineates the subdivisions of the branches, such as predictive analytics, personalized treatment, medical imaging, and operational efficiency. Under each of these, all of them emphasize how machine learning is revolutionizing the way healthcare operates-from very early detection of some diseases to administrative activity automation presently in the trend of healthier, smarter, and effective healthcare delivery.

1.2 Current Trends and Challenges

The state of affairs of machine learning in health care highlights its rapid evolution and across the board application. Federated learning is being developed as a privacy-preserving method for data analysis to foster sharing between institutions without disclosing confidential patient information (Gong Wu, 2022). Alligator is similar to its conventional counterparts, improvements in NLP facilitate effective manipulation and processing of unstructured clinical notes and sentiment analysis to enhance patient care (Naik Acharya, 2022). Real-time monitoring systems facilitated by IoT devices increase patient involvement and management of chronic disease, leading to a healthcare that is more proactive and patient centered (Xu Yang, 2020). These are great advances upon which many challenges exist. Ethical issues like algorithmic bias and technology inequality with the application of AI need to be addressed much more seriously by the concerned scholars (Choudhury & Dhar, 2023; Vayena & Blasimme, 2018). Privacy and safety of data, as issues, remain critical within big data-sharing systems (Liu et al., 2020). In addition, reproducibility of AI model validation is lacking and the difference in the progress of research and their translation to clinical implementation prevents an easy expansion (Park Han, 2018). Overcoming these challenges will be the first step toward realizing the full benefits of ML in health care.

Current trends in Machine Learning for healthcare

- Predictive Analytics: For early detection and effective planning for treating diseases.
- Personalized Medicine: Personalized therapy according to both genetic and clinical data.
- Artificial Intelligence in Medical Imaging: For improved diagnostic accuracy for X-ray, MRI, and CT scan images.
- Natural Language Processing in Healthcare: Automating clinical documentation and extracting insights from patient records.

Challenges in Machine Learning for Healthcare

- Data Privacy and Security: Compliance with regulations, namely HIPAA and GDPR.
- Bias in Data: Inequities created because of unrepresentative datasets.
- Model Interpretability: The critical need for healthcare professionals to understand how decisions made by ML can be understood.
- Integration Issues: Barriers to infrastructures in terms of how they can incorporate ML into existing healthcare workflows.

2. KEY MACHINE LEARNING TECHNIQUES IN HEALTHCARE

Machine learning (ML) has become a revolutionary tool in health care, providing new solutions for diagnosis, therapy, and patient care. Using data-driven methods, ML methods solve sophisticated problems ranging from predictive analysis to individualized medicine. Such methods are generally grouped by supervised, unsupervised, and reinforcement learning respectively, and appropriate for individual health care applications and provide different advantages. Supervised learning, the most popular method, is the core of the tasks that need labeled data. This encompasses disease prediction, medical imaging analysis, and risk stratifications of patients. For example, algorithms, namely, random forests and neural networks, are used on patient records and laboratory results to predict heart disease or diabetes with high accuracy. Tools powered by supervised learning also support radiologists by detecting anomalies in medical imaging, streamlining diagnostic workflows (Bauer et al., 2022). In contrast, unsupervised learning has its strength on finding hidden patterns in unlabeled data, and is very suitable on patient segmentation and the anomaly detection. Clustering methods such as K-means or DBSCAN facilitates the aggregation of patients on the basis of similar health characteristics, which opens opportunities for targeted interventions and tailor-made care. In the meantime, RL is gaining its momentum for applications, such as personalized treatment strategy optimization and hospital resources management. Through the use of real-time feedback these system's dynamically adjust to changing patient requirements, benefit outcomes, and effectiveness (Haque et al., 2022). On their own, these machine learning methods are the foundation of current AI-based healthcare advancements, which could lead toward a smarter, more responsive healthcare system.

2.1 Supervised Learning Applications

Supervised learning with labeled data is of prime importance in health care, providing predictive and analytical functions. Algorithms such as Support Vector Machine (SVM), Random Forests and Deep Neural Networks have a key role to play in the diagnosis of cancers, diabetes and cardiovascular disease, etc. (Esteva et al., 2017) showed the ability of supervised learning for reaching a level of agreement in classifying skin cancer reaching as high as that of dermatologists and also its capacity to complement the expert knowledge of clinicians. Based on a patient's history, laboratory, and imaging data such models offer early and precise diagnosis in order to improve the patient's outcome. Supervised learning is perhaps the most typical application of medical images, in which it is applied to complex imaging data to identify pathologies. Specifically in the case of radiological imaging, e.g., supervised algorithms can detect tumors or fractures on X-rays, CT scans, and MRIs, respectively, which translates to fewer diagnostic errors and enhanced reliability (Bauer et al., 2022). Another significant use case is the prediction of treatment response (i.e., the assessment of risk for readmission or the prediction of patients' recovery trajectories) based on historical data.

2.2 Unsupervised Learning in Patient Segmentation

In healthcare applications where the underlying latent patterns also need to be extracted without any information (i. e., unsupervised patient segmentation). Clustering methods, for example, K-means and DBSCAN, remodel patients based on alike valued health measures in order to provide specific health interventions. For example, (Huang et al., 2018) explained the promise of unsupervised learning for population stratification of disease risk prediction and preventive medicine advice, using genetic markers and lifestyle phenotype. Besides segmentation, unsupervised learning algorithms are applied to the task of anomaly detection since they detect outliers in patient data potentially representing rare diseases or medical file inaccuracies. Dimensionality reduction such as Principal Component Analysis (PCA) creates smaller data sets of the large healthcare data and therefore can be transformed into clinically useful data. These skills, including, but not limited to, the use of IoT-enabled devices, enable continual monitoring and real-time query, which lead to precision medicine.

2.3 Reinforcement Learning for Personalized Medicine

Reinforcement learning (RL) is transforming personalized medicine with the creation of closed loop, real-time adaptive treatment algorithms. Unlike static conventional techniques, RL models have dynamic abilities (e.g., dynamically responding to the dosage of medication in chronic diseases such as diabetes) allowing an optimal patient care with respect to time (Haque et al., 2022). This ensures that treatment will always be fine-tuned and modified in a patient-specific way in order to optimize treatment effectiveness. In particular, RL is also maturing in the case of resource optimization in health applications. RL algorithms, e.g., are implemented in ICUs to efficiently schedule human and material resources (staff, equipment) in order to deliver high-priority life-support resources (Cohen and Phillips, 1987, 1988). Yet it is only possible to transfer RL to objective decision making in ethical sensitive areas like healthcare with good overall and interpretability because such functions are needed in clinical practice, essentially providing a road to safe and clinically viable applications.

Table 1 presents an overview of the comparison between supervised, unsupervised, and reinforcement learning approaches in health care. It is off by one option with respect to data needs, main tasks, algorithms, benefits, and drawbacks of each method. The table also shows in the field the practical application examples of obtained learning, how these methods can be used to help diagnosing disease, grouping patients, and planning individual treatments.

Table 1. Comparison of Supervised, Unsupervised, and Reinforcement Learning in Healthcare

Aspect	Supervised Learning	Unsupervised Learning	Reinforcement Learning
Definition	Learns from labeled data by mapping inputs to outputs.	Learn patterns and structures from unlabeled data.	Learns optimal actions through trial-and-error feedback from the environment.
Input Data	Requires labeled datasets.	Uses unlabeled datasets.	Operates with states, actions, and rewards.
Key Tasks	Classification (e.g., disease diagnosis), Regression (e.g., outcome prediction).	Clustering (e.g., patient segmentation), Dimensionality Reduction (e.g., simplifying genomic data).	Decision-making (e.g., personalized treatment plans, resource allocation).
Algorithms	SVM, Decision Trees, Neural Networks, Random Forests.	K-Means, DBSCAN, PCA, Hierarchical Clustering.	Q-Learning, Deep Q-Networks, Policy Gradient Methods.
Data Requirements	Requires extensive labeled data.	Can work without labels but needs large, diverse datasets.	Requires a defined reward structure and iterative training.
Applications	Predicting diseases, analyzing medical imaging, prognosis modeling.	Patient subgrouping, anomaly detection, genetic data clustering.	Dynamic dosage adjustment, ICU resource management, adaptive treatments.
Advantages	High accuracy with sufficient data, clear interpretability.	Identifies hidden patterns and structures; no labeling required.	Learns complex strategies, adapts dynamically to real-time conditions.
Challenges	Expensive and time-consuming data labeling.	Difficulty in interpreting results and evaluating performance.	Computationally intensive; risk of unsafe actions without proper validation.
Example in Healthcare	Diagnosing diabetes using clinical records.	Clustering patients based on lifestyle and genetic markers.	Optimizing stroke rehabilitation plans.

3. APPLICATIONS OF MACHINE LEARNING IN HEALTHCARE

ML is revolutionizing healthcare through innovative diagnostic, therapeutic, and operational efficiency. Its ability to process and analyse large data sets enables early diagnosis and precise prognosis, and healthcare thus shifts from being reactive to predictive and personalised. ML algorithms are also widely used in disease diagnosis and prediction, in understanding patients' vulnerability to cancer, diabetes or cardiovascular diseases. For instance, (Esteva et al., 2017) demonstrated the promise of ML in skin cancer diagnosis, to predict dermatoscope-equivalent accuracy in skin cancer detection, thereby changing the diagnostic accuracy. Using such data, these systems produce actionable intelligence that can be used for early intervention with the promise of improving patient outcomes (Deo, 2015). Adding to the diagnosis role, ML contributes substantially to facilitating drug discovery which historically has been a tedious and costly process. Algorithms are able to predict the behaviour, potency, and toxicity of molecules, and thus reduce the time spent in the search to identify potential drug candidates (Kumar Sharma, 2023). Other key applications are providing personalized treatment regimens, in which ML agents use patient data to predict the best efficacy and efficiency of the treatment (Haque et al., 2022). Beyond clinical care, ML stands out for remote patient monitoring with Internet of Things (IoT)-sensing devices, real-time vitals monitoring and response that can improve the accessibility and quality of care (Huang et al., 2018).

Table 2 summarizes the applications of machine learning in healthcare: disease diagnosis, medical imaging, drug development, personalized treatment, and remote patient monitoring. It indicates the improvements in accuracy in diagnosis, speed in drug development, individualism of treatments, and global real-time monitoring. Efficient healthcare is much more personalized and monitored.

Table 2. The Applications of Machine Learning in Healthcare

Application Area	Description
Disease Diagnosis and Prediction	In recent times, ML has found increasing acceptance in surgery in predicting diseases after analyzing medical history, genetics, or biomarkers data. In this way, an improvement in diagnostic accuracy may be brought about by early interventions when it is happening. Some ML paradigms such as deep learning and Support Vector Machines help predict diseases, including but not limited to cancer, diabetes, and some cardiovascular diseases.
Medical Imaging and Diagnostics	Using ML capabilities, enhanced medical imaging gains by automatically reading X-rays, CT scans, or MRIs for abnormalities. Such systems would assist radiographs by presenting a high-precision evaluation and an additional support scheme in planning surgery so far. So far, deep learning techniques have been successfully applied in segmentation and diagnosis of medical images.
Drug Discovery and Development	This way, ML speeds up drug development through the analysis of molecular data to identify candidate molecules for use in new drugs and the ability to predict their efficacy. Early stages in drug development are shortened, thereby reducing time and cost. ML also comes in handy in the repurposing of existing drugs for new diseases that otherwise would provide quicker routes to therapeutic solutions.
Personalized Treatment Plans	ML helps to customize treatment regimens according to personal health data such as genetics and clinical history. Adaptive learning models may optimize the dosage for chronic diseases like diabetes and hypertension while leading to better outcomes and fewer side effects.
Remote Patient Monitoring	Remote monitoring systems incorporated with medical IoT devices will now leverage ML to track each patient's vital signs and predict threats to health (like arrhythmia or hypoglycemia). These systems allow intervention in real time while also being part of chronic disease management. This means that fewer patients will be admitted to the hospital again.

4. INTEGRATION OF MACHINE LEARNING WITH EMERGING TECHNOLOGIES

Emerging technologies combined with machine learning (ML) tend to be more impactful in delivering innovative solutions for healthcare problems. Integration into such technologies as IoT and blockchain enhances ML's processing, analyzing, and securing data, besides delivering actionable insight in real time. For example, IoT devices can collect and store massive amounts of patient data and run ML models to analyze and possibly predict potential health risks. In the same light, ML will be complementing the secure decentralized architecture of blockchain by guaranteeing the integrity of sensitive medical data that will serve as input in training and decision making (Haque et al., 2022; Huang et al., 2018).

At this point, it further revolutionizes telemedicine and remote surgeries with ML convergence along with augmented realities (AR) and 5G towards diagnosis and treatment of patients at a distance. As a case in point, an ML algorithm could be trained by AR data in an operating room to guide surgical procedures with reduced errors and improved precision. With the application of such technologies, the provision of healthcare services is widely scaled and without compromising quality service delivery in the most underserved regions.

4.2 Role of IoT in Healthcare Machine Learning

IoT devices have a significant utility within a healthcare context where they provide real-time, continuous data streams (e.g., heart rate, glucose streams, activity parameters). The analysis is fed into different ML algorithms to differentiate outliers, predict health outcomes and advise on preventative measures. Devices as wearable contain sensors from which patient information is transferred to ML models, and training is done to identify patterns and trigger alarms for clinicians in an emergency situation (i.e., arrhythmia, respiratory compromise) (Huang et al., 2018).

Furthermore, IoT-ML integration is vital for chronic disease management. For diabetic patients, smart sensors monitor glucose values and automatically propose individual insulin dosage recommendations by taking ML-based predictive models. This continuous hijacking of IoT facilitates fewer hospital visits, more adherence to self-care, and more self-treatment of diseases by patients. However, problems such as information privacy and device interoperability still need to be addressed in order to realize IoT application in medicine.

Figure 2. Network diagram showing IoT-enabled devices transmitting data to ML systems.

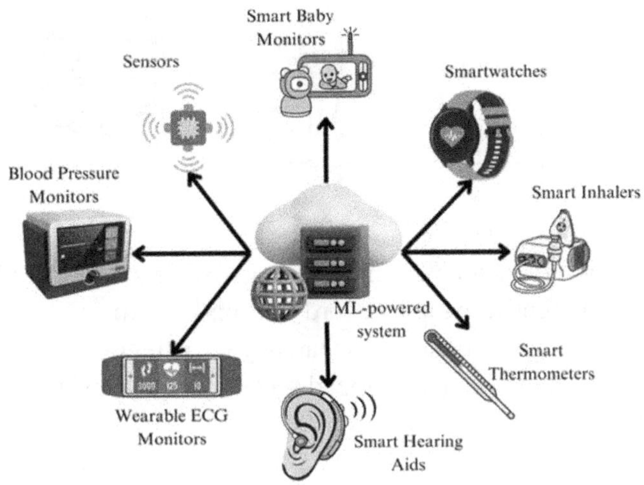

The real-time data from a patient is being collected from IoT-enabled devices as shown in Figure 2, includes wearable health trackers and medical sensors, and is then transmittable to machine learning systems. These ML systems learn from this data to derive insights that can be used for predictive analytics, early diagnosis, or personalized treatment. Thus, the very effective continuous monitoring and timely interventions that both IoT and ML can bring to healthcare are emphasized.

4.3 Blockchain for Secure Healthcare Data

Blockchain technology solves the problem of securely and transparently working with health data. Because of its decentralized, tamper proof nature, blockchain allows ML models to be trained with data that is, in turn, auditable and trustworthy. The importance of this especially in privacy, preserving patient data and in compliance with the law such as HIPAA and GDPR (Gong Wu, 2022) is also relevant.

In the field of healthcare, blockchain enhances interoperability of systems through a secular, cryptographically secure electronic ledger for storing patient information, clinical notes and medications. ML models, on one hand, are in a position to make use of this information that is trusted for analysis, resulting in more efficient prediction and decision. Moreover, tasks embodied in the smart contracts developed on blockchain can be automated (e.g., insurance claim or drug prescription) and thereby minimize the administrative costs associated and the possible errors. With this integration, it can establish trust among its stakeholders that is the foundation of collaborative health ecosystems.

Figure 3. Integration of Blockchain in Securing ML Models and Patient Data

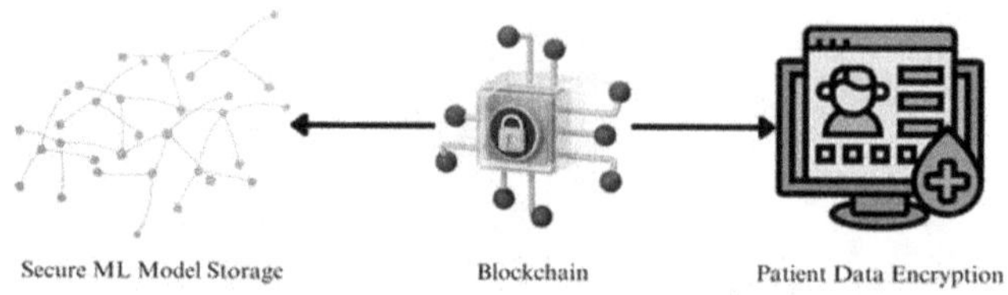

Figure 3 depicts integration of machine learning security models with the pharmacy industry using the blockchain technology. The entire patient record and updates to models will be immutable to a blockchain. It assures, therefore, integrity and transparency of patient records and model updates. This framework promotes trust and pre-empts unauthorized access, thereby ensuring data privacy compliance in health м шина applications.

5. ADVANCEMENTS IN NATURAL LANGUAGE PROCESSING (NLP) IN HEALTHCARE

Some things here entail-the improvements of NLP application in health making computers able to analyze unstructured text data for important insights. The list of applications includes clinical text mining, disease phenotype extraction, and automated diagnosis systems among others with the aim of improving healthcare efficiencies and decisions. On a larger scale, NLP models are capable of processing enormous patient records and viewing these in terms of trends, anomalies, and possibly even diseases, thus aiding in predictive analytics by gathering prognostic knowledge about diseases. Such applications promote data-driven healthcare systems, thus resulting in lower resource wastage by (Naik and Acharya, 2022) outcomes. Such are possibilities with NLP, such as having virtual health assistants and chatbots interact with patients. Thus, appointment scheduling, adherence reminders, or symptom description aids patients in connection and lessens administrative overhead. And with the combined scope of artificial intelligence technologies, especially machine learning, it can cover greater extents of healthcare challenges.

5.1 Automated Clinical Documentation

The automated clinical documentation makes use of NLP technologies to streamline and enhance the process of maintaining accurate medical records. Examples of such systems include speech-to-text transcription and structured generation of data which extracts all critical information from the interaction of physician and patient and transforms it into short organized formats. This moves away from human documentation errors and allows manpower to be dedicated to patients. The NLP-enabled documentation provides for consistency, minimization of redundancies, and easy integration into electronic health records (EHRs) (Johnson et al., 2016).These further immediate transcription tools analyze spoken words and contextualize them into summaries, prescriptions, and progress notes. This speeds up the process of documentation as well as adherence to regulations. Advances in the power and understanding of a language make NLP document clearing rethink the management of clinical data within the health system.

Figure 4. Workflow diagram illustrating how NLP generates clinical notes from patient interactions

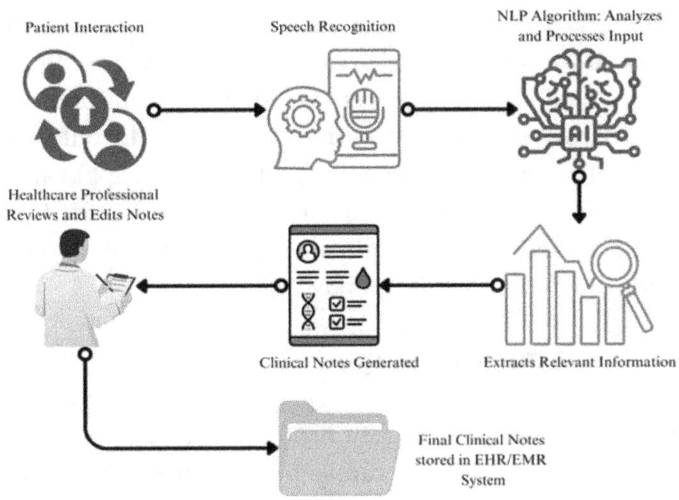

Figure 4 shows the process by which Natural Language Processing (NLP) converts communication of the patients into structured clinical notes. Some of the steps here are given voice or text by the patient, listening by speech-to-text conversion, extraction of the relevant information through NLP algorithms, and generation of structured clinical notes. This makes possible faster documentation and relieves the healthcare provider of administrative tasks, thus resulting in an efficient workflow.

5.2 Sentiment Analysis for Patient Feedback

It has found its way to become a very important instrument for understanding the patient's satisfaction and effectively enabling worsening healthcare services. This area of artificial intelligence is used to analyze the online reviews, responses given in the surveys, and the feedback provided by the patient, and this will devise possible trends in public opinions to highlight improvement areas. For example, the systems used machine learning models to categorize the feedback into three sentiments- positive, negative or neutral; these will help the healthcare providers address the grievances in advance (Naik and Acharya, 2022). It enables organizations to measure themselves against competitors and impact targeted quality improvements, for example, better staff behaviour or certain procedural refinements. It helps in real-time processing of unstructured text inputs making sure that the patient does not have to wait long when it comes to addressing complaints. The real aim of all sentiment analysis is to bring healthcare services to be patient-centric, alongside making sure that high standards of care are given.

6. CASE STUDIES AND SUCCESS STORIES

Case studies and success stories demonstrate how transformative machine learning and artificial intelligence can be in the healthcare field. For instance, IBM Watson for Oncology has thus far examined the patient records and suggested evidence-based cancer treatments. Use of contact management and automated follow-ups through AI-enabled chatbots which saved lives as they are programmed with different answers based on symptoms to cater for patients that need urgent help. AI cuts through millions of research papers, clinical trials, and mountains of studies as well as records, helping oncologists find evidence supporting their decisions (Naik & Acharya, 2022). One is about the successful prediction of major kidney injuries using the AI model developed by Google's DeepMind, which could predict such disorders 48 hours before its occurrence, hence resulting in a much better outcome for the patients (Gong & Wu, 2022). These case studies depict the possibility that these ML applications deliver toward more accurate diagnoses and streaming of resources with enhanced operational efficiencies. They are, at the same time, examples in the real world that could provide the impetus needed for the wider adoption of these technologies in health systems across the globe.

Case Study 1: IBM Watson for Oncology

IBM Watson for Oncology integrates advanced machine learning algorithms on a vast repository of medical knowledge to individualize cancer treatment management. NLP makes use of unstructured data from research papers, clinical guidelines, and patient records. Watson assesses tumor types, genetic mutations, and clinical history and recommends the most suitable treatment options. Thus, this tool has fast-tracked decision-making and eradicated errors at Manipal Comprehensive Cancer Center to sharpen oncology practices. By improving the comprehension of the newly introduced medical advancements behind its suggestions, it empowers oncologists to make informed data-driven decisions that will, at the end, bring about improved outcomes for patients.

Lessons Learned: The success shown by IBM Watson in Oncology confirms that there is value in its use with the knowledge base of artificial intelligence for clinical decision support. It shows that AI can improve precision of treatment planning. However, privacy considerations about patient data and continuous validation of AI recommendations in clinical settings are two major areas to be addressed. Data transparency and reliability of AI-driven insights must be ensured for universal adoption across the healthcare sector.

Case Study 2: Google DeepMind for Acute Kidney Injury (AKI)

Google DeepMind's AKI predictive model is able to transform the very essence of how preventive healthcare is and will be: the real-world demonstration of AI in saving lives. It uses the most developed deep neural networks-having proven ability-to analyze patient data: blood pressure trends and certain electrolyte levels among others-for assessing AKI risk. In an actual trial with the U.S. Department of Veterans Affairs, the system flagged a patient as high risk two days in advance through alerts for the health professionals concerned to conduct timely interventions such as fluid management or dialysis. Such early detection then essentially contributed to reducing the mortality rate and healthcare costs, thus validating predictive analytics as a means of preventing life-threatening conditions like AKI (Gong & Wu, 2022).

Lessons Learned: This case shows that early diagnosis and prevention capture the true beauty of AI; predictive analytics conquers everything. While promising in terms of what the technology can accomplish, needless to say, certain concerns to do with data quality and the algorithmic transparency for those in the clinic take the lead for trust by those in health and patients alike and continuous evaluation and improvement of the model to be integrated into clinical practice.

Case Study 3: AI-Powered Radiology for Breast Cancer Detection

The AI model developed by Google for mammogram analysis has transformed the detection of breast cancer. Traditional mammograms have a tendency to yield false positives and negatives, resulting in unnecessary biopsies or missed diagnoses. The Google model was trained on more than 90,000 mammograms and therefore detects some subtleties that remain undetectable by radiologists. The clinical trials with 25,000 women yielded an improvement in the detection rate of 9.4%, while false positives were reduced by 5.7%. This has not only improved diagnostic accuracy but also been integrated into radiology workflows all over the world (Esteva et al., 2017).

Lessons Learned: The AI model for mammography developed by Google presents proof for the potentially large relevance of deep learning in the analysis of medical images and, in particular, regarding achieving a greater precision in diagnosis. The world beyond such tools is fraught with ethical considerations. Radiologists may not lose their jobs but feel unrealistic hope in AI that may render them obsolete. Moreover, the continuous validation and recalibration of models for various patient populations should be monitored. Trust should be developed in AI through transparent engagement of health professionals and patients alike.

6.1 Lessons Learned from Real-World Implementations

In real-world applications of AI to healthcare, certain critical lessons emerged that can serve to guide future efforts in this arena. Such lessons include data integration and data quality challenges. The machine learning model IBM Watson for Oncology or the prediction model for AKI humanized by Google DeepMind draws heavily on the consistent high-quality data from various internal and external sources. Standardization of data and issues about silos can also cause adverse effects on these systems. Accurate integration, cleansing, and structuring of data are fundamental in this area to improve the accuracy and effectiveness of AI models. However, the ethical side of this is more on privacy issues as far as patient involvement is concerned and security of sensitive data. AI systems will have to be compliant with privacy regulations such as HIPAA, be transparent and interpretable to limit potential biases associated with them-to retain trust in the technology. The other lesson learned from actual deployment is that human-AI collaboration is vital. AI must augment, not replace, the skills of clinicians. AI-powered radiology and predictive analytics Artificial intelligence can enhance clinical decision-making through its integration into clinical workflow-enhanced and more accurate and speedy information. However, clinical judgment will always validate and direct final decisions because they should be evidence informed. On top of it all, there should be scalability and adaptability to a new healthcare environment for an AI system to be considered successful. Predictive analytics can be linear with chronic heart failure and AKI, whereby AI systems can evolve with new data and the changing healthcare arena. Last, but not least, developing how those within the healthcare profession can trust AI tools is also critical to their successful adoption.

Figure 5. Lessons Learned from Real-World Implementations of Machine Learning in Healthcare

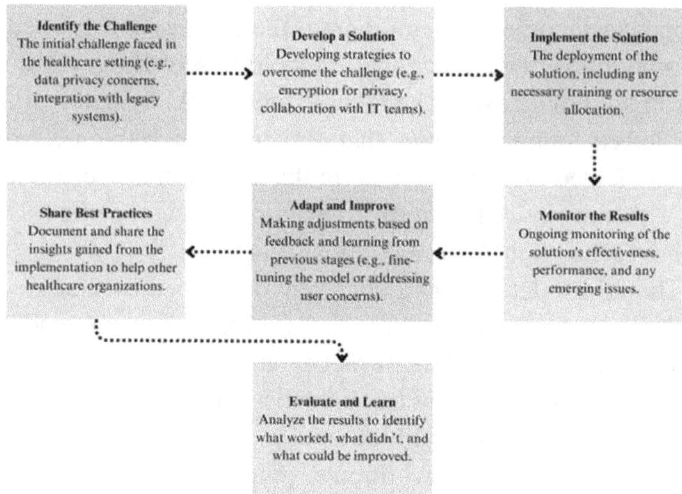

Figure 5 shows the high-level learnings from a real-life field deployment of machine learning in healthcare. Performance issues of data privacy, integration with legacy systems, and model reliability form the general problems that were transcended by means of supplying good-encrypted data storage; continued retraining of the models; and collaboration between departments. These lessons highlight the importance of good planning and adaptability in any successful ML implementation.

7. ETHICAL AND REGULATORY CONSIDERATIONS

As artificial intelligence technology is being developed in the field of health, it creates new ethical dilemmas as well as regulations that need to be balanced between high innovation and compliance to policy matters. One of such ethical dilemmas is the informed consent of the patients for their data to be used in training and analysis of the AI systems. Patients should be sufficiently informed about use of their data, even as it respects their autonomy and rights. The innovative frameworks and regulations, such as General Data Protection Regulation (GDPR) and Health Insurance Portability and Accountability Act, address various transparency aspects meant to translate into trust from stakeholders. Complying with such laws means that AI does not write over the rights of patients but promotes innovations in health care.

Another major consideration involves accountability and liability around the decisions generated by AI. It becomes difficult to identify who might be responsible when wrong diagnoses or recommendations result from AI models. The removed institutions and healthcare providers should work toward establishing dynamic accountability frameworks, with them as endorsers of the model and betters of the process. Also, ethical standards demand that algorithmic interpretability be ensured to maintain ethical standards. The explainability of models should give clinicians explainable results based on the model's inputs to eliminate questions raised about the AI.

Equally critical is pondering the possible socioeconomic implications of AI in healthcare. Advanced AI systems may inadvertently widen the gap between high-resource and low-resource healthcare settings, as not all facilities can afford cutting-edge technology. Policies must uphold equitable access to AI tools such that these tools will not be beneficial to just some patients but to all, regardless of location or economic standing. Public participation aligns with the encouragement of open-source AI development and public-private partnerships in democratizing healthcare innovation.

7.1 Data Privacy and Security

The sensitivity of patient data makes data privacy and security the most vital thing in AI-powered healthcare. Its broad application requires the establishment of excellent measures to safeguard it from breaches and unauthorized access into the system. The use of encryption techniques and secure data transfer protocols along with anonymization of patient records are some of the well-considered practices in preventing violations to privacy regulations without denying availability of the data for AI training. Federated learning has potential in this case, by allowing model training onto distributed data without compromising privacy (Gong and Wu, 2022). However, an increased dependence on interconnected systems also creates a possible opportunity for cyber threats. Hackers can penetrate a healthcare institution employing stolen credentials with the hopes of exploiting security holes in the institution's AI infrastructure. Periodic audits, penetration tests, and the addition of blockchain technologies into the system can help improve defense. Data integrity and traceability provided by blockchain give that secure environment for storing and sharing healthcare information.

Another concern is patient trust in the privacy and security of AI systems. This includes educating patients about the assurances undertaken in keeping their data safe to bring about transparency and confidence. They need to mention policies that will respond to misuse or breach in data and provide fast actions to minimize damage from possible events.

7.2 Bias and Fairness in AI Models

Bias in AI may be one of the most alarm bells among all other alerting issues regarding the ones related to health. Almost always, bias is created by using imbalanced data whereby certain masses of people groups would be favored above others. A common example includes poor performance in case-diagnosing conditions more affecting women in models that were developed or learned from men. Such forms of bias call for assembling datasets that reflect diversity and representation relevant to intended target populations. Keeping track of maximized fairness will also include the evaluation of AI models with the metrics for fairness. Some of them include techniques like re-sampling, re-weighting, and adversarial debiasing for bias-fixating processes during training. Reporting model performance between the demographics needs to be complemented with appropriate information on identification of disparities or enough treatment of intervention mechanisms. Also, the input of all the professional aspects outside AI will go a long way in providing a holistic input in fairness in AI.

It also provides a picture of broader systemic failures that currently characterize healthcare—for example, the differential availability of diagnostic tools or treatments. It should be integrated into each stage of the process, from collection to deployment. AI ethics boards will thus have a significant role in conducting systematic reviews for biases of models against the criteria for justice and equity.

Table 3 depicts several types of biases which occur in healthcare datasets along with sampling, measurement, and labeling bias and their relative impact on model predictions. The focus is on the ways through which these biases lead to incorrect or unfair outcomes on a large scale, especially on those cases underrepresented in terms of their proportions. Moreover, the table spells out the importance of removing these biases for making machine learning models in health much more reliable and equitable.

Table 3. Common biases in datasets and their impact on model predictions

Bias Type	Description	Impact on Model Predictions
Sampling Bias	Sampling bias occurs-this is a state that happens when the data sample does not represent the entire population.	Over-represented or underrepresented groups can thus lead to inaccurate predictions from the model for those under-represented groups.
Label Bias	It comes about as a result of mislabeling or wrongly assigning labels in a dataset.	The model will, therefore, learn a wrong thing as it will have been trained on fraud or misled data, which will later reflect in its inference at a large extent inaccuracy as well as a generalization error.
Selection Bias	Occurs when there is a higher likelihood of including an individual in a dataset relative to others or group members.	The model might then give biased results and preferences to the features of the over-represented population resulting in imprecise conclusions and recommendations for the others.
Measurement Bias	When the data collection tools systematically bias the data collected, then it is said to have sampling bias.	The model may learn wrong or vague data, resulting in incorrect predictions or overfitting erroneous patterns.
Confirmation Bias	When data is chosen to fit a hypothesis or preconceived idea, it is called sample bias.	Therefore, the model may cast off a number of critical data points that counter the hypothesis, which results in skewed predictions, which support the initial assumption rather than mirror reality.
Cultural Bias	Different sources of cultural, linguistic, or prejudicial data.	A culture and linguistically biased model can lead to biased outcomes in healthcare by performing very well in a particular cultural setup and failing to do so accurately or even fairly for people from different cultural setups.
Historical Bias	This happens when global data harks back to old prejudices or stereotypes.	Models based on past societal biases may lead to bias predictions or decision making, which would adversely affect some groups such as women or minorities.
Algorithmic Bias	This happens when the model architecture or the learning algorithm favors certain patterns.	Systematic errors or unfair predictions on the basis of certain features such as race, gender, or age may still occur even when those features are not relevant to the task.

8. ADVANTAGES OF MACHINE LEARNING IN HEALTHCARE

Machine learning (ML) has made healthcare precision, efficiency, and accessibility in medical practices a real possibility. This is achieved using data-driven algorithms that permit much more accurate diagnosis, prediction about patient outcomes, and personalized treatments compared with manual ones. Such potential lies in disease detection at early stages through oncology, radiology, and cardiology, where traditional methods often fail. It has also enabled clinicians to make some previously unreachable insight known by giving them the ability to analyze complex datasets, genetic information, and medical imaging.

Another very important merit of ML is improving efficiency in healthcare operations. Automate administrative work generally, but even certain patient-specific ones removing entirely unnecessary burdens off health care providers while timing patient intervention in getting care. In addition, IoT with wearables has introduced continuous monitoring of patients and enabled proactive intervention. This action has been a good breakthrough for increasing access to healthcare especially in more remote locations or those underserved for health care equity.

Key Advantages:

- Enhanced Diagnostic Precision: ML based tools improve diagnostic accuracy in disease identification and decrease the errors in clinically used domains, i.e., radiology and pathology.
- Personalized Treatment Plans: That will allow better treatment response by integration analysis of the patients' genetic, lifestyle and clinical data.
- Predictive Analytics: Offers the early diagnosis and the option of preventive actions for clinicians.
- Improved Operational Efficiency: Offers integrated management of patient records, appointment scheduling and billing which increases efficiencies and minimizes errors.
- Remote Patient Monitoring: Enables the remote long-term health monitoring provided by IoT-enabled devices that, in turn, support chronic disease management.
- Accelerated Drug Discovery: And it indicates on the large scale dataset which potential drugs and also predicts the efficacy, which helps accelerate the drug development timeline.
- Cost Reduction: Reduces healthcare cost through less unnecessary procedures, less hospitalization, and less administrative work.
- Data-Driven Decision Support: Provides clinicians with actionable data, which can be rapidly and more effectively used for medical decision making.

9. CHALLENGES AND FUTURE DIRECTIONS

AI brought challenges for healthcare, which need focused solutions to release the technology's complete potentiality. Data availability and quality is the primary challenge, for data to get fragmented across many systems and differ widely in formats and quality. The question increasingly becomes how to harmonize these for full-fledged AI training. In addition, small amounts of labeled medical data hinder supervised learning models, thereby pushing innovation such as semi-supervised or unsupervised learning. Then there are also the challenges in the legal and ethical domain as the evolutionary frameworks are not able to catch up with the race of rapid technological advancements. Global regulations for AI-in-healthcare should become clearer for safety along with transparency and accountability. However, training and deploying the more advanced AI models-such as deep neural networks-require exorbitant computation resources for either training or execution that are significant barriers in resource-constrained settings.

Looking toward the future, we will run multi-modal AI systems that ingest different data types such as medical imaging, genomics, and electronic health records (EHRs). Edge computing promises to enable on-device AI processing of data to make it available right in the healthcare device at the moment, without having to transmit it elsewhere, especially in remote or rural communities. Such roadblocks would enable favorable chances for generalizing AI throughout everybody's healthcare system.

9.1 Interpretability and Explainability

After revealing the app that treats hassle in the recruitment of employees in an organization, artificial intelligence has again quarreled to fly in the face of converting all data into any language, fictional or dramatized. The software breach continues. The irony of interpreting AI into human text has been hard and uneasy for modern researchers. (Lee et al., 2020) in the interview emphasize three areas: interpretability, explainability, and generality. All three are important in the transformation of models in medicine. A model needs to transform itself into a patient-specific treatment, thus requiring justification of the interpretation process that will be used by patients to link the model with a treatment. The insightful models must give consideration to readjusting the factor of interest at the treatment level to be specified in terms of patient probability.

Interpretability and explainability are determinants for acceptance of AI in clinical practice. AI must provide a message for justifying its decisions. Black-box models- such as deep learning systems- have a high degree of opacity and often fail to justify the conclusions they come to. Abstractive or interpretable arguments like SHAP and LIME were meanwhile invented for providing insights on model behavior. Explainable AI (XAI) is especially critical for the high-stake era involving oncologists and cardiologists. The decision they are making then would directly impact lives. Hence, XAI would narrow down from model predictions made available on processes with the human-readable explanation to clinical reasoning. One such example can be drawn when using a decision tree model to predict a patient's risk of diabetes, relying on significance such as BMI, age, glucose levels, and other factors, allowing them to validate it against the clinician's knowledge. Thus, to have some interpretability, it is often necessary to give up the degree of model complexity and performance. It will be an important challenge for the future, however, because the most complex AI models will still be well above a balance between the accuracy and transparency of their predictions. Research in future should delineate interesting specific interpretations that fit with clinical workflows.

9.2 Scalability and Integration in Clinical Workflows

Deploying artificial intelligence within different clinical settings has been a challenge around scalability. In fact, AI systems often fail when transforming from the tightly controlled experimental environment to an actual health institution. Data format differences, infrastructure variation, and training levels of staff culminate in bottlenecks that prevent the seamless integration of AI in clinical practices. Nonetheless, such hurdles can be overcome through custom AI solutions catering to the specific clinical workflow. A much more integrated interaction during the AI tool integration should also consider how these tools fit into the existing healthcare systems like EHR systems. For example, bridging the gaps as highlighted within HL7 FHIR (Fast Healthcare Interoperability Resources) aims at ensuring the smooth flow of data from AI application to clinical systems. Scalable AI tools would also require a capability for incremental learning hence evolving over time with the additions of new patient data and medical knowledge.

Involving healthcare professionals into the design and deployment phase will cause better alignment of the tools with clinical needs. Feedback loops and updates of AI using repeated iterations can optimize the performance of AI against clinician satisfaction. Real scalability through cloud-hosted AI and forming partnerships with health providers will exponentially expand adoption.

9.3 Potential of Federated Learning

Federated learning is one of the changing paradigms to resolve the issues related to patient privacy in healthcare. The patient data is not put together for training AI models but decentralizes learning with all data residing in the local devices with the only model updates being shared. This is especially useful in institutional environments as most of them do not allow sharing of data due to legal and ethical issues. One of the possible applications of FL is training predictive models in multiple hospitals where patient privacy is the leading concern. This can be done by aggregating insights into a federated learning framework that aggregates distributed datasets for improved diagnostic accuracy on rare diseases. For example, Gong & Wu, 2022, show how data security can be guaranteed by FL while allowing advancement in collaboration concerning AI. However, despite the advantages mentioned above, federated learning still brings communication overhead and model-convergence challenges. Effective aggregation techniques along with secure communication protocols are helpful in optimizing the overall performance of these systems. As the federated learning matures, its ability to democratize AI training across healthcare systems would reinvent collaborative medical research and innovation in AI.

10. CONCLUSION

The advent of machine learning in medicine is an enormous step towards the emergence of more precise, personalized and data-driven medical applications. Machine learning has proven to be effective not only in disease prediction, automated diagnostics, but also in remote patient monitoring, and as a result has been able to transform the way care is provided in health care contexts. These algorithms give their specific contribution that leads to a quicker and more precise selection, and that in the end facilitates an optimal patient care, a reduction of the health workers' workload. As machine learning technologies continue to be developed, their influence on both the accuracy of medicine, as well as efficiency of operations, will continue to increase. However, for stakeholder trust to be developed, strong ethical, transparent, and equitable implementation is essential.

Machine learning provides a unique opportunity to improve the quality of healthcare delivery through predictive analytics for chronic diseases, enhanced imaging methods, and personal recommendations in treatment. It has presented tools for clinicians that can work through volumes of data in real-time for insights once unattainable. Emerging technologies, such as federated learning and edge computing, now present new options for innovating in addressing privacy issues while enabling decentralized healthcare solutions. But all the same, there remain pretty big challenges. Data fragmentation, lack of interoperability, and even biases in AI models have rendered machine learning far from fulfilling its promises. Broadly ethical issues around data privacy and security as well as scalability and seamless integration with clinical workflows accompany all these grandfathered practical challenges. It takes all stakeholders, including policymakers, researchers, and healthcare professionals, concertedly to address them to ensure robust, fair, and equitable machine learning solutions.

Indeed, the future of machine learning in health is changing as the technology advances toward predictive, preventive, and personalized medicine. In the next several decades, machine learning models are expected to connect seamlessly with morally-neutral or subjective IoT devices, wellness wearables, and genome data to build complete patient profiles that make real-time decisions. Federated learning and blockchain technologies can address various privacy issues while allowing collaboration beyond borders and between health systems worldwide. Concurrently, since AI models will start to become more interpretable, the integration of these models in regular clinical practice will further establish clinician trust and decision-making. Multi-modal AI systems that will synthesize different datasets are established to open up insights that humans currently cannot understand and generate breakthroughs in new ways to diagnose and treat hard-to-diagnose complex diseases. Innovate and collaborate further, and machine learning will enhance the delivery of health care, as well as change the perspective on human health.

REFERENCES

Ahmed, M. U., Begum, S., & Funk, P. (2016). Artificial intelligence in health and medicine: Where do we stand? *International Journal of Medical Informatics*, *84*(1), 74–86.

Arora, A., Ranjan, P., & Srivastava, R. K. (2023). Application of machine learning in medical diagnostics: A systematic review. *Journal of Medical Systems*, *47*(3), 17–29.

Bauer, C. R., Reddy, K. A., & Singh, M. (2022). Deep learning in medical imaging: Emerging applications and challenges. *Computer Methods and Programs in Biomedicine*, *227*, 107–122.

Ben-Israel, D., Jacobs, W. B., Casha, S., Lang, E., & Clarke, D. B. (2021). The impact of machine learning on patient care: A systematic review. *Neurosurgery*, *87*(1), 14–24.

Choudhury, T., & Dhar, P. (2023). AI in healthcare: Ethical dilemmas and regulatory challenges. *Ethics, Medicine, and Public Health*, *24*, 100–118.

Deo, R. C. (2015). Machine learning in medicine. *Circulation*, *132*(20), 1920–1930. DOI: 10.1161/CIRCULATIONAHA.115.001593 PMID: 26572668

Dilsizian, S. E., & Siegel, E. L. (2014). Artificial intelligence in medicine and cardiac imaging. *Cardiology Clinics*, *32*(2), 225–234. PMID: 24793799

Esteva, A., Kuprel, B., Novoa, R. A., Ko, J., Swetter, S. M., Blau, H. M., & Thrun, S. (2017). Dermatologist-level classification of skin cancer with deep neural networks. *Nature*, *542*(7639), 115–118. DOI: 10.1038/nature21056 PMID: 28117445

Gong, C., & Wu, J. (2022). Federated learning in healthcare: A review and future directions. *Journal of Biomedical Informatics*, *128*, 104026.

Haque, A., Guo, M., & Albayda, J. (2022). Emerging applications of reinforcement learning in personalized medicine. *Nature Machine Intelligence*, *4*(5), 371–382.

Huang, Z., Lu, X., & Duan, H. (2018). Health information sharing in IoT healthcare: Machine learning techniques and privacy concerns. *Computers in Biology and Medicine*, *96*, 90–101.

Jiang, F., Jiang, Y., Zhi, H., Dong, Y., Li, H., Ma, S., Wang, Y., Dong, Q., Shen, H., & Wang, Y. (2017). Artificial Intelligence in Healthcare: Past, Present, and Future. *Stroke and Vascular Neurology*, *2*(4), 230–243. DOI: 10.1136/svn-2017-000101 PMID: 29507784

Johnson, A. E. W., Pollard, T. J., & Mark, R. G. (2016). Reproducibility in critical care: A vision for improving healthcare. *Critical Care Medicine*, *44*(1), e102–e109.

Kang, H., & Park, Y. (2021). Predictive analytics for chronic disease management using AI. *Healthcare Analytics*, *3*(2), 53–65.

Kelly, C. J., Karthikesalingam, A., Suleyman, M., Corrado, G., & King, D. (2019). Key challenges for delivering clinical impact with artificial intelligence. *BMC Medicine*, *17*(1), 195. DOI: 10.1186/s12916-019-1426-2 PMID: 31665002

Kishor Kumar Reddy, C., Daduvy, A., Madana Mohana, R., Assiri, B., Shuaib, M., Alam, S., & Abdullah Sheneamer, M. (2024). Enhancing Precision Agriculture and Land Cover Classification: A Self –Attention 3D Convolutional Neural Network Approach for Hyperspectral Image Analysis. *IEEE Access : Practical Innovations, Open Solutions*, *12*, 125592–125608. Advance online publication. DOI: 10.1109/ACCESS.2024.3420089

Kumar, S., & Sharma, A. (2023). Machine learning algorithms for drug discovery and development. *Journal of Cheminformatics*, *15*(4), 41–55.

Lee, J. H., & Jeong, K. (2021). AI-driven medical imaging: Trends and future outlook. *Medical Image Analysis*, *75*, 102301.

Liu, Y., Wei, S., & Zhang, X. (2020). Privacy-preserving healthcare using blockchain and AI. *Journal of Medical Systems*, *44*(5), 78–91.

McKinney, S. M., Sieniek, M., Godbole, V., Godwin, J., Antropova, N., Ashrafian, H., Back, T., Chesus, M., Corrado, G. S., Darzi, A., Etemadi, M., Garcia-Vicente, F., Gilbert, F. J., Halling-Brown, M., Hassabis, D., Jansen, S., Karthikesalingam, A., Kelly, C. J., King, D., & Shetty, S. (2020). International evaluation of an AI system for breast cancer screening. *Nature*, *577*(7788), 89–94. DOI: 10.1038/s41586-019-1799-6 PMID: 31894144

Monika Singh, T., Kishor Kumar Reddy, C., Ramana Murthy, B. V., Nag, A., & Doss, S. (2025). AI and Education: Bridging the Gap to Personalized, Efficient, and Accessible Learning. In M. Ouaissa, M. Ouaissa, H. Lamaazi, M. El Hamlaoui, & K. Reddy C. (Eds.), Internet of Behavior-Based Computational Intelligence for Smart Education Systems (pp. 131-160). IGI Global. DOI: 10.4018/979-8-3693-8151-9.ch005

Naik, N., & Acharya, U. R. (2022). Role of natural language processing in healthcare data analysis. *Computer Methods and Programs in Biomedicine*, *227*, 106924.

Obermeyer, Z., & Emanuel, E. J. (2016). Predicting the future—Big data, machine learning, and clinical medicine. *The New England Journal of Medicine*, *375*(13), 1216–1219. DOI: 10.1056/NEJMp1606181 PMID: 27682033

Park, S. H., & Han, K. (2018). Methodologic guide for evaluating clinical performance and effect of AI in medical imaging. *Radiology*, *286*(3), 800–809. DOI: 10.1148/radiol.2017171920 PMID: 29309734

Rajkomar, A., Dean, J., & Kohane, I. (2019). Machine Learning in Medicine. *The New England Journal of Medicine*, *380*(14), 1347–1358. DOI: 10.1056/NEJMra1814259 PMID: 30943338

Reddy, C. K. K., Rangarajan, A., Rangarajan, D., Shuaib, M., Jeribi, F., & Alam, S. (2024). A Transfer Learning Approach: Early Prediction of Alzheimer's Disease on US Healthy Aging Dataset. *Mathematics*, *12*(14), 2204. DOI: 10.3390/math12142204

Reddy, K. K., Badam, R., Alam, S., & Shuaib, M. (2024). IoT Driven Accessibility:A Refreshable OCR-Braille Solution for Visually Impaired and Deaf-Blind Users through WSN. *JETECH Elsevier*, *2*(April), 128–137. Advance online publication. DOI: 10.1016/j.ject.2024.04.007

Shameer, K., Johnson, K. W., Glicksberg, B. S., Dudley, J. T., & Sengupta, P. P. (2018). Machine Learning in Cardiovascular Medicine: Are We There Yet? *Heart (British Cardiac Society), 104*(14), 1156–1164. DOI: 10.1136/heartjnl-2017-311198 PMID: 29352006

Singh, T. M., & Lippert, K. (2024). Digital Twins in Human Activity Prediction on Gait Using Extreme Gradient Boosting Local Binary Pattern: Healthcare 6.0. In Dubey, A., Kumar Reddy, C., Doss, S., & Hanafiah, M. (Eds.), *Exploring the Advancements and Future Directions of Digital Twins in Healthcare 6.0* (pp. 240–261). IGI Global., DOI: 10.4018/979-8-3693-5893-1.ch012

Topol, E. (2019). High-performance medicine: The convergence of human and artificial intelligence. *Nature Medicine, 25*(1), 44–56. DOI: 10.1038/s41591-018-0300-7 PMID: 30617339

Vayena, E., & Blasimme, A. (2018). Challenges in the ethics of AI in healthcare. *Nature Medicine, 24*(9), 1303–1305.

Wang, F., & Preininger, A. (2019). AI in healthcare: Applications, challenges, and future directions. *Computers in Biology and Medicine, 112*, 103–119.

Xu, J., & Yang, P. (2020). Real-time monitoring in healthcare with machine learning techniques. *Journal of Artificial Intelligence in Medicine, 106*, 101865. Topol, E. J. (2019). *Deep Medicine: How Artificial Intelligence Can Make Healthcare Human Again.* Basic Books.

Yu, K. H., Beam, A. L., & Kohane, I. S. (2018). Artificial Intelligence in Healthcare. *Nature Biomedical Engineering, 2*(10), 719–731. DOI: 10.1038/s41551-018-0305-z PMID: 31015651

Chapter 4
Advanced Machine Learning Techniques Driving Innovation in Healthcare Systems and Personalized Medicine

M. Arul Sankar
Mahendra Engineering College, India

G. Balachandran
Jeppiaar Engineering College, India

S. Ramesh
SRM Institute of Science and Technology, India

R. Bhavani
Sathyabama Institute of Science and Technology, India

Umesha Raddy
East West Institute of Technology, India

Raj Kumar Masih
Jazan University, Saudi Arabia

ABSTRACT

Collecting, organizing, analyzing, and managing health data is the focus of health information management. Computer Science, Data Analytics, Information Science, Medicine, Business, And Information Management are all parts of it. A new topic within healthcare, machine learning (ML) is rapidly developing. They provide faster and more accurate analysis of health data. Artificial intelligence (AI) is a crucial area within software engineering. Drawing on knowledge gained from prior experiences or lessons learned, it provides a simplified solution to these problems of the present. As a field, software engineering makes use of specialized machine learning computations. Machine learning techniques such as Recurrent Neural Networks, Decision Trees, Naive Bayes Classifier, Ensemble Vector Machine, and Linear discriminant Analysis are introduced in this chapter. The methods are all laid out in great detail, allowing the reader to come up with their solutions to the problems provided.

DOI: 10.4018/979-8-3373-1022-0.ch004

1. INTRODUCTION

There has been a recent increase in the amount of digital healthcare data. The patient's details, demographics, test results, doctor's prescription, and other relevant data are included in this set. Researchers may use this data to understand better the health problems facing the population now and, perhaps, to foretell such problems in the future. Keeping track of all the growing amounts of digital health information is no easy feat. In order to keep patient information private, secure, and usable, the organization needs to have the appropriate application and tool. This contributes to the long-term objectives of efficient data management, high-quality treatment, and the avoidance of wasteful spending. Informatics can bridge the gap between paper health records and digital technology, which is becoming more important as the number of digital records grows. Using these resources, doctors may better keep track of their patients' medical histories. The doctor and the administrative staff can then zero in on the most important details thanks to the recorded information.

1.1 Health Information Management

Health information management focuses on collecting, organizing, analyzing, and managing health data. It also includes data analytics, computer science, information science, medicine, business, and information management. These areas contribute to the enhancement of the system's quality by delivering high-quality care in a timely manner. In the hospital, instead of using paper, staff members utilize electronic devices to document patient Information. These devices facilitate both the collection of data and its processing for use by inpatients.

Managed health data should be revised regularly to reflect the most recent developments in data analytics, confidentiality, safety, information governance, and interoperability.

- Protecting sensitive electronic health records from unauthorized access is of the utmost importance.
- Incorporating new rules, panels, and structures for the organization's data management is an important part of information governance.
- Interoperability: The capacity for businesses and stakeholders to communicate data effectively.
- Data analytics: analyzing raw data to make decisions in real-time.

1.2 Goal of ML in Healthcare

The goal of machine learning, a subfield of AI, is to enable computers to learn from data in order to perform tasks such as prediction and action generation without human intervention. Figure 1 shows how machine learning might change healthcare in a revolutionary way, affecting diagnosis, treatment, and illness prevention. The following are a few examples of possible medical uses for machine learning:

- Predictive analytics: Machine learning algorithms may examine data from electronic health records, claims data, and other sources to forecast the probability of certain health outcomes, such as the beginning of chronic illnesses or hospital readmissions. This may aid medical professionals in determining which individuals pose the greatest risk of complications and in taking preventative measures.

- Diagnosis and treatment: Machine learning algorithms can be trained to examine medical pictures, such as X-rays or CT scans, to aid in diagnosis or choose the best course of therapy.
- Personalized medicine: Machine learning can be used to determine which therapies will have the best chance of success based on a patient's unique traits, such as genetics and medical history.
- Clinical decision support: By incorporating machine learning algorithms into clinical decision-support systems, healthcare practitioners may enhance the quality of patient care through more informed decision-making.
- Population health management: Data from huge populations may be analyzed using machine learning to find patterns and trends that might guide the creation of public health programs.

In healthcare, machine learning has the ability to increase efficiency, decrease expenses, and improve patient outcomes. Although machine learning has been around for a while, the current deluge of data generated by healthcare organizations has brought it into the spotlight. More than 80% of healthcare business executives have an AI strategy, and 86% of healthcare companies employ ML technologies in some way, according to one survey. In the broader realm of artificial intelligence, ML plays a significant role (Rahman et al., 2024). Mathematical learning is characterized as "the capacity of a computer to reproduce intelligent human behavior." To make choices based on fresh data that has comparable traits or variables, algorithms are taught to learn from existing data. An essential component of information science that needs to be applied to different ML models is the interaction of many fields, particularly computer science, statistics, and mathematics. In spite of our superior intellect, we are fallible due to our short-term memory limitations. An opportunity to apply machine learning to assist humans in making decisions that take into consideration a great deal of contextual information arises when the exponential growth of data is coupled with the increasing processing power of computers. Heart failure care, clinical decision assistance in clinical medicine, and medical imaging are just a few of the recent medical fields in which to apply ML. ML is more concerned with a model's predictive power than more conventional hypothesis-driven statistical analysis (Chua et al., 2023). For a long time, epidemiologic approaches have been the backbone of healthcare data collection. The lack of efficient integration between the two disciplines is a serious barrier, particularly when data scientists and epidemiologists work as a team. ML approaches provide new ways of answering diverse questions. Additionally, it has been said that, despite the wide variety of terminology used in various fields, terms that are equivalent or nearly so are often used interchangeably. Suppose they are made aware that ML uses these notions with a new framework in mind. In that case, epidemiologists and statisticians should have no trouble understanding them because they have long utilized them in hypothesis-driven research. Clinicians, public health doctors, pathologists, as well as radiologists are among the other medical experts who have more experience with hypothesis-driven research instead of ML algorithms. Therefore, it's important to demonstrate how the two distinct but connected fields have common conceptual ground. In this written overview, we will try to give you a rundown of several important ML ideas and how far they may go in healthcare. Classification of machine learning models and the specifics of the available algorithms are the main points of discussion. If you want to make a smart choice, this methodological review will give you a rundown of all the important ML algorithms.

2. MACHINE LEARNING IN HEALTHCARE MARKET OVERVIEW

The World Health Organization predicts a tenfold increase in the need for healthcare professionals by 2030. Machine learning technologies powered by artificial intelligence have the potential to increase healthcare providers' time to devote to each patient's unique needs while simultaneously reducing the burden on already overburdened healthcare systems.

Figure 1. MI / ML Current Market

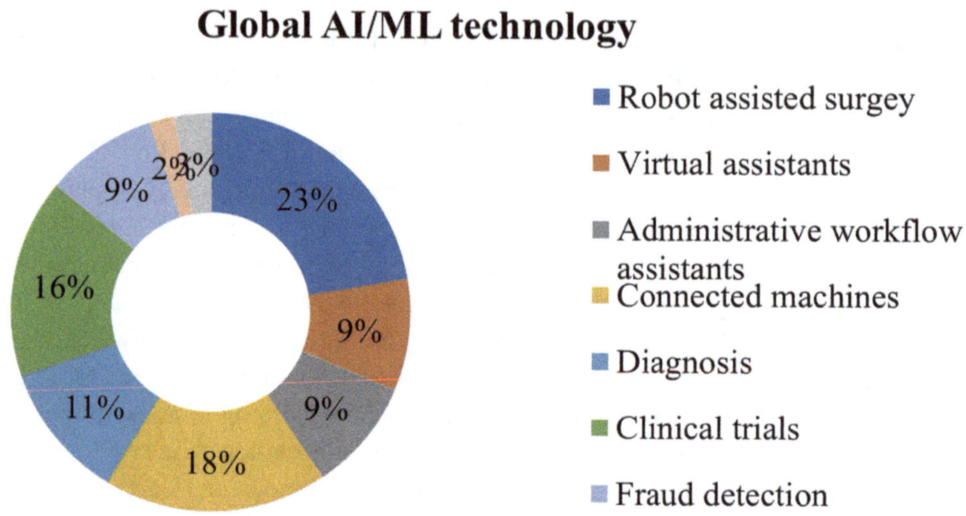

2.1 ML Applications for Healthcare

The use of machine learning is enabling research institutes, firms, and startups to revolutionize healthcare by developing innovative solutions in areas such as personalized medication and diagnostics:

2.1.1 Disease Diagnosis and Prediction

In the past, doctors had to rely on their intuition, years of expertise, and the tests that were available to them when diagnosing patients. However, machine learning is rapidly changing the diagnostics industry as a whole due to its superior speed and ability to detect subtle associations and trends in large datasets. In radiology, for instance, specialized machine learning models can analyze X-rays, MRIs, and CT scans to pinpoint abnormalities like tumors or lesions with pinpoint accuracy (Reddy et al., 2024). Early identification is crucial for good treatment outcomes along with patient survival in illnesses like cancer or cardiovascular problems, making these models especially beneficial for early-stage diagnosis. Machine learning is being used for more than just diagnoses; it is also being used to forecast the likelihood of a patient having a given illness, as well as its commencement and development, by analyzing personal data such as lifestyle variables, genetic predispositions, and prior medical problems. By doing so, healthcare practitioners may enhance patient outcomes via personalized treatment, the implementation of preventive measures, and monitoring tactics prior to the onset of symptoms.

2.1.2 Research labs

Machine learning may enhance hypothesis testing and provide light on the true mechanism of a disease in a laboratory setting. By analyzing large amounts of complex data, algorithms can model the course of illness, allowing scientists better to understand both the onset and treatment of various disorders. Predicting a patient's response to individual medications allows for more tailored treatment plans, which is particularly helpful for illnesses like cancer. In addition, researchers may use machine learning to create a hypothesis model, which can subsequently be refined and repeated repeatedly according to the changing data. This method has the potential to speed up the creation of innovative solutions by increasing the precision of predictions and fostering better cooperation between doctors and data scientists.

2.1.3 Personalized medicine and treatment plans

The advent of personalized medicine is among the most encouraging trends in contemporary healthcare. Machine learning can analyze patient data to help healthcare practitioners forecast the most successful treatment choice while minimizing the risk of bad reactions. This means that patients won't have to adopt a one-size-fits-all strategy. When treating cancer, for example, the results could vary greatly from patient to patient, making this method very useful. Customized treatment programs are also flexible and evolving as a result of machine learning models' inherent capacity to learn from fresh data (Sanchez et al., 2022). Especially helpful in managing chronic diseases like hypertension or diabetes, the model can suggest dosage or medication adjustments based on treatment efficacy, meaning the treatment is continuously optimized to suit the patient's evolving condition and ensure it remains effective. One further benefit of personalized treatment plans powered by machine learning is their ability to anticipate when patients may go off course and then implement interventions like reminders or follow-up visits to keep them on track.

2.1.4 Predictive analytics for patient outcomes

Predictive analytics may predict the chances of disease progression and the likelihood of complications during hospital admission/readmission by analyzing EHRs and other data sources like genetic information as well as wearable devices with machine learning algorithms (Kishor Kumar Reddy et al., 2025). This allows medical professionals to proactively address an opportunity for health issues before they grow into critical, ensuring that interventions are timely, targeted, and effective (Sabry et al., 2022). When it comes to healthcare, predictive analytics is most often used for:

- **Chronic disease management:** By analyzing a patient's past data and present health indicators, models may detect when their condition is starting to worsen. This allows doctors to adjust their medication, suggest lifestyle modifications, or boost monitoring.
- **Treatment response (mainly in oncology):** Machine learning techniques can forecast the efficacy of chemotherapy regimens and targeted medicines by analyzing data from individuals with comparable characteristics. This lessens the need for a process of trial and error, which may lead to ineffective treatment and unneeded adverse effects.

- **Post-surgical care:** Patients at increased risk for postoperative problems, including infections and blood clots, may be identified by analyzing preexisting diseases, surgical complexity, and recovery data models. These factors help to determine which patients will have lengthier recovery durations. By doing so, healthcare practitioners may lessen the likelihood of readmission and enhance recovery outcomes via preventive measures.
- **Medication management:** Medical professionals may better serve their patients by prescribing medications with the lowest risk of adverse effects based on predictions of how individuals with specific genetic profiles would react to such medicines.
- **Preventive care:** Healthcare practitioners can take preventative actions for patients who, due to personal variables, including family history, lifestyle choices, and early warning signals, are at high risk of acquiring chronic illnesses. This improves health in the long run and lessens the burden of chronic illnesses on individuals and the healthcare system as a whole.

2.1.5 Drug discovery and development

Researchers are finding that machine learning is useful for medication development since it helps them find novel treatments more precisely and predicts how safe and successful they will be via:

- Predicting the interactions between chemicals and distinct target proteins and enzymes by analyzing intricate biological data, including genetic information, structures of protein, and molecular interactions.
- To guarantee the drug's safety for patients, it is necessary to model and forecast how changes to its chemical structure would impact its efficacy. Additionally, this results in medications with a better chance of success during clinical trials.
- Looking at results from previous clinical trials to make educated guesses about the new drug's efficacy and safety. By revealing acceptable patient categories, dosage regimens, and possible adverse effects, this research may help improve the trial's design, making it operate more efficiently and successfully.

Machine learning analysis of current medication data may find chances for repurposing and forecast possible new medicinal applications for existing chemicals.

2.1.6 Improving operational efficiency

In addition to enhancing direct patient care, machine learning has the potential to streamline healthcare operations, save costs, and increase efficiency—all without sacrificing quality of care:

- Machine learning may assist healthcare institutions in cutting costs and discovering the most effective sources for high-quality, cost-effective products through supply chain management. This involves anticipating demand for supplies, optimizing inventory levels, and eliminating waste.
- The unpredictability of patient admissions is a common problem in healthcare settings, particularly hospitals. It may cause overstaffing or understaffing, which in turn can squander resources or put patients at risk. In order to foretell the need for services in the future, machine learning models

may examine past data like patient admission rates, seasonal patterns, and the health patterns of the local population.

- Patient flow management: Effective patient flow management depends on eliminating delays and improving the flow of treatment. Data like patient demographics, admission trends, and treatment durations may be analyzed by machine learning to forecast and control patient flow. Triaging patients in Emergency procedures by analyzing their symptoms and medical history to prioritize those most in need, optimizing surgical scheduling, or monitoring bed availability are all areas where this may assist in alleviating bottlenecks.
- Administrative duties: Scheduling appointments, creating invoices, and managing patients are all tedious and error-prone when done by hand. Machine learning algorithms may automate these processes, which benefits all parties involved by decreasing paperwork, increasing payment cycles, and decreasing appointment wait times.

2.2. Challenges in Implementing ML Models in Healthcare

Using ML algorithms in healthcare raises many issues, which specialists discuss.

- To generalize the model's conclusions to a larger population, machine learning models need high-quality data.
- The development of efficient data management strategies at all levels is, therefore, a prerequisite for integrating ML models into healthcare. Furthermore, it is necessary to develop data processing using ML pipelines that include product front ends that are easy to use.
- With the help of these pipelines, raw data may be transformed into datasets suitable for training ML models. To put the data to good use, the right people need to come up with a data governance plan.
- Another major problem is that, unless you employ models like decision trees, which enable straightforward interpretation, ML-based predictions seldom provide explanations for the forecast.
- Legal processes lack efficiency in the event of a probable mistake while using an ML model to forecast a health consequence. The intricacy of legal processes in various nations makes this statement rather tough to implement in reality.

3. REVIEW OF STUDIES

Building an intelligent healthcare system while protecting patients' privacy is the primary goal of the Federated Learning technique, as stated in (Hegde et al., 2023). That research looks at two FL-based algorithms, Logistic Regression and Artificial Neural Network. Three hospitals collaborated on the development of the FL-ANN and FL-LR frameworks, which were then tested separately using datasets related to diabetes and chronic kidney disease. Performance measurements like FL Process Time are used to compare these frameworks. In terms of FL-Process Time, the research found that the FL-LR structure performed better than FL-ANN. An improved accuracy of 98.12% and an FL Processing Time of 10.5 seconds are produced by the FL-LR using the CKD dataset. Using a maximum FL Procedure Time of 846.9 seconds, FL-ANN achieved 97.66% accuracy on the diabetes dataset.

The review in (Shehab et al., 2022) discusses the limitations of current diagnostic tools in comparison to ML's promise for early illness identification. From 2015 to 2024, it follows the growth of ML approaches and examines different ML algorithms applied in sectors including cancer, diabetes, and heart disease. Concerning data privacy, in particular, the evaluation delves into ethical and technological hurdles. As for future directions, they suggest combining ensemble learning with deep learning models. That paper is important because it provides a good summary of ML in early illness identification, which may improve diagnostic accuracy, decrease healthcare expenditures, and improve patient outcomes.

Protecting private medical information and other resources requires a strong security system, as stated in (Wazid et al., 2023). Machine learning and deep learning models have their uses, and ensemble-based models show promise for eliminating security risks (Yadav et al., 2025). Here, they provide an innovative ensemble-based ML-envisioned strategy for the EIDS-HS, or Industry 5.0-driven healthcare system, to identify various forms of infiltration. They assess the reliability, precision, recall, F1-score, computational complexity, and other important performance metrics as they test the suggested EIDS-HS on a benchmark dataset. The proposed EIDS-HS has been thoroughly tested and shown to be secure against a wide range of potential threats. The key performance metrics also show that EIDS-HS outperforms the state-of-the-art intrusion detection techniques.

The purpose of that review article is to assess the current ethical frameworks for medical ML and provide a thorough summary of their effectiveness in dealing with ethical issues (Javed et al., 2023). In particular, that study delves into the prevalent ethical frameworks that govern healthcare ML, illuminating key issues such as data security, informed consent, equality, and patient autonomy. Statistical tools for bias identification, quantitative measures, and qualitative theme analysis are all used to tackle these difficulties. Applications in telemedicine, remote patient monitoring, and systems for clinical decision support provide more context and insight (Singh et al., 2022). Existing ethical frameworks are used to assess each scenario and find any gaps or restrictions. They provide practical suggestions for developing ethical standards based on their thorough analysis and research. Finally, the study highlights the critical need for strong ethical frameworks to govern ML applications in delicate healthcare settings and summarizes important results. New frameworks for ethics that can accommodate changing technology and moral conundrums in healthcare ML should be the subject of future research.

Classification, early-stage detection, and diabetes prediction using a machine learning-based technique are suggested in (Butt et al., 2021). Plus, it shows a possible IoT diabetes monitoring device that a healthy person or someone with diabetes may use to keep tabs on their blood glucose levels. Three distinct classifiers—logistic regression, random forest, and multilayer perceptron—have been used for diabetes categorization. Their prediction study has made use of linear regression, moving averages, and long short-term memory. An industry-standard PIMA Indian Diabetes dataset is used for experimental assessment. Among the classifiers tested, MLP achieved the highest accuracy rate of 86.08%, while LSTM significantly improved diabetes prediction accuracy to 87.26%. The suggested strategy is shown to be adaptable in numerous public healthcare applications by a comparison examination with current state-of-the-art approaches.

The purpose of that research is to examine the potential applications of artificial intelligence and machine learning in healthcare, the difficulties in implementing these applications, and the ethical considerations that arise from the broad use of AI in the healthcare system, all the while studying the rules and laws that govern that field. Research Approach: To outline the difficulties and ethical considerations of using AI and ML in healthcare, that paper uses qualitative methods to examine different uses of these technologies and their effects on patient care. Findings: The results show that the amount of data gathered by the healthcare business has grown significantly in recent years. As of 2020, the world's data production will reach forty zettabytes, with organized data increasing at a rate of 40% annually and unstructured data at a rate of over 80%. Industries like healthcare, which place a premium on protecting individuals' privacy, security, and personal information, are compelled to implement effective data governance practices in response to rising regulatory and compliance demands (Hegde et al., 2023). Healthcare businesses are increasingly using AI along with machine learning technologies to make sense of the data generated by the data explosion and make sure it's accessible when needed (Nadakuditi et al., 2024).

An overview of ML's use in two important healthcare applications, activity recognition, and vital sign monitoring, is given in the paper (Ahmed & Cho, 2023). Radar has the potential to revolutionize healthcare by allowing for the prediction of several chronic respiratory and cardiac disorders via vital sign monitoring. Since being unable to carry out even the most basic of tasks may cause immense distress, activity recognition is another popular use. Radar hardware, Commercial radars, and healthcare radar history are all covered in the article. Then, the article moves on to discuss how healthcare radars have used ML. The article continues by explaining how healthcare radars may use ML to circumvent the shortcomings of traditional radar data processing chains. New generative ML ideas for healthcare radars are also discussed in passing in the piece. Among other intriguing discoveries, it was found that ML is used to overcome the limits of old algorithms rather than to replace them when it comes to vital sign monitoring entirely. Activity recognition, in contrast, is ML-dependent at all times. CNNs and SVMs are the two most used methods in these domains. Data augmentation is one area where generative AI is poised to make a big splash in the near future.

To create non-biased supervised machine learning models, the dataset is pre-processed in the present research (Khan & Alkhathami, 2024). The models include Logistic Regression, Perceptron, Random Forest, Adaptive Boosting, and Deep Neural Network. Additional analysis of these models is conducted by removing characteristics with strong correlation, decreasing the number of dimensions, lowering the likelihood of overfitting, and expediting the training process. With an estimated accuracy of 99.55% under both restricted and entire feature space, Random Forest was determined to perform ideally across binary along with multiclass detection of IoT Attacks (Kaza et al., 2024)That development was accompanied by a decrease in computing reaction time, which is critical for detecting and responding to attacks in real-time.

Examines how healthcare-specific full-stack development techniques could benefit from AI and ML in (Gurusamy & Mohamed, 2021). Developers may build smart systems that can analyze massive volumes of medical data, provide individualized treatment suggestions, automate administrative duties, and enhance patient care as a whole by using AI and ML algorithms. Highlighting the revolutionary potential of these technologies, that article explores important methods, obstacles, and possibilities related to full-stack building for healthcare apps that use AI and ML.

Beginning with a theoretical representation of the pipeline of ML-HCAs' conception, development, and deployment, as well as the parallel pipeline of assessment and supervision activities at each level, a systematic method for detecting ML-HCA ethical problems is outlined in (Char et al., 2020). On top of that model, they overlay important concerns that bring up problems of value, in addition to ethical considerations found mostly in a literature study, as well as some unexamined ethical considerations. A multi-disciplinary team of varied stakeholders will need to work together to comprehend and then handle the ethical consequences of ML-HCAs, and that pipeline model approach will be helpful for systematic ethical evaluations of ML-HCAs from creation to implementation (Singh et al., 2025) (Ganiya et al., 2024).

ML is a subfield of AI that enables computers to acquire knowledge and skills via observation and experimentation rather than manual coding. The goal is to create algorithms that can learn from data efficiently (Karthik, Aalam, et al., 2024). Here, learning is collecting data from many sources, analyzing it, finding patterns, and then using those patterns to make better judgments going forward. The main goal is to make robots capable of learning autonomously (Karthik, Hamatta, et al., 2024), without any help from people. No matter where you go or what you do, data will be created in today's environment. Humans have produced one billion gigabytes, or exabytes, of data up to 2005. From 1,200 exabytes in 2010 to 7,900 exabytes in 2015 and an expected 40,900 exabytes in 2020, the data created has grown exponentially. The amount of data being produced is increasing at an exponential pace and will keep doing so (Poloju & Rajaram, 2024). Machine learning is quickly becoming a promising new area of study within the healthcare sector. They provide faster and more accurate analysis of health data. Machine learning has many potential uses in the medical field, including:

- Disease diagnosis;
- medication development forecasting;
- medical image analysis;
- smart health systems;
- data collection via crowdsourcing

The clinic's accounting department uses the Decision Support System to monitor charges, AR, AP, and AP payments. Additionally, this strategy aids in maintaining the patient's insurance coverage and various return options. This company offers a variety of healthcare-related DSS modules. By providing clinicians with a picture of a patient's health problems or by revealing patient histories, decision support systems aid in illness inquiry (Maguluri et al., 2024)A web-based structure integrated with computerized patient/therapeutic records also provides assistance in determining a patient's condition and a guide that suggests when to take the right medication at the right time.

4. ML STUDIES: PIPELINE

- Strategies for data collecting: Whether in real-time or using retrospective datasets, data gathering is an essential part of every research study involving human subjects. Using the right tactics results in effective and focused research.
- Input features: In ML approaches, the most essential thing is to pick and extract characteristics that will help the model produce better results. The features with the greatest influence may be employed.
- Metrics for Prediction and Classification: The number of instances to examine, the sorts of cases, the type of datasets, the type of research, and so on are eight separate factors. Table 4 shows the values that the authors have provided for the several language variables that match the study's measure. For metrics to be better understood, the values of each parametric characteristic are identified according to the linguistic variables. This metric value is useful for further categorizing the characteristics into their potential subtypes.

Figure 2. ML Data Pipeline Model

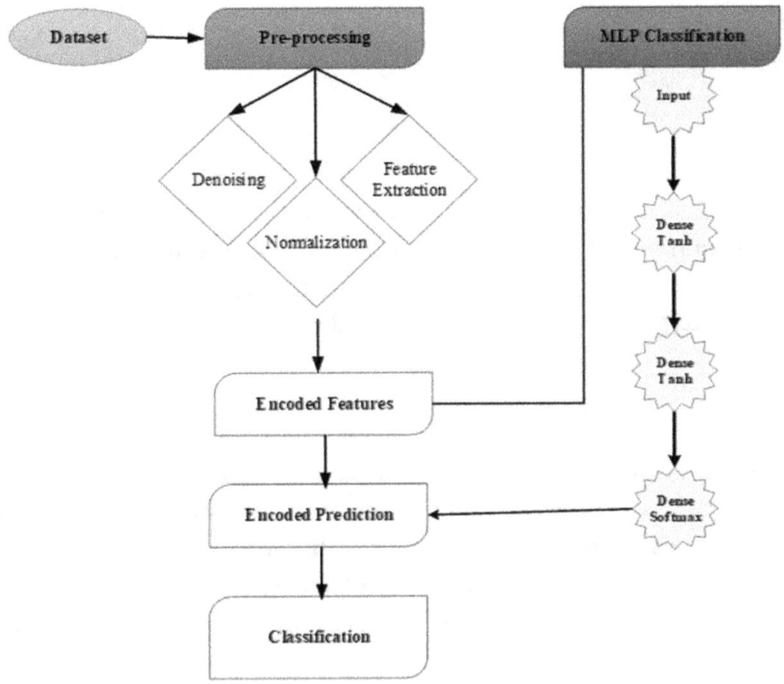

A. Supervised Machine Learning

During training, the algorithm incorporates this knowledge into an exercise that correlates inputs with corresponding outcomes. In supervised learning, the classification problem is a typical starting point (Chiranjeevi & Rajaram, 2024).

B. Semi-supervised Learning

Finding the optimal classifier from both labeled and unlabeled data is what it's all about. It transfers strong classification performance utilizing unlabeled data. Only a small number of presumptions are necessary for this approach to work (Kalaivani et al., 2023).

C. Unsupervised Machine Learning

In unsupervised learning, no training is applied to the labels. Unsupervised learning uses techniques including clustering, hierarchical clustering, fuzzy clustering, K-means clustering, and association rule mining. In this case, a cluster is subdivided according to the availability of labeled but trained data. These methods are used to build a framework with data samples.

D. Reinforcement Learning

The computer application facilitates this learning by providing access to the dynamic setting in order to accomplish a predetermined objective. The software receives feedback in the form of prizes and penalties as it overcomes its weaknesses.

Some of the algorithms include:

(i). LR

For general binary classification issues, logistic regression's standard prediction approach works well. LGR's idea is to take the logit of an odds ratio and convert it to its natural logarithm. Its primary function is to examine the interplay between independent and dependent variables. There are only two possible values for the anticipated variable Y: yes (1) and no (0).

(ii). RF

The original Random Forest (RF) methodology used a classification with regression tree (CART) based on the bagging method and bootstrap aggregation as its classifier. RF is an ensemble method. It constructs the CART tree at random, picking variables to divide at each node. When evaluating random forest performance, the out-of-bag (OOB) fault is calculated as the average of the errors made by each weak sample when an approximation test error is used. Finally, in order to increase the random forest's amplitude and determine the relevance of factors, each tree was constructed on node impurity.

(iii). MARS

A nonparametric statistical approach called MARS was created by Friedman et al. (Friedman, 1991) in the field of physics. Automatically creating a criteria model and separating linear-regression slopes to go through several complicated data sets and build prediction models is the capability of this flexible regression processing. Multiple intervals of the space of independent variables are used to adopt approximate nonlinearity using linear regression slopes. The optimal MARS model begins with a forward approach that builds a large number of potential basic functions and knots to overfit the data. In the second step, we generated the optimum combination using the generalized cross-validation criteria (GCV). In addition to not having to take into account the distribution for demand function or errors, MARS may handle missing data by using dummy variables.

Figure 3. ML Algorithms for Healthcare

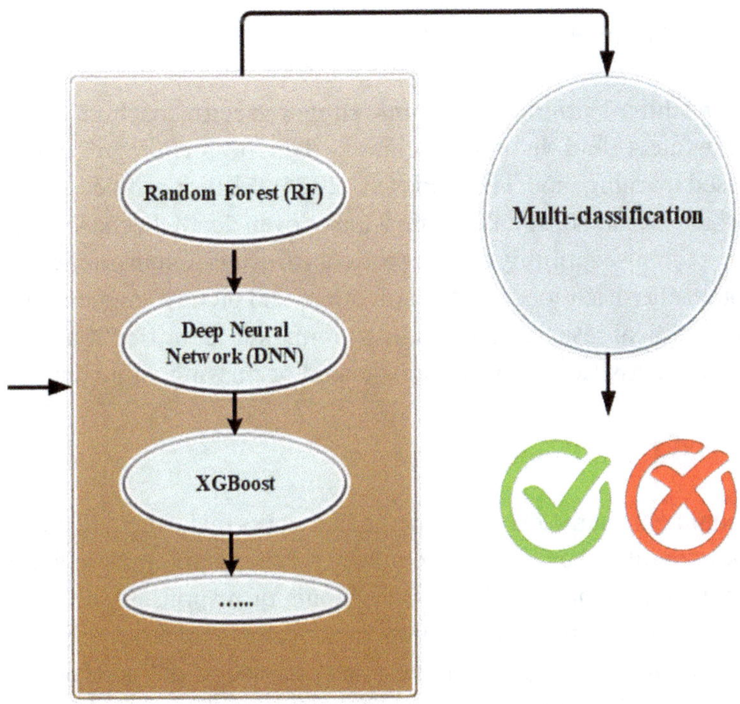

(iv). CART

In 1984, the classification, as well as the regression-tree method, was created by Breiman et al. (Steinberg, 2009). A set of rules is produced by the CART algorithm by use of recursion. The impurity is determined by applying the Gini index to each attribute segmentation, after which CART constructs a maximum tree to binary split the two subsets into both directions halves. Analysis of nodes with leaf nodes begins at the root. To find the segmented traits and values, we employ the least Gini index. Then, when each node has two exclusive offspring, the parent node may split them in half and continue calculating iteratively until the decision tree is built.

(v). XGBoost

In order to solve classification and regression issues, XGBoost employs a gradient-boosting decision tree (GBDT) technique. During the building of each tree layer, the greedy technique maximizes the objective function's maximum gain. In order to build a tree, the algorithm iteratively adds trees and splits their features (Ango et al., 2024). With each new tree, the algorithm learns a different function to fit the residual from the previous forecast. Lastly, the accuracy rate is better when numerous learners are joined together to generate the final prediction, as opposed to just one learner. To address the issue of overfitting, XGBoost employs regularization terms to manage the model's complexity. At the same time, objective function optimization calculates pseudo residues using the second derivative of the Taylor expansion loss function.

(vi). Support Vector Machine

When it comes to machine learning algorithms, support vector machines (SVMs) are perhaps the most employed in the medical field. In order to classify data, perform regression, and identify outliers, SVMs use the supervised learning model (Guido et al., 2024). Millions of people have been able to avoid serious side effects, which include hospital readmission or even death, because of this algorithm's recent application in predicting the susceptibility of heart patients to drugs. Other applications of Support Vector Machines include protein classification, text classification, and picture segmentation. SVMs have extensive use in clinical and medical research for imaging biomarker identification, cancer and neurological illness diagnosis, and data classification from unbalanced or missing value datasets.

(vii). Neural Networks

The adaptive and nonlinear characteristics of neural networks make them ideal algorithms for processing data. The network integrates the many interconnected processing units in a multi-layered structure. Network properties include the ability to learn from inputs or responses, self-organization, and adaptability. Brain networks accept environmental inputs in the same manner as the brain systems of humans or other higher-level creatures. The replicating neurons in a neural network process the incoming data in the same way as neurons in living organisms do. If necessary, the network's output may be sent back into the network to enhance the existing system.

Data conceptualization, (c) data association, (d) categorization, and (a) prediction are the four main domains of ANN's application. Among the many types of prediction, networks are directed random search, perceptron, and backpropagation. Classification networks include learning vector quantization, probabilistic neural networks, and counter propagation networks; the Hopfield system, Boltzmann machine, Hamming system, and bi-directional associative memory address difficulties involving data associations. Networks such as self-organizing maps and adaptive resonance networks have been shown to be more appropriate for data conceptualization. An important function that ANNs have been performing in decision-making is the ability to make all-encompassing choices. Decisions must be made via evolution, which is a time-consuming process. The development may be very brief, depending on the assignment's trajectory, which is, in turn, affected by feedback from choices made in earlier phases. Another kind of evolution is the long-term kind, which develops the change gradually throughout a person's lifetime. No matter how long or short the evolution is, ANN has to be able to use input from past judgments to alter present preference settings.

Perception is one of several popular and easy ways to create neural networks. Around the 1960s, Frank Rosenblatt created the perception networks. A single binary output is produced by perception from several binary inputs. The input might be anything from 1 to an unlimited number.

Figure 4. Example of a basic perception network

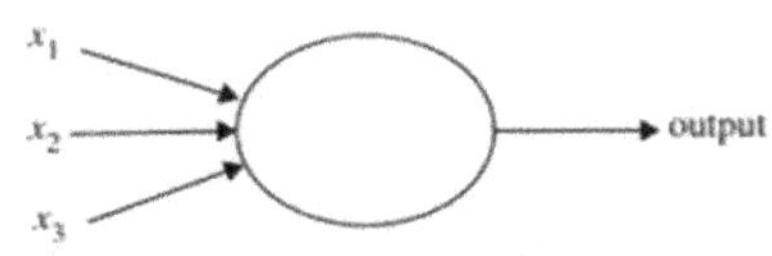

It is possible to determine the perception network's output via

$$\text{Output} = \begin{cases} 0 \text{ if } \sum_j w_j x_j \leq \text{threshold} \\ 1 \text{ if } \sum_j w_j x_j > \text{threshold} \end{cases}$$

where $w_1, w_2, \ldots$ are actual values that represent the weights, and they indicate the relative relevance of the inputs to the output rate. A value is used to assess the output label, whthe sum over j of , open paren w sub j, x sub j, close paren. he output will be set to 0 if the value is equal to or lower than the threshold and to 1 if it is higher than the threshold. A neuronal parameter, such as a threshold, is a real number as well.

(viii). Fuzzy for Intelligent Decision Making

In 1965, Lotfi A. Zadeh put out the concept of fuzzy logic or FL (ZADEH, 1996). To aid in decision-making, fuzzy logic (FL) mimics human reasoning. By giving each input a value between zero and one, fuzzy logic may capture the concept of uncertainty. False is represented by the binary number 0 and positive by the binary number 1. Mathematical techniques are often used to construct the range of values among extremes, which are then processed by computers in order to attain human-like thinking. Applying FL may help bridge the gap between quantitative and qualitative modeling. While a FL model's input-output mapping is quantitative, the system is internally controlled by a set of qualitative language rules. The universe's elements, which include every conceivable element for a connected issue, are used to build the fuzzy set. In a base set, x is the total amount of elements, and the universe is determined by the membership function μA(x).

The following membership functions have been identified for different applications: triangle, trapezoidal, Γ-, S-, exponential, and Gaussian functions. Fuzzy inference refers to the method of finding the input-output mapping using fuzzy logic. Rules are used to make decisions inside the mapping. Fuzzification and defuzzification are two steps in fuzzy inference. Fuzzy rules provide the foundation for the expertise and expertise needed to relate input parameters to output variables. Mamdani fuzzy rules and Takagi-Sugeno fuzzy rules are the two main types of these rules. Fuzzifiers, inference engines, defuzzifiers, and fuzzy rule bases are the building blocks of an inference system, sometimes called a fuzzy expert system. The rule's base module receives the fuzzified values from the crisp inputs. Conditional IF-THEN statements regulate the output variable and are used to create the rules. We apply the rules to the fuzzy values and then assess the results as fuzzy values. The fuzzy values are de-fuzzified and transformed back into crisp values in order to make them usable in the actual world. FL has been recognized as an effective decision-making tool because of its capabilities, which include:

- The ability to handle nonlinear challenges as a result of universal approximation,
- more options for defining uncertainty, a consistent and redundant rule base and rules, and so on.
- Problems with complicated mathematical models may have their exact answers found using simple models and imprecise approximation.

5. BENEFITS OF MACHINE LEARNING IN HEALTHCARE

- **Improving Patient Care -** Personalized medicine uses machine learning to tailor treatments to individual patients, which improves treatment efficacy, decreases side effects, and enhances the patient experience. With the ability to track patients' vitals in real-time, algorithms using machine learning may aid in the treatment of chronic diseases and the early identification of possible health problems, all of which contribute to better long-term health outcomes.
- **Earlier diagnosis**- Machine learning algorithms have been developed to detect early symptoms of illness, improving patient outcomes and increasing the likelihood of successful treatments.
- **Reducing healthcare costs**- One way to lower healthcare expenses without sacrificing quality is to increase operational efficiency, decrease mistakes, and improve patient outcomes.
- **Enhancing data privacy and security -** A big worry as healthcare moves towards digitization is the security of critical patient data. In order to comply with data protection rules such as GDPR, machine learning models anonymized patient data while preserving the data's usefulness for research and analysis. On top of that, healthcare organizations may be instantly notified of any breaches or illegal access using sophisticated machine learning algorithms.
- **Drug development**—Machine learning is speeding up the process of discovering and developing new drugs by optimizing certain steps.

6. IMPLICATIONS TO PRACTICE

It may enhance the detection of drug-related illnesses from brain pictures by using image processing, segmentation, and ML approaches. It is equally important to create a tailored model using behavioral analysis for various mental disorders. Using ML technology, a person's condition may be diagnosed with more precision and speed. Observations of structural and functional variations in the brain may aid in the diagnosis of such disorders in the fields of psychology and neuroscience. The addition of a digital hotline would further cut down on expenses and save time. Despite some elements disagreeing, neurobiological abnormalities may be connected with drug abuse-related psychological illnesses. When diagnosing diseases does not always need a great deal of unique subjective and qualitative information, the multi-model method works well. Disorderly behaviors brought on by substances may affect several areas of the brain, including the control and sensory centers, the reward circuits, the impulses, the density of gray matter, the compulsive behavior center, and the neural dysfunctional networks.

7. LIMITATIONS AND FUTURE DIRECTIONS

In light of the work methodology they used and the outcomes they reported, the researchers identified several research deficiencies and obstacles. These problems may be better addressed, and addiction therapy may evolve in the future with the help of machine learning. Researchers need to figure out how to do longitudinal studies with many multivariate endpoints that contribute to addiction problems, even if there aren't many articles on the subject. The primary and exclusive way to diagnose drug use disorders is via clinical examinations. In order to find a workable answer, researchers may use ML techniques and other forms of artificial intelligence. There was a difference in the performance of the ML models when using state-of-the-art approaches for feature identification, validation, and extraction, as well as when using empirical data from various sources. It would be beneficial to discuss findings from other studies on topics including COVID-19, retinopathy, neurological disorders, and mental health. In order to build and test their models, researchers utilize their data sets in unique ways. The current model's performance must be taken into account in order to build a master dataset for ML transfer learning (Reddy C et al., 2024). Thus, screening for drug misuse at an earlier stage leads to more successful treatment outcomes. We now have a better grasp of the multi-dimensional patterns of behavior and medicine thanks to ML models. Scalability, appropriateness for engineering, and computing are the reasons for their utilization. It would seem that computer technology has the potential to solve the problem of mental health issues caused by substance abuse. To help direct future studies, below are a few drawbacks of ML approaches:

- No Pre-trained ML Model Available: Medical image processing is difficult and time-consuming, but diagnostic systems may make use of pre-built models that can be adjusted and incorporated. The distribution and performance of medical pictures would result in reduced expenses, time, and resources.
- Validation and mistakes: Drug usage habits are not universal, and writers have found this to be a challenge. Small datasets and case-based studies, no matter how well they are verified, will always include variance and jitter. Misdiagnosis is a common problem with these models when their practicality is raised.
- Greater longitudinal research is required: It is possible to conduct more effective analyses using integrated imaging and other data. Despite the difficulties of classifying individuals, longitudinal studies nevertheless provide helpful information.
- Drug-specific group studies: as drug addiction is a risk factor for many mental health issues, this kind of research would be excellent. Substance misuse may impact the mental health of people from all walks of life and economic backgrounds. To better understand the societal effects of addiction, it is helpful to examine data and demographic groupings in isolation. As the paper points out, ML applications are always evolving, which allows for these kinds of research gaps to exist.
- In the pursuit of more robust computations and outcomes, the paramount component of ethics may be disregarded, leading to questions of interpretability. Applying ML prediction to studies of human substance addiction may lead to inaccurate labeling of subjects as drug users. Consequently, it was not possible to apply ML findings to clinical procedures and instruments since they were too far removed from the study locations (Chinthala et al., 2022).
- An unreliable dataset on drug abuse prevents digital healthcare systems from automating and using data-driven diagnostics, a novel approach to data analysis that uses digital interventions.

- Not much is known about early-onset prediction: We can anticipate the subsequent stage of drug usage based on the data that is already available. This is why geographically specific studies based on gender and conducted on-site are necessary. At several points along the conclusion process, it is essential to validate multi-disciplinary information.

8. CONCLUSION

Potentially revolutionary to the status quo of healthcare service delivery is the use of machine learning for healthcare forecasting. Machine learning has many applications in healthcare, including as improving the accuracy of diagnoses, streamlining decision-making, and automating administrative tasks. Data privacy concerns, ethical considerations, and the need for stringent validation and regulation are just a few of the potential obstacles to machine learning in the health industry. Last but not least, a thorough understanding of the complex and ever-changing healthcare system, collaboration between healthcare professionals and data scientists, and the responsible and ethical utilization of machine learning are all necessary for machine learning to completely benefit medicine.

REFERENCES

Ahmed, S., & Cho, S. H. (2023). Machine learning for healthcare radars: Recent progresses in human vital sign measurement and activity recognition. *IEEE Communications Surveys and Tutorials*, *26*(1), 461–495. DOI: 10.1109/COMST.2023.3334269

Ango, R., Masih, R. K., Reddy, C. K. K., Shuaib, M., Singh, M., & Alam, S. (2024). Fraud Detection in Banking using the Kaggle Credit Card Dataset and XGBoost Model. *2024 International Conference on IoT Based Control Networks and Intelligent Systems (ICICNIS)*, 968–973. DOI: 10.1109/ICICNIS64247.2024.10823227

Butt, U. M., Letchmunan, S., Ali, M., Hassan, F. H., Baqir, A., & Sherazi, H. H. R. (2021). Machine learning based diabetes classification and prediction for healthcare applications. *Journal of Healthcare Engineering*, *2021*(1), 9930985. DOI: 10.1155/2021/9930985 PMID: 34631003

Char, D. S., Abràmoff, M. D., & Feudtner, C. (2020). Identifying ethical considerations for machine learning healthcare applications. *The American Journal of Bioethics*, *20*(11), 7–17. DOI: 10.1080/15265161.2020.1819469 PMID: 33103967

Chinthala, K. K. R., Thakur, M. S., Shuaib, M., & Alam, S. (2022). Prospects of Computational Intelligence in Society: Human-Centric Solutions, Challenges, and Research Areas. *Journal of Computational and Cognitive Engineering*.

Chiranjeevi, P., & Rajaram, A. (2024). A smart recommender model based on learning method for sentiment classification. *Multimedia Tools and Applications*, •••, 1–21. DOI: 10.1007/s11042-024-20347-z

Chua, M., Kim, D., Choi, J., Lee, N. G., Deshpande, V., Schwab, J., Lev, M. H., Gonzalez, R. G., Gee, M. S., & Do, S. (2023). Tackling prediction uncertainty in machine learning for healthcare. *Nature Biomedical Engineering*, *7*(6), 711–718. DOI: 10.1038/s41551-022-00988-x PMID: 36581695

Friedman, J. H. (1991). Multivariate adaptive regression splines. *Annals of Statistics*, *19*(1), 1–67.

Ganiya, R. K., Veeraiah, D., Thatha, V. N., Rao, K. S., Rao, J. N., Manjith, R., & Rajaram, A. (2024). Revolutionizing vascular health through the temporal convolutional transformer for drug screening and model evolution. *Biomedical Signal Processing and Control*, *95*, 106390. DOI: 10.1016/j.bspc.2024.106390

Guido, R., Ferrisi, S., Lofaro, D., & Conforti, D. (2024). An overview on the advancements of support vector machine models in healthcare applications: A review. *Information (Basel)*, *15*(4), 235. DOI: 10.3390/info15040235

Gurusamy, A., & Mohamed, I. A. (2021). The role of AI and machine learning in full stack development for healthcare applications. *Journal of Knowledge Learning and Science Technology ISSN: 2959-6386 (Online)*, *1*(1), 116–123.

Hegde, M. G., Shenoy, P. D., & Venugopal, K. R. (2023). A Comparative Study of Neural Network and Machine Learning on Privacy Preserving Federated Learning for Healthcare Applications. *2023 IEEE Technology & Engineering Management Conference-Asia Pacific (TEMSCON-ASPAC)*, 1–6.

Javed, H., Muqeet, H. A., Javed, T., Rehman, A. U., & Sadiq, R. (2023). Ethical frameworks for machine learning in sensitive healthcare applications. *IEEE Access : Practical Innovations, Open Solutions*, *12*, 16233–16254. DOI: 10.1109/ACCESS.2023.3340884

Kalaivani, K., Kshirsagarr, P. R., Sirisha Devi, J., Bandela, S. R., Colak, I., Nageswara Rao, J., & Rajaram, A. (2023). Prediction of biomedical signals using deep learning techniques. *Journal of Intelligent & Fuzzy Systems*, *44*(6), 9769–9782. DOI: 10.3233/JIFS-230399

Karthik, A., Aalam, S. S., Sivakumar, M., Sundari, M. V. R., Rose, J. D., Elangovan, M., & Rajaram, A. (2024). Improving brain tumor treatment with better imaging and real-time therapy using quantum dots. *Biomedical Signal Processing and Control*, *95*, 106286. DOI: 10.1016/j.bspc.2024.106286

Karthik, A., Hamatta, H. S. A., Patthi, S., Krubakaran, C., Pradhan, A. K., Rachapudi, V., Shuaib, M., & Rajaram, A. (2024). Ensemble-based multimodal medical imaging fusion for tumor segmentation. *Biomedical Signal Processing and Control*, *96*, 106550. DOI: 10.1016/j.bspc.2024.106550

Kaza, V. S., Alamer, A., Alam, S., Shuaib, M., Basudan, S., & Sheneamer, A. (2024). Detecting and forecasting cryptojacking attack trends in Internet of Things and wireless sensor networks devices. *PeerJ. Computer Science*, *10*, e2491. DOI: 10.7717/peerj-cs.2491 PMID: 39650421

Khan, M. M., & Alkhathami, M. (2024). Anomaly detection in IoT-based healthcare: Machine learning for enhanced security. *Scientific Reports*, *14*(1), 5872. DOI: 10.1038/s41598-024-56126-x PMID: 38467709

Kishor Kumar Reddy, C., Kaza, V. S., Madana Mohana, R., Alhameed, M., Jeribi, F., Alam, S., & Shuaib, M. (2025). Detecting anomalies in smart wearables for hypertension: A deep learning mechanism. *Frontiers in Public Health*, *12*, 1426168. DOI: 10.3389/fpubh.2024.1426168 PMID: 39850864

Maguluri, L. P., Chouhan, K., Balamurali, R., Rani, R., Hashmi, A., Kiran, A., & Rajaram, A. (2024). Adversarial deep learning for improved abdominal organ segmentation in CT scans. *Multimedia Tools and Applications*, *83*(35), 82107–82129. DOI: 10.1007/s11042-024-18578-1

Nadakuditi, S., Kumar, B., & Kumar, T. (2024). AI and Machine Learning in Healthcare-Applications, Challenges and Ethics. *International Journal of Health Sciences*, *7*(4), 36–43. DOI: 10.47941/ijhs.1949

Poloju, N., & Rajaram, A. (2024). Transformation with yolo tiny network architecture for multimodal fusion in lung disease classification. *Cybernetics and Systems*, •••, 1–22. DOI: 10.1080/01969722.2024.2343992

Rahman, A., Debnath, T., Kundu, D., Khan, M. S. I., Aishi, A. A., Sazzad, S., Sayduzzaman, M., & Band, S. S. (2024). Machine learning and deep learning-based approach in smart healthcare: Recent advances, applications, challenges and opportunities. *AIMS Public Health*, *11*(1), 58–109. DOI: 10.3934/publichealth.2024004 PMID: 38617415

Reddy, C. K. K., Rangarajan, A., Rangarajan, D., Shuaib, M., Jeribi, F., & Alam, S. (2024). A transfer learning approach: Early prediction of Alzheimer's disease on US healthy aging dataset. *Mathematics*, *12*(14), 2204. DOI: 10.3390/math12142204

Reddy, C. K. K., Reddy, P. A., Janapati, H., Assiri, B., Shuaib, M., Alam, S., & Sheneamer, A. (2024). A fine-tuned vision transformer based enhanced multi-class brain tumor classification using MRI scan imagery. *Frontiers in Oncology*, *14*, 1400341. DOI: 10.3389/fonc.2024.1400341 PMID: 39091923

Sabry, F., Eltaras, T., Labda, W., Alzoubi, K., & Malluhi, Q. (2022). Machine learning for healthcare wearable devices: The big picture. *Journal of Healthcare Engineering*, *2022*(1), 4653923. DOI: 10.1155/2022/4653923 PMID: 35480146

Sanchez, P., Voisey, J. P., Xia, T., Watson, H. I., O'Neil, A. Q., & Tsaftaris, S. A. (2022). Causal machine learning for healthcare and precision medicine. *Royal Society Open Science*, *9*(8), 220638. DOI: 10.1098/rsos.220638 PMID: 35950198

Shehab, M., Abualigah, L., Shambour, Q., Abu-Hashem, M. A., Shambour, M. K. Y., Alsalibi, A. I., & Gandomi, A. H. (2022). Machine learning in medical applications: A review of state-of-the-art methods. *Computers in Biology and Medicine*, *145*, 105458. DOI: 10.1016/j.compbiomed.2022.105458 PMID: 35364311

Singh, A., Joshi, K., Alam, S., Bharany, S., Shuaib, M., & Ahmad, S. (2022). Internet of Things-Based Integrated Remote Electronic Health Surveillance and Alert System: A Review. *2022 IEEE International Conference on Current Development in Engineering and Technology (CCET)*, 1–6. DOI: 10.1109/CCET56606.2022.10080629

Singh, A., Nagabhooshanam, N., Kumar, R., Verma, R., Mohanasundaram, S., Manjith, R., & Rajaram, A. (2025). Deep learning based coronary artery disease detection and segmentation using ultrasound imaging with adaptive gated SCNN models. *Biomedical Signal Processing and Control*, *105*, 107637. DOI: 10.1016/j.bspc.2025.107637

Steinberg, D. (2009). CART: classification and regression trees. In *The top ten algorithms in data mining* (pp. 193–216). Chapman and Hall/CRC. DOI: 10.1201/9781420089653.ch10

Wazid, M., Singh, J., Das, A. K., & Rodrigues, J. J. P. C. (2023). An ensemble-based machine learning-envisioned intrusion detection in industry 5.0-driven healthcare applications. *IEEE Transactions on Consumer Electronics*, *70*(1), 1903–1912. DOI: 10.1109/TCE.2023.3318850

Yadav, G., Bokhari, M. U., Alzahrani, S. I., Alam, S., & Shuaib, M. (2025). Emotion-Aware Ensemble Learning (EAEL): Revolutionizing Mental Health Diagnosis of Corporate Professionals via Intelligent Integration of Multi-Modal Data Sources and Ensemble Techniques. *IEEE Access : Practical Innovations, Open Solutions*, *13*, 11494–11516. DOI: 10.1109/ACCESS.2025.3529032

Zadeh, L. A. (1996). Fuzzy logic, neural networks, and soft computing. In Fuzzy sets, fuzzy logic, and fuzzy systems: selected papers by Lotfi A Zadeh (pp. 775-782).

Chapter 5
Harnessing Predictive Analytics for Proactive Healthcare and Improved Patient Outcomes

S. Ramesh
https://orcid.org/0009-0002-5087-6265
SRM Institute of Science and Technology, India

R. Bhavani
Sathyabama Institute of Science and Technology, India

G. C. Jagan
Jeppiaar Engineering College, India

A. Rajaram
E.G.S. Pillay Engineering College, India

A. Rasheedha
Sri Ramakrisha Engineering College, India

Noor A. Ibraheem
University of Baghdad, Iraq

V. Remya
Sri Sairam Engineering College, India

ABSTRACT

Improving patient risk score structures, anticipating the start of illness, and optimizing hospital operations are just a few examples of the practical insights that may be generated by applying machine learning to electronic health records (EHRs). Better patient outcomes, more efficient operations, and better decision-making are all possible thanks to predictive analytics in healthcare. Discover the ways this technology revolutionizes patient care by facilitating early intervention, cutting expenses, and enhancing overall efficiency. There is a promising gap in the literature about statistical models that take use of the diversity and depth of data obtained from HER. We review the benefits of machine learning over more conventional analytical techniques and provide an outline of its use in clinical settings in this chapter. We outline the practical and methodological difficulties when applying machine learning in both academia and industry. As a conclusion, we provide our thoughts on potential machine learning uses in the future that might have far-reaching effects on healthcare.

DOI: 10.4018/979-8-3373-1022-0.ch005

1. INTRODUCTION

Better patient care and more positive outcomes are both made possible by predictive modeling in healthcare. It can determine which sick people are in the greatest danger and would benefit most from treatment. Additionally, predictive analytics explores insights from trends in inpatient data to build successful marketing, forecast product safety with optimized dosage, guide clinical trial concepts, and a whole lot more. Predictive analytics is a tool that healthcare companies may use to improve efficiency, foresee patient requirements, and generate forecasts about future health patterns by analyzing both current and historical data (Islam et al., 2020). Many data sources within the healthcare ecosystem, including electronic health records (EHR), insurance records, administrative files, and others, are fed into predictive analytics systems. Statistical modeling, data extraction, and machine learning are the tools used in this advanced analytics genre to provide fresh insights. These findings have wide-ranging applications for healthcare organizations, including the treatment of chronic diseases and the reduction of hospital readmission rates. A variety of predictive analytics techniques are available, each with its own unique purpose: to analyze past data, find patterns, track trends, and extrapolate future outcomes. Classification, clustering, and time series models are among the most popular types of predictive analytics models (Obijuru et al., 2024). The healthcare industry often uses classification models to forecast health insurance fraud, improve patient health, and reduce the cost of healthcare services. Cluster models allow for the profiling and evaluation of people according to variables like age, number of inpatient hospitalizations, likelihood of needing an emergency room visit within the next twelve months, etc. Monthly ER visits or yearly medical bills are two examples of data that may be plotted using time series models; by assisting companies in anticipating when, when, and how treatment should be given, predictive analytics—regardless of the model used—can lead to higher operational efficiency, enhanced patient safety, and improved patient outcomes (Khan et al., 2024). Systems for predicting and avoiding the most prevalent and expensive diagnoses, improved accuracy in forecasting duration of stay, and assistance for doctors in personalizing treatments are all outcomes of health systems' use of predictive analytics. Individual patients have access to a plethora of resources that may help medical professionals improve patient care, including health apps, fitness trackers, wearable gadgets, and medical monitors. Predictive analytics technologies may be used to evaluate data from various sources, allowing for the provision of more tailored healthcare (Gates et al., 2024). Healthcare providers and groups have significantly benefited from technological advancements, which have revolutionized the delivery of healthcare. There is a deluge of data that may be used to enhance health outcomes because of the digitalization of healthcare records and the introduction of technology. With the use of predictive analytics, healthcare organizations and doctors may examine data, spot patterns, and tailor treatment to each individual patient.

Figure 1. IoT Model for Predictive Analytics

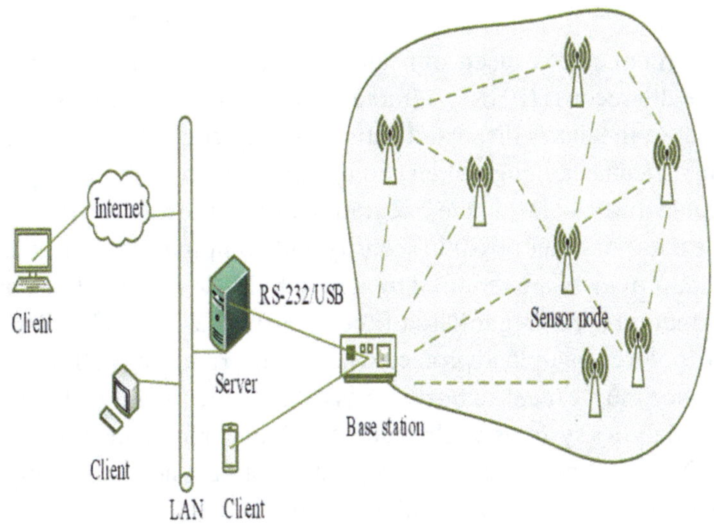

1.1 Use of Predictive Analytics in Healthcare

While healthcare organizations produce vast quantities of data, they face significant challenges in turning that data into actionable insights that might enhance patient outcomes. The goal of healthcare data analytics is to improve the management of both patient care and overall operations. Its many applications include studying how to save healthcare costs, improve patient care, and even anticipate disease outbreaks (Cano-Marin et al., 2023). On a more macro level, analytics may assist healthcare businesses in streamlining internal processes, maximizing resource use, and enhancing care team coordination and efficiency (Rojas et al., 2022). The following sectors of healthcare are greatly affected by data analytics' capacity to turn raw healthcare information into practical insights:

- Clinical decision support
- Quicker, more accurate diagnosis of medical conditions
- High success rates of surgeries and medications
- Automation of hospital administrative processes
- Clinical research
- Development of new treatments
- Discovery of new drugs
- Prediction and prevention of diseases

1.2 Challenges and limitations of implementing predictive analytics in healthcare

There are several interconnected aspects of healthcare services, such as insurance and the delivery of treatment. Electronic health records (EHRs), remote patient monitoring (RPM) devices, imaging equipment, etc., all contribute to the data's dispersed nature (Reddy et al., 2024). Because of this, healthcare organizations have a significant challenge when attempting data integration; they will need the assistance of data specialists to guide the data during the integration procedure and verify that predictive algorithms are feeding on accurate data. Another possible security and compliance risk is data storage (Al-Talafheh et al., 2024). Healthcare providers are required to adhere to HIPAA regulations and safeguard patients' Protected Health Information (PHI) regardless of the data storage method they use: cloud, on-premise, or hybrid. For instance, before you upload protected health information (PHI) to a cloud service, you and the provider of that service must execute a business associate agreement. It should be noted that the data used to train predictive analytics systems might restrict their accuracy. Machine learning algorithms were able to forecast COVID-19 patient outcomes using historical data accurately, but there is no assurance that such models will always be right (Khubrani & Alam, 2021).

2. RELATED PREDICTIVE ANALYTICS MODEL FOR HEALTHCARE

Explores the fundamental algorithms and methods used in healthcare prediction analytics, including data mining, statistical modeling, and machine learning, in (Alharthi, 2018). They go into the many uses of this technology, which include better patient classification for risk assessment, illness prevention via focused therapies, and healthcare systems' ability to allocate resources optimally. However, data privacy and algorithmic biases are critical ethical considerations that must be carefully considered before predictive analytics are used. That study highlights the groundbreaking potential of predictive analytics in healthcare, opening the path for a future of proactive medicine and individualized treatment. It also suggests that regulatory frameworks may need to be adjusted to guarantee the responsible use of that technology.

In order to collect and analyze health information from wearables in real-time, identify abnormalities, and anticipate possible health problems before they become serious, complex algorithms have been developed, as shown in (Etli et al., 2024). With performance metrics showing an accuracy of 94.8%, an RMSE of 0.208, and an MAE of 0.406, the suggested approach displays a high degree of accuracy. These findings demonstrate that the proposed algorithms are capable of detecting even the most minute changes in health parameters, which allows for faster treatments and better patient outcomes. The results show that real-time analytics and wearable health monitors may help close the information gap and provide valuable insights, leading to a more proactive and individualized approach to healthcare.

Looking at the potential benefits, current challenges, and impact on patient care, the review paper (Rahim et al., 2025)investigates data analytics' use in healthcare settings. Predictive analytics for early disease detection, personalized treatment regimens generated from patient data, and public health supervision are just a few of the benefits that data analytics may provide. Additional topics covered in the paper include healthcare analytics, data privacy, and interoperability. It discusses how data analytics could improve medical outcomes and treatment quality, and it evaluates strategies for overcoming these challenges. With a median of 5.5 and an average of 0.430, the suggested strategy makes use of a 90%

probability proportion for a positive test outcome (LR+). Predictive models that help with early illness detection and tailored medication are evaluated and enhanced using these measures. While data analytics has many potential advantages in healthcare, the results show that many obstacles must be overcome before it can have a maximum effect on patient results (Rahim et al., 2025).

Figure 2. Predictive Analytic Model in Healthcare

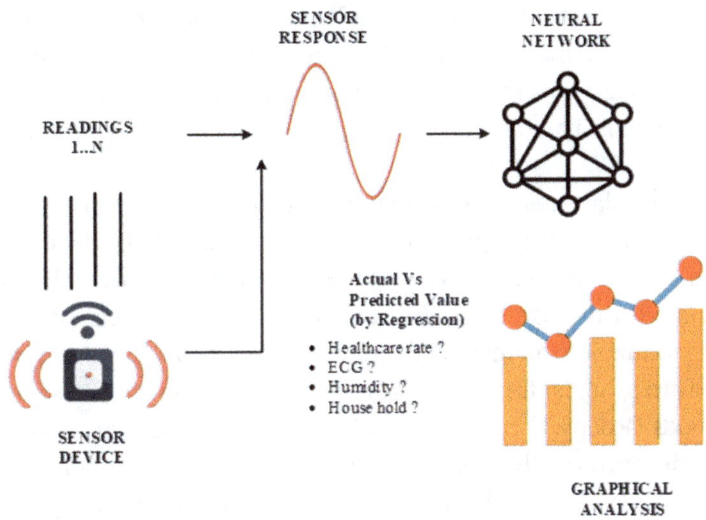

Studying how Eli Lilly uses AI and predictive analytics, the authors of (Ibikunle et al., 2024)investigate the game-changing impact on healthcare market forecasts. Insights powered by artificial intelligence are quickly becoming indispensable for predicting market trends, gauging the effects of new regulations, and improving product differentiation in the cutthroat international healthcare industry. Machine learning methods and massive datasets allow AI to see connections and trends that human forecasters would miss, giving businesses such as Eli Lilly a better picture of how the market will behave in the future. Using legislative changes like the U.S. Inflation Reduction Act as an example, the research delves into how AI improves decision-making by forecasting healthcare industry developments. Pharmaceutical businesses have both possibilities and problems as a result of that legal shift, which aims to decrease medicine costs and increase market access. With the help of AI, businesses can predict how these changes to regulations would affect their bottom line and modify their marketing approach appropriately. To illustrate the point, pharmaceutical corporations may use predictive analytics to foresee future price pressures on individual products, which allows them to create profitable pricing models that are competitive.

That paper delves into the unrealized possibilities of predictive analytics in healthcare and social work, with a focus on early intervention approaches, as discussed in (Kumar & Suthar, 2024). Predictive analytics is becoming more popular in many fields, although it has seen very little specialized use in social work. By conducting a comprehensive literature analysis and outlining the potential benefits and limitations of using predictive analytics in hospital social work, that research aims to address that gap. The results of that study provide important new insights for social work practitioners and policymakers, and they add to the current conversation about predictive analytics' role in healthcare.

That article summarizes the revolutionary impact of data analytics on healthcare, particularly as it pertains to patient outcome prediction models, in (Pendyala, 2024). The goal of the study is introduced in the introduction, which also covers the significance of data analysis in healthcare. It draws attention to the many forms of healthcare data, the difficulties in collecting and managing that data, and the development of data analytics in that sector. Next, we'll take a look at predictive modeling's function in healthcare, highlighting its importance in bettering patient outcomes and the typical methods used for that purpose. Electronic health records, smartwatches, genetic and genomic information, and social determinants of health are some of the data sources included in the article, which is a predictive modeling tool. Ethical issues, data pretreatment, model selection, validation methods, and the whole predictive model development process are covered. Personalized treatment planning, early illness identification, hospital resource management, patient engagement, and other predictive model applications are also included in the study.

Examines the many ways data analytics is changing healthcare, with an emphasis on patient-centric approaches and how they affect service provision, in (Ibeh et al., 2024). An enormous amount of data has been created in the healthcare industry due to the introduction of wearable devices and electronic health records (EHRs). With the use of sophisticated analytics, medical professionals may improve patient care by drawing valuable conclusions from that data. Utilizing customized health data to maximize preventative measures, adjust treatment strategies, and anticipate illness outcomes is at the heart of patient-centric methods (Reddy C et al., 2024). That paper explores the approaches used in patient-centric statistical analysis, specifically looking at how AI, predictive modeling, and machine learning algorithms are used to provide individualized healthcare treatments. In addition, the examination delves into how data analytics have revolutionized healthcare delivery. Essential components of healthcare administration include maximizing the efficiency of operational procedures, the allocation of resources, and the discovery of cost-effective treatments. Healthcare systems may achieve operational efficiency, waste reduction, and better resource allocation by using data analytics.

Healthcare decision-making, risk assessment, and care optimization may all be significantly improved with the use of predictive analytics, as discussed in the study (Edoh et al., 2024). By analyzing large amounts of data, predictive analytics can determine which patients are most likely to acquire long-term health problems and then use that information to fine-tune their treatment plans. Predictive models may enhance patient outcomes and effectiveness in healthcare settings by combining diverse data sources, such as genetic information, wearable technologies, and electronic health records. Despite the benefits, the article brings attention to important concerns such as the security and privacy of data, prediction model biases, and the need for strong regulatory frameworks. The study highlights the significance of continuing research to enhance data integration, refine prediction models, and address ethical concerns in order to guarantee fair healthcare delivery. Ultimately, that article argues that a more effective and responsive healthcare system may be achieved by a deliberate approach to using predictive analytics.

That paper explores the uses of FL in smart health systems, specifically how it may be integrated with wearables, the IoT, and remote monitoring to enable decentralized data processing in real time for predictive analytics and individualized treatment (Abbas et al., 2024). Security threats such as adversarial assaults and data poisoning, along with model inversion, are among the important issues it resolves. It also addresses concerns about data heterogeneity, flexibility, and interoperability across systems. Not only that, but the assessment also stresses the need for new privacy-preserving technologies like secure multiparty computing and differential privacy to get beyond FL's shortcomings. If they want FL to become more widely used in healthcare and improve its efficiency and accuracy, they must overcome these obstacles. At the end of the day, FL has the ability to revolutionize healthcare by creating safe, data-driven systems. That might lead to better results for patients, more efficient operations, and complete control over one's own data.

By classifying AI predictive models according to their ability to proactively estimate the progression of a patient's illness and its possible impact, prioritize patient readmissions, and create effective personalized treatment plans, (Hossain et al., 2024) hopes to address the adoption of combined AI in healthcare organizations and improve patient health. Avoiding unnecessary testing, making better use of resources, and reducing hospital stays are three of the most significant cost reductions identified by the study. Based on quantitative data from healthcare systems and actual situations, the authors of that paper provide solid conclusions for AI-driven predictive analytics (Singh et al., 2025) (Ganiya et al., 2024). Also, it shows that healthcare organizations that have used AI have achieved their goal of a 25% decrease in operational costs and an improvement in patient outcomes, with readmission rates lowered by 15% to 20%. In addition, the ethical implications of using AI in healthcare are discussed, with a focus on protecting patients' personal data (Karthik, Aalam, et al., 2024) (Karthik, Hamatta, et al., 2024). As far as they are aware, that research is the first of its kind to conduct a comprehensive analysis of AI in healthcare and to provide concrete recommendations for expanding their understanding of AI's potential to improve patient outcomes while reducing healthcare expenditures.

3. PREDICTIVE ANALYTICS MODELS FOR HEALTHCARE

A wide variety of statistical methods, including information mining, predictive modeling, and ML, are part of predictive analytics. These methods sift through and attempt to comprehend factual data, both current and historical, in order to make predictions about the future. Predictive healthcare mathematical frameworks in use today search for opportunities and threats by tracing their origins in past data (Karthik et al., 2025). Models guide decision-making for individual candidate communication by recognizing linkages among multiple variables, which allows for qualitative evaluation of risk connected to a given set of situations (Poloju & Rajaram, 2024). A subfield of statistics known as “predictive methodology” is used to make inferences about future trends and regular patterns of behavior based on previously collected data (Maguluri et al., 2024). Predictive scores are provided for several entities, including medical patients, products, cars, and equipment, in order to identify processes that impact numerous entities. We have a model for analyzing medical reports, identifying drugs, smart hospital record systems, etc., as an example of a patient's sickness (Syamala et al., 2024) .

The mathematical technique of predictive modeling (also known as predictive analytics) involves the use of data mining, machine learning, and statistical approaches to find patterns in data and to determine the likelihood of certain events (Kalaivani et al., 2023). If we know how something has behaved in the past, we can use predictive modeling to figure out what's likely to happen next.

Figure 3. Predictive Analytics Flowchart

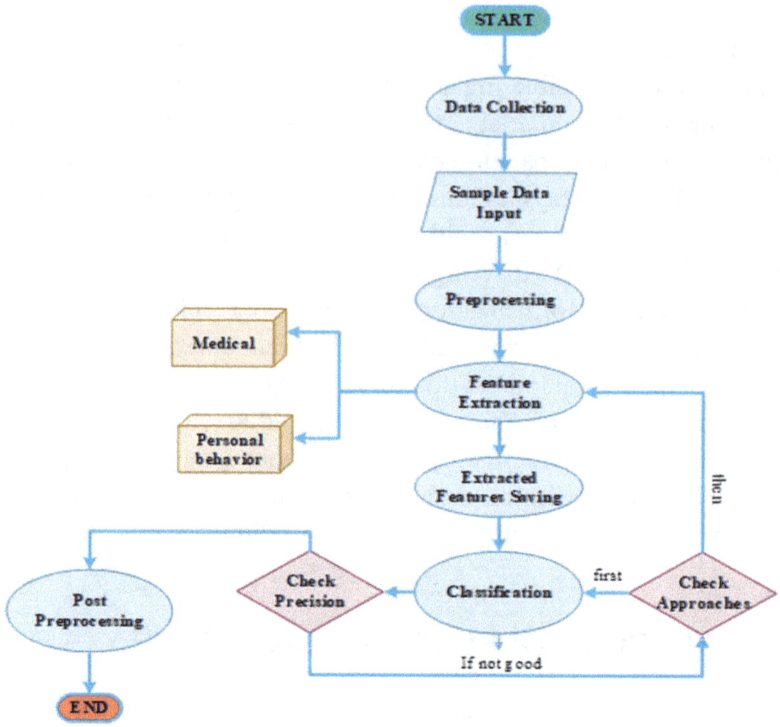

Applying algorithms to data in order to make predictions is what predictive modeling is all about. Due to its iterative nature, the method trains the simulation in a way that is best suited to achieving the aim of achieving business objectives. There are many analytical modeling steps involved in predictive modeling:

- Data collection and cleaning: It ensures accurate forecasts by extracting just the important information by obtaining data from diverse sources and then using cleansing procedures to eliminate noise.
- Making a simple chart and carefully analyzing your data should be your first steps before beginning to construct your model. It is critical to comprehend data behavior and establish correlations between variables. It becomes challenging to construct an effective model without this insight. You may discover a lot, however, if you put in the time. By laying the groundwork for future research and model creation, this method may provide substantial clarity into the current issue and its solutions.

Standardization

The size of the monitored data for different sensors varied greatly, as shown in Figure 7. Inputting this data directly into a network framework would cause the input characteristics to be unevenly weighted, which would prevent the model from converging. As a result, according to Formula (14), this work takes the monitoring data from each of the sensors in Table 3 and applies mean subtraction with variance normalization to it separately.

$$X^* = \frac{X - \mu}{\sigma}$$

The normalized data is represented as X^*, while X stands for the original sensor information, μ is the mean of every sample for one sensor, and σ is the standard deviation of every sample for one sensor. The process of convergence of gradient descent to the best solution is accelerated, and the accuracy and precision of prediction outputs are improved by data standardization.

- Sometimes, the data is well-suited to a certain algorithm or model, which allows for the construction of a prediction model. The optimal course of action is not always black and white. It is recommended that you run many algorithms and compare their results as you study the data. Find some test information and apply some categorization rules to see how well the model performs.
- Make use of the model in all of your company operations: If you want the model to assist your healthcare organization in enhancing patient care, you need to incorporate it into your processes.

Table 1. Data Cleaning Model

Type of Error	Definition	Possible Causes
Missing data	There are gaps in a patient's record where healthcare was provided but not documented, making the record incomplete.	The patient's lack of health insurance prevents them from seeking medical attention. If a patient discontinues visiting their doctor or insurance company, there will be no one to follow up with them. Problems with insurance claim processing, such as: - Inaccurate data entry into the database - The linking of records is incomplete; that is, records for the same patient are not connected. The patient's lack of health insurance prevents them from seeking medical attention.
Missing data not missing at random	Unobserved environmental or patient-specific variables are the root cause of data gaps in medical records.	Regardless of how they will be, patients do not seek medical attention. A doctor gives the wrong diagnosis to a patient.
Outcome or exposure misclassification	Improper categorization of patients according to their illness status or their exposure status (e.g., medical treatment, risk factor for disease)	mistakes or omits information while documenting a patient's visit in a note - Personnel at a healthcare facility or clinic fails to submit an insurance claim, miscodes a patient's diagnosis or treatment,

Prognostic modeling is a tool of predictive analytics. In order to predict healthcare trends, it often employs a machine learning algorithm. These models may be evaluated for new values using the data they were trained on, and they can anticipate the outcomes that will benefit a firm (Ango et al., 2024). Two types of prediction models exist. Here are the following:

- Regression Models
- Classification Models

(i). Regression Models

Predicting an actual value is the job of regression models. For Simple Linear Regression, the formula is,

$$Y = B0 + B1 * X$$

A line in two-dimensional space may be represented by Equation 1. In this case, "X" is an independent variable that changes the dependent variable "Y," and "Y" is the dependent variable that describes the relationship between the two variables. Likewise, ' BI ' is the coefficient for the ' X '; it tells how each change in ' X-1 ' changes ' Y '. The constant word "B 0," describes Y's base value. Finding the line that matches the data the best is really what it is.

To find the line that fits the data best, the ordinary least squares approach is employed. It states that there should be no more than a minimal number for the sum of squared discrepancies between the 'Y' values in the dataset and their online counterparts. Optimal fitting is achieved by locating the line that minimizes the sum (Yadav et al., 2025).

(a). Multiple Linear Regressions

The outcome of a response variable may be determined by using multiple linear regression, a statistical measure, as shown in Eq. 2.

$$W = A0 + A1 * F1 + A2 * F2 + \cdots + An * Fn$$

'W' stands for our dependent variable, whereas F1, F2,...Fn represents our independent variables.

Dummy Variable: A fake variable, also called a pointer variable, framework variable, one-hot encoding, or Boolean marker, is a variable in measurements in econometrics that can take on the binary values of 0 or 1. Its purpose is to indicate the absence or proximity of an uncontrolled condition that could change the outcome.

Dummy Variable Trap: Think about the property "city name," which might be anything from London to Delhi. Divide this category column into two columns that contain binary values, i.e., 0 or 1 (D1) for Delhi and D2) for London. We may see that 1 – D1 is always equal to D2 if we understand that D1 is valued at 0, then it stands to reason that D2 would be valued at 1, and vice versa. This constraint prevents the model from differentiating between the impacts of D1 → 1 and D2. The dummy variable's trap describes this situation. So it won't function correctly. So, we can't include both D1 along with D2 in our model; instead, we need to choose one and leave it out. For example, if you have 4 variables, take out 1 and put in 3, and if you have 100 variables, put in 99.

The p-value: For a specific measurable model in factual speculative evaluation, the p-value, likelihood esteem, or asymptotic centrality is the probability that, if the defective theory were true, the measurable summary (for instance, the example, the mean difference between two observed groups) would be stronger than or equal to the actual observed outcomes.

It is something that is well-known in the context of several independent variables in multiple linear regression. The old adage goes something like, "The more garbage you put into a model, the more garbage it will produce." In other words, carefully choosing which independent variables to include in your model is essential if you want to produce a decent model. There are going to be useless qualities; therefore, it seems that not all of them need to be considered when building a model.

3.2 Classification Models

Neural Network-Based Negative Selection Algorithm

There has been a lot of study into using neural networks in IoT platforms. Our method relies on a straightforward neural network methodology that employs supervised learning and binary classification; specifically, it is based on perceptrons. The collection is appropriately divided into linearly separable subsets using this binary classification procedure. The input x is converted to one binary number. Here is the input function f(x):

$$f(x) = \begin{cases} 1 \text{ if } w \cdot x + b > 0 \\ 0 \text{ otherwise} \end{cases}$$

" " is identified as a weight vector, " b " is identified as bias, and " $w - x$ " is assumed in Eq. (7.2)

$$\sum_i^m w_i \cdot x_i$$

A dot product is "." and "m" is the number of inputs. In a similar vein, feed-forward neural networks may handle problems in a wide variety of classes. In this method, the activation function with the number of hidden layers is used to solve a large number of neurons using distinct layers. It will be assumed that the input is error-free in categorization, so the suggested method may be simplified. The idea behind a negative selection algorithm comes from the way immune systems in mammals distinguish between self and non-self.

The algorithm proposes a strategy based on the notion of non-self-discriminating. Anomaly, while self-pattern detection methods that discriminate come after this one. There are two sets of input, as we've already established. N represents the normal set of data, whereas A stands for the anomaly set. C stands for the whole dataset, were

$$C = NA$$

After that, we looked at how the honeybee algorithm works and why it might be useful for the project.

The NA object is defined as normal in Eq. (7.3), and the categories that follow the equation are used to categorize NA as either an attack set or a normal set:

$$D = (f, M)$$

Where "f" stands for the classification function. Many sets of detectors make up "M". We use the honeybee algorithm for optimization so that we may continue to provide a safe optimization method.

Table 2. Performance Metrics for evaluation of Predictive Analytics

Performance Measure	Definition	Formula or Plot
Accuracy	The ratio of a model's accurate classifications (both positive and negative) to the overall amount of predictions	$A = \frac{TP + TN}{TP + TN + TN}$
Specificity (also called the true negative rate)	The ratio of the overall amount of negative class members in the data (including both true negatives and false positives) to the total number of proper negative classifications (true negatives)	S=NN/(N+fP)
Negative predictive value	The ratio of the entire number of negative classifications (including both true and false negatives) to the total number of accurate negative classifications	NPV=TN/(NN+FN)
Precision (also called positive predictive value)	The ratio of all positive classifications (including false positives) to the total number of right classifications (true positives)	P or PPV $= \frac{\mathrm{Tp}}{TPFP}$
Recall (also called sensitivity or the true positive rate)	The number of positive class members in the data divided by the total number of valid positive classifications (true positives)	$R = \frac{TP}{TPT/N}$

4. DISCUSSION

Continuous monitoring of vital indicators, including respiration rate, cardiovascular health, sleep duration, and glucose levels, is made possible by wearable technology. Artificial intelligence systems may examine this data in real time to spot out-of-the-ordinary occurrences that point to developing health problems like uncontrolled blood sugar levels, cardiac arrhythmias, or respiratory diseases. Even before an individual realizes there's an issue, the wearable may notify doctors and other healthcare practitioners of any suspicious activity, allowing for prompt intervention. One example is the annual impact on millions of individuals by atrial fibrillation. But it's common for the illness to go undiagnosed and untreated. By using remote electrocardiogram (ECG) recordings, wearables can keep an eye on irregular heart rhythms and facilitate effective and rapid cardiac therapy. Patients are also able to take charge of their own health care with the help of AI. They will be able to make better choices on their health and treatment plans with access to up-to-the-minute information. It may be as easy as receiving a notification to keep the volume at a reasonable level while using AirPods. Even in the most serious instances, AI systems may help patients stay healthy and cut down on hospital visits by reminding them to take their meds at the right times, suggesting ways to exercise differently, and arranging for follow-up consultations or blood tests. In order to ensure that healthcare services run smoothly, AI systems use predictive modeling to find any inefficiencies and bottlenecks. To avoid overscheduling of personnel and resources (such as procedural containers, MRI scanning devices, X-ray devices, etc.), the system may, for example, forecast when patient admissions would be at their highest volume and suggest optimal appointment booking slots. In addition to preventing shortages and expensive overstocks, this predictive capacity guarantees that healthcare facilities retain the proper quantity of inventory, including medications, cotton swabs, surgical gowns, masks, and more. Further, AI deep learning models reduce administrative burdens by automating regular operations like patient registration, invoicing, and claims processing. They provide them with the ability to manage money better and essential patient records. Overall quality and sustainability of healthcare institutions are enhanced when facilities run at peak efficiency, allowing them to care for more individuals in a given time utilizing the right resources.

5. CONCLUSION

Using statistical analysis in healthcare has huge, far-reaching advantages. Healthcare has the potential to become more efficient, effective, and patient-centered with the help of predictive analytics, which might improve patient care and outcomes, save costs, and make customized medicine a reality. Given the nascent nature of predictive analytics, there is much room for growth in the area, especially as it pertains to healthcare. However, preliminary findings indicate that predictive analytics may significantly enhance healthcare delivery in terms of both efficiency and quality. With the ever-changing landscape of technology, predictive analytics have the potential to revolutionize healthcare by enhancing health outcomes and opening up new avenues for improvement.

REFERENCES

Abbas, S. R., Abbas, Z., Zahir, A., & Lee, S. W. (2024). Federated Learning in Smart Healthcare: A Comprehensive Review on Privacy, Security, and Predictive Analytics with IoT Integration. *Health Care*, *12*(24), 2587. PMID: 39766014

Al-Talafheh, K., Aplop, F., Al-Yousef, A., Obiedat, M., & Khazaaleh, M. (2024). Predictive Big Data Analytics Capability Model to Enhancing Healthcare Organization Performance. *International Journal of Advances in Soft Computing & Its Applications*, *16*(3), 149–165. DOI: 10.15849/IJASCA.241130.09

Alharthi, H. (2018). Healthcare predictive analytics: An overview with a focus on Saudi Arabia. *Journal of Infection and Public Health*, *11*(6), 749–756. DOI: 10.1016/j.jiph.2018.02.005 PMID: 29526444

Ango, R., Masih, R. K., Reddy, C. K. K., Shuaib, M., Singh, M., & Alam, S. (2024). Fraud Detection in Banking using the Kaggle Credit Card Dataset and XGBoost Model. *2024 International Conference on IoT Based Control Networks and Intelligent Systems (ICICNIS)*, 968–973. DOI: 10.1109/ICICNIS64247.2024.10823227

Cano-Marin, E., Mora-Cantallops, M., & Sanchez-Alonso, S. (2023). The power of big data analytics over fake news: A scientometric review of Twitter as a predictive system in healthcare. *Technological Forecasting and Social Change*, *190*, 122386. DOI: 10.1016/j.techfore.2023.122386

Chiranjeevi, P., & Rajaram, A. (2024). A smart recommender model based on learning method for sentiment classification. *Multimedia Tools and Applications*, •••, 1–21. DOI: 10.1007/s11042-024-20347-z

Edoh, N. L., Chigboh, V. M., Zouo, S. J., & Olamijuwon, J. (2024). *Improving healthcare decision-making with predictive analytics: A conceptual approach to patient risk assessment and care optimization.*

Etli, D., Djurovic, A., & Lark, J. (2024). The Future of Personalized Healthcare: AI-Driven Wearables For Real-Time Health Monitoring And Predictive Analytics. *Current Research in Health Sciences*, *2*(2), 10–14.

Ganiya, R. K., Veeraiah, D., Thatha, V. N., Rao, K. S., Rao, J. N., Manjith, R., & Rajaram, A. (2024). Revolutionizing vascular health through the temporal convolutional transformer for drug screening and model evolution. *Biomedical Signal Processing and Control*, *95*, 106390. DOI: 10.1016/j.bspc.2024.106390

Gates, J. D., Yulianti, Y., & Pangilinan, G. A. (2024). Big data analytics for predictive insights in healthcare. *International Transactions on Artificial Intelligence*, *3*(1), 54–63. DOI: 10.33050/italic.v3i1.622

Hossain, S., Ahmed, A., Khadka, U., Sarkar, S., & Khan, N. (2024). AI-driven Predictive Analytics, Healthcare Outcomes, Cost Reduction, Machine Learning, Patient Monitoring. *AIJMR-Advanced International Journal of Multidisciplinary Research, 2*(5).

Ibeh, C. V., Elufioye, O. A., Olorunsogo, T., Asuzu, O. F., Nduubuisi, N. L., & Daraojimba, A. I. (2024). Data analytics in healthcare: A review of patient-centric approaches and healthcare delivery. *World Journal of Advanced Research and Reviews*, *21*(02), 1750–1760. DOI: 10.30574/wjarr.2024.21.2.0246

Ibikunle, O. E., Usuemerai, P. A., Abass, L. A., Alemede, V., Nwankwo, E. I., & Mbata, A. O. (2024). Artificial intelligence in healthcare forecasting: Enhancing market strategy with predictive analytics. *International Journal of Applied Research in Social Sciences*, *6*(10).

Islam, M., Usman, M., Mahmood, A., Abbasi, A. A., & Song, O.-Y. (2020). Predictive analytics framework for accurate estimation of child mortality rates for Internet of Things enabled smart healthcare systems. *International Journal of Distributed Sensor Networks*, *16*(5), 1550147720928897. DOI: 10.1177/1550147720928897

Kalaivani, K., Kshirsagarr, P. R., Sirisha Devi, J., Bandela, S. R., Colak, I., Nageswara Rao, J., & Rajaram, A. (2023). Prediction of biomedical signals using deep learning techniques. *Journal of Intelligent & Fuzzy Systems*, *44*(6), 9769–9782. DOI: 10.3233/JIFS-230399

Karthik, A., Aalam, S. S., Sivakumar, M., Sundari, M. V. R., Rose, J. D., Elangovan, M., & Rajaram, A. (2024). Improving brain tumor treatment with better imaging and real-time therapy using quantum dots. *Biomedical Signal Processing and Control*, *95*, 106286. DOI: 10.1016/j.bspc.2024.106286

Karthik, A., Hamatta, H. S. A., Patthi, S., Krubakaran, C., Pradhan, A. K., Rachapudi, V., Shuaib, M., & Rajaram, A. (2024). Ensemble-based multimodal medical imaging fusion for tumor segmentation. *Biomedical Signal Processing and Control*, *96*, 106550. DOI: 10.1016/j.bspc.2024.106550

Karthik, A., Sahoo, S. K., Kumar, A., Patel, N., Chinnaraj, P., Maguluri, L. P., & Rajaram, A. (2025). Unified approach for accurate brain tumor Multi-Classification and segmentation through fusion of advanced methodologies. *Biomedical Signal Processing and Control*, *100*, 106872. DOI: 10.1016/j.bspc.2024.106872

Khan, A., Zubair, S., Shuaib, M., Sheneamer, A., Alam, S., & Assiri, B. (2024). Development of a robust parallel and multi-composite machine learning model for improved diagnosis of Alzheimer's disease: Correlation with dementia-associated drug usage and AT (N) protein biomarkers. *Frontiers in Neuroscience*, *18*, 1391465. DOI: 10.3389/fnins.2024.1391465 PMID: 39308946

Khubrani, M. M., & Alam, S. (2021). A detailed review of blockchain-based applications for protection against pandemic like COVID-19. *Telkomnika*, *19*(4), 1185–1196. DOI: 10.12928/telkomnika.v19i4.18465

Kumar, D., & Suthar, N. (2024). Predictive analytics and early intervention in healthcare social work: A scoping review. *Social Work in Health Care*, *63*(4–5), 208–229. DOI: 10.1080/00981389.2024.2316700 PMID: 38349783

Maguluri, L. P., Chouhan, K., Balamurali, R., Rani, R., Hashmi, A., Kiran, A., & Rajaram, A. (2024). Adversarial deep learning for improved abdominal organ segmentation in CT scans. *Multimedia Tools and Applications*, *83*(35), 82107–82129. DOI: 10.1007/s11042-024-18578-1

Obijuru, A., Arowoogun, J. O., Onwumere, C., Odilibe, I. P., Anyanwu, E. C., & Daraojimba, A. I. (2024). Big data analytics in healthcare: A review of recent advances and potential for personalized medicine. *International Medical Science Research Journal*, *4*(2), 170–182. DOI: 10.51594/imsrj.v4i2.810

Pendyala, S. K. (2024). Healthcare Data Analytics: Leveraging Predictive Analytics For Improved Patient Outcomes. *International Journal Of Computer Engineering And Technology (Ijcet)*, *15*(6), 548–565.

Poloju, N., & Rajaram, A. (2024). Transformation with yolo tiny network architecture for multimodal fusion in lung disease classification. *Cybernetics and Systems*, •••, 1–22. DOI: 10.1080/01969722.2024.2343992

Rahim, M. J., Afroz, A., & Akinola, O. (2025). Predictive Analytics in Healthcare: Big Data, Better Decisions. *International Journal of Scientific Research and Modern Technology*, *4*(1), 1–21.

Reddy, C. K. K., Rangarajan, A., Rangarajan, D., Shuaib, M., Jeribi, F., & Alam, S. (2024). A transfer learning approach: Early prediction of Alzheimer's disease on US healthy aging dataset. *Mathematics*, *12*(14), 2204. DOI: 10.3390/math12142204

Reddy, C. K. K., Reddy, P. A., Janapati, H., Assiri, B., Shuaib, M., Alam, S., & Sheneamer, A. (2024). A fine-tuned vision transformer based enhanced multi-class brain tumor classification using MRI scan imagery. *Frontiers in Oncology*, *14*, 1400341. DOI: 10.3389/fonc.2024.1400341 PMID: 39091923

Rojas, J. C., Rohweder, G., Guptill, J., Arora, V. M., & Umscheid, C. A. (2022). Predictive analytics programs at large healthcare systems in the USA: A national survey. *Journal of General Internal Medicine*, *37*(15), 4015–4017. DOI: 10.1007/s11606-022-07517-1 PMID: 35396657

Singh, A., Nagabhooshanam, N., Kumar, R., Verma, R., Mohanasundaram, S., Manjith, R., & Rajaram, A. (2025). Deep learning based coronary artery disease detection and segmentation using ultrasound imaging with adaptive gated SCNN models. *Biomedical Signal Processing and Control*, *105*, 107637. DOI: 10.1016/j.bspc.2025.107637

Syamala, M., Chandrasekaran, R., Balamurali, R., Rani, R., Hashmi, A., Kiran, A., & Rajaram, A. (2024). Evaluating generative adversarial networks for virtual contrast-enhanced kidney segmentation using Res-UNet in non-contrast CT images. *Multimedia Tools and Applications*, •••, 1–24. DOI: 10.1007/s11042-024-19626-6

Yadav, G., Bokhari, M. U., Alzahrani, S. I., Alam, S., & Shuaib, M. (2025). Emotion-Aware Ensemble Learning (EAEL): Revolutionizing Mental Health Diagnosis of Corporate Professionals via Intelligent Integration of Multi-Modal Data Sources and Ensemble Techniques. *IEEE Access : Practical Innovations, Open Solutions*, *13*, 11494–11516. DOI: 10.1109/ACCESS.2025.3529032

Chapter 6
Innovative Approaches to Remote Health Monitoring Systems for Enhanced Patient Care and Accessibility

Manjunath G. Asuti
https://orcid.org/0009-0003-4855-4563
BNM Institute of Technology, India

S. Ramesh
SRM Institute of Science and Technology, India

D. Prabakar
SRM Institute of Science and Technology, India

G. Balachandran
Jeppiaar Engineering College, India

T. Anuja
Jeppiaar Engineering College, India

A. Rajaram
E.G.S. Pillay Engineering College, India

Haider Khalaf Jabbar
University of Misan, Iraq

ABSTRACT

Real-time remote patient monitoring, enabled by the integration of biosensors and multi-hop Internet of Things (IoT) networks, marks a transformative shift in modern healthcare. Biosensors placed throughout healthcare environments transmit vital data via interconnected microcontrollers to centralized servers using secure cloud infrastructure. Emphasizing systems developed for elderly care, this study categorizes key architectures, examines deployment challenges, and identifies opportunities for further innovation. Remote health monitoring solutions enhance continuous care, support independent living, and ensure rapid medical response through real-time access to patient data. By leveraging IoT and cloud connectivity, these systems promise to overcome traditional care limitations and elevate healthcare accessibility and quality.

DOI: 10.4018/979-8-3373-1022-0.ch006

1. INTRODUCTION

An advancement in technology, the Internet of Things (IoT), enables electrical devices and sensors to exchange data and connect over the web. It exemplifies the IoT's rise as a game-changing force, linking and sharing data across heterogeneous systems. This integration creates a unified digital-physical ecosystem, with devices dynamically interacting via the internet. In healthcare, IoT has catalyzed innovations in remote diagnostics, wearable health monitors, fitness tracking, and telemedicine platforms. These technologies support health education, disease management, and coordinated care delivery. Scientometric analyses affirm IoT's increasing prominence in biomedical research and healthcare system design (Rehman et al., 2024).

Remote health monitoring systems—central to IoT in healthcare—leverage biosensors, microcontrollers, and wireless body area networks (WBANs) to capture vital parameters such as heart rate, blood oxygen saturation, ECG signals, and body temperature. These sensors transmit data via short-range communication protocols like Bluetooth Low Energy (BLE), Zigbee, and 6LoWPAN to edge devices or fog nodes (Shuaib et al., 2023). Data is then aggregated, filtered, and pre-processed at the network edge using lightweight microprocessors before being pushed to centralized cloud platforms for advanced analytics and storage. Cloud-based engines, often integrated with AI algorithms, enable anomaly detection, predictive diagnostics, and automated alerts—forming a closed feedback loop between patient and provider (A. Singh et al., 2022).

A typical architecture comprises multi-hop sensor networks, local gateways, fog computing nodes, and cloud APIs for medical dashboards or EHR integration. MQTT and CoAP are frequently adopted for real-time, lightweight data transmission, while RESTful APIs ensure interoperability with existing healthcare information systems. These systems empower clinicians to monitor patients continuously outside hospital environments—particularly beneficial for chronic disease management, geriatric care, and post-operative recovery (Alam et al., 2023).

Nevertheless, the deployment of such systems is not without challenges. Hardware failures, power interruptions, or unstable network coverage can result in data loss or temporal blind spots in monitoring. Furthermore, ensuring data security, integrity, and HIPAA-compliant transmission across IoT layers remains a complex task. Adaptive fault tolerance, context-aware computing, encryption protocols, and redundancy through hybrid edge-cloud architectures are essential countermeasures.

This chapter explores the layered architecture, communication strategies, sensor configurations, and data pipelines that underpin remote health monitoring solutions. It also delves into emerging challenges—such as latency, energy efficiency, and patient privacy—and identifies future directions for scalable, intelligent, and context-adaptive IoT-based healthcare systems.

2 REMOTE HEALTHCARE SYSTEM MODEL

By recording every aspect and action, Internet of Things (IoT) devices allow doctors to monitor the condition of older patients. Information is shared with staff members and nurses who provide care for elderly individuals (Carter et al., 2021). IoT will enable people with impairments to connect their home healthcare gadgets. Hence, doctors may occasionally monitor their patients' conditions. The data that is created and gathered, however, is vulnerable to a number of dangers. Attacks provide hackers with full leadership and management (C&C), which disrupts the equipment. In the healthcare business, these assaults may deplete the power of sensors, leading to their failure or perhaps bringing down the whole IoT network.

2.1 Integration of Biosensors with IoT

In the field of real-time surveillance of patients in hospitals, the combination of biosensors and multi-hop IoT systems is quickly becoming a foundational component in the revolution of healthcare services (Karmakar et al., 2022). The capacity to install several biosensors in various parts of healthcare institutions and have them all linked together via multi-hop IoT systems is what drives this integration. By strategically placing sensors in various locations, healthcare providers may keep tabs on patients in multiple wards, critical care facilities, and even outlying places all at once, giving them a complete picture of their health. This combination can revolutionize how standard hospital services handle real-time remote monitoring of patient activities, which is a testament to its significance. Biosensors with multi-hop connectivity may provide vital signs in real time over great distances, freeing healthcare practitioners from geographical limitations. Improved patient outcomes, earlier action in the case of abnormalities, and more efficient healthcare delivery are all possible results of this (V. K. Singh et al., 2023). Integrating biosensors and multi-hop Internet of Things (IoT) systems in hospitals has the potential to revolutionize healthcare by creating a more connected and responsive system. This system would allow for real-time remote patient monitoring, thereby eliminating the restrictions of conventional healthcare.

2.2 Medical Data Collection

Smart healthcare sensors, such as those that monitor heart rate and brain activity, gather information about patients. Gathering, analyzing, and keeping tabs on medical data is what it's all about. In the medical data collection layer, several gadgets are used to gather data initially. Sensors, mobile phones, wearable tech, and cameras are all examples of such gadgets (Peyroteo et al., 2021). Phase two entails data analysis, which records and examines each action taken by a senior patient. After that, the data is processed and stored on a secure server. The ability to remotely monitor and automatically record healthcare data, such as a patient's medical history and current state

2.3 Medical Data Applications

When it comes to the Internet of Things, the conventional application layer is in charge of processing data, storing it, and creating user interfaces. Comparatively, healthcare-specific apps, data, and services are the domain of the medical application layer (Bellino et al., 2022). For instance, EHRs that store patient information, platforms for remote consultations, tools for real-time monitoring, medical resources, medical treatment, diagnosticians, and so on. In addition, medical records are organized and maintained by the medical application layer. This layer guarantees the transmission of valid, secure, confidential, and trustworthy patient data via the communication system. The following protocols are examples of application layers: SecureMQTT, WebSockets, RESTful, Hypertext Transfer Protocol, Message Queuing Telemetry Transport (MQTT), and CoAP. The use case determines the most suitable IoT protocol (Sharma et al., 2022).

Figure 1. Data collection in healthcare

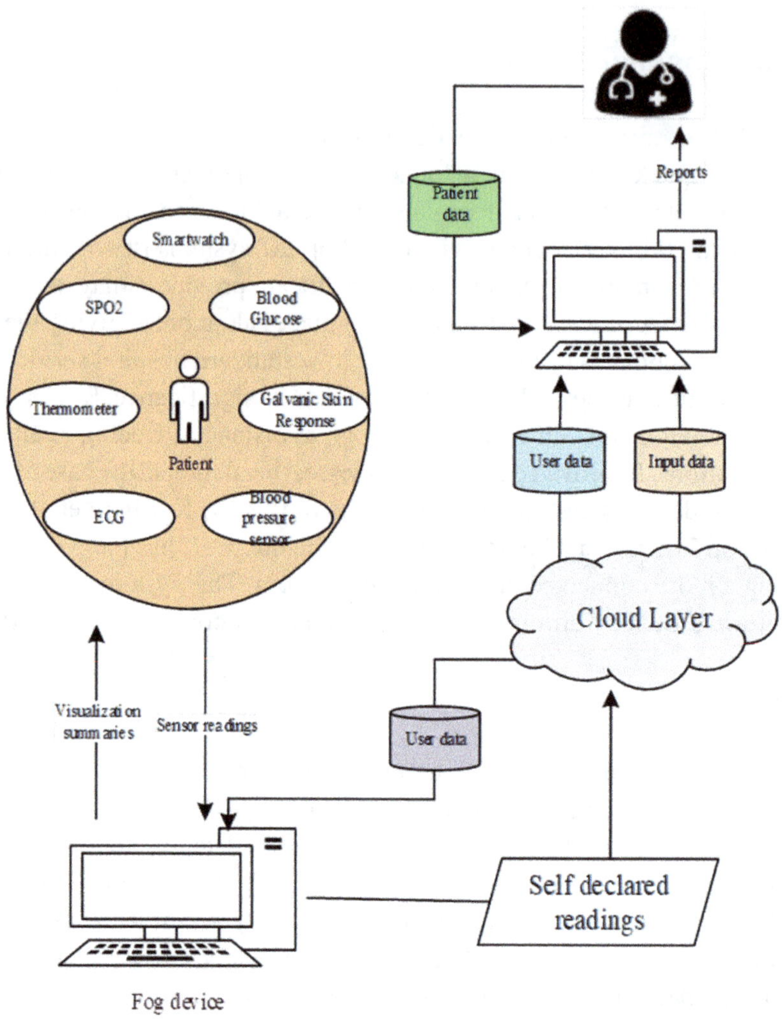

3 CHALLENGES OF REMOTE MONITORING SYSTEMS

3.1 Network Latency

Due to the centralization and remote deployment of cloud servers, network latency becomes a significant issue for end users. As mentioned, latency on the network is much reduced with fog gateways since they are located close to end users' devices. Using the WiFi infrastructure for a healthcare application, the experiment conducted reveals that latency is 21 ms in Fog and 161 ms in the cloud. Network latency is greater in MEC than in Fog because user devices connect to the network server at the base station.

3.2 Internet Bandwidth Utilization

In remote health monitoring and other similar applications, fog gateways along with MEC servers may process and save data locally, allowing for just the summary data to be broadcast via the cloud. This is because health monitoring sensors often generate enormous volumes of data. Because of this, the amount of bandwidth used via the Internet is drastically decreased. Figure 1 shows the difference in bandwidth consumption between different technologies' topologies.

3.3 Power Consumption

When compared to the cloud computing method, FC and MEC perform far better in terms of power usage. In comparison to MEC and cloud computing, distributed architectures like Fog use less power, as Hartmann highlighted. Refining sensor data locally also decreases data transported via the cloud, which in turn decreases power consumption, which is very important for healthcare applications.

3.4. Execution Time

According to the analysis, cloud computing offers an abundance of storage space and processing power. According to the needs of data processing, cloud computing may also be able to expand resources on demand. Because of this, analyzing the massive amounts of data produced by health apps requires extremely little time to run. The execution time to analyze data is greater in MEC because servers with base stations have comparatively limited resources. On top of that, fog devices often have low power consumption, but their processing and storage capacity cause them to have longer execution times.

3.5. Context Awareness

One of the key ideas used in health apps is context awareness, which allows users to make use of data like a patient's location, the whereabouts of other nearby patients, and environmental resources. As a result, partnerships might enable MEC platforms to implement real-time context-aware applications, such as remote health monitoring, allowing for improved decision-making. Fog computing often uses equipment like routers and switches, which have a limited view of the system. Therefore, their context awareness isn't as good as MEC's. The capacity for communication between the nodes, however, makes this problem less severe. Cloud computing, in contrast, lacks context awareness due to its design as an independent server linked to the Internet.

3.6. Real-Time Compatibility

The cloud computing method bypasses data filtering by transmitting health sensor readings straight to remote computers in the cloud. Cloud computing is not useful for real-time applications because of this reason. With the use of fog computing, health apps may swiftly react to undesired occurrences by detecting them in real time and analyzing the data locally. Solutions that seek to provide rapid reactions to crucial circumstances in healthcare settings are a part of the real-time feedback gathering. In order to detect falls and communicate this information to caregivers, the authors used a real-time signal-processing technique. Fog servers gather and analyze all health information by executing these algorithms at the network's border. Another method that is suggested to keep an eye on stroke-related falls is using a real-time analytical system. Any of the uses above cannot proceed without an immediate reaction from caretakers or actuators.

4. CURRENT REMOTE HEALTH MONITORING SYSTEMS

The goal of Coman et al. (2024) is to discuss and investigate intelligent approaches to diet-related illness management by utilizing cutting-edge technology like connected care, the IoMT, and RHMS to combat the increasing incidence of these conditions. Case studies that focus on specialized RHMS capabilities showcase that technique as exceptional. By presenting a new assessment approach and their customization for proactive treatment of illnesses impacted by dietary habits, the research hopes to illustrate an opportunity for three RHMS. An innovative viewpoint in healthcare, the RO-SmartAging System takes a holistic view of aging by integrating the effects of food on the body throughout time. New insights into healthcare evaluations are provided by the NeuroPredict Platform, which uses complicated neuroinformatics to improve their knowledge of the relationships among brain health, nutrition, and general wellness. An innovative method for illness management, the HepatoConect system monitors liver function in real-time and uses that information to provide patients with tailored dietary suggestions. These innovative solutions go beyond what is normally possible in healthcare by using state-of-the-art technology.

A Cloud Access Security Broker approach is suggested in Javed et al. (2023) that (a) records all operations done on user data and (b) stores these records in a private blockchain that can be accessed by the patients who own the data. Patients can access their data via queries on the blockchain, monitor its transfer, and get notifications in the event that their data is accessible via an administrator or transferred from the cloud. Here, we put into practice a web app that takes in patients' medical information, a CASB that safely saves those records in the cloud, and a private blockchain that records every activity that takes place in the app's and the CASB's backend in real-time. We test the system's robustness and efficiency with different patient loads and scenarios.

According to Schütz et al. (2022), the majority of the existing literature on digital assessments has concentrated on studying the use of a small number of particular measures collected via mobile devices. On the other hand, that kind of technology may not be the best option, particularly for long-term uses in older people, and it might exacerbate the digital divide. Given the success of genomics and other large-scale systems biology methods in precision medicine, it is reasonable to assume that they may have a similar impact on remote health monitoring. We provide and explain a zero-interaction digital exhaust in that context, which is a collection of 1268 digital measurements, including a person's behavior, physiology, and activities. That set is based solely on zero-interaction sensing technologies and is contactless, which makes it more accessible to older folks. Then, by using the generated digital exhaust on real-world data, we show that it is possible to create several digital clinical outcome evaluations that are relevant to aging. When combined with state-of-the-art machine learning, these evaluations are very effective, often competing with mobile methods. Last but not least, we stress the potential of that large-scale strategy for the discovery of new digital biomarkers.

The paper delves into the many issues and potential benefits that come from that confluence (B. Singh & Kaunert, 2024). The investigation provides valuable insights into developing successful legal frameworks by examining patient data privacy, rules regarding medical devices, and liability problems.

The article also muses on the possible long-term effects of these innovations, such as better patient care, remote surveillance, and streamlined healthcare delivery. That project aims to create a future in healthcare that is both creative and focused on the needs of patients by integrating technology and legislation in a manner that protects their rights and privacy. That research study takes a close look at the health monitoring systems that use IoT and 5G technologies, and it investigates the legal considerations that come with their adoption. Focusing on the privacy, regulatory, and ethical issues raised by these technologies, that article seeks to provide a thorough legal examination of the possibilities and threats posed by their use in healthcare.

The purpose of that research is to look at what's new with remote health surveillance systems (Dalloul et al., 2023). Antenna designs, tiny implanted antennas, on-body wearable solutions, and flexible detection and imaging systems are just a few of the many topics covered in that extensive article. Their studies additionally explore the methodologies used by monitoring systems, such as channel characteristic analysis, wireless capsule endoscopy developments, and imaging and sensing technology insights. There is hope that these developments will lead to more precise and efficient monitoring, which in turn will improve patients' health outcomes.

An HBR-Radio-based passive (bi-static) radar health monitoring system is shown in Ahmed et al. (2023). To do remote health monitoring, HBR-Radio makes use of ambient radio frequency disturbance detection. HBR-Radio is a method for monitoring vital signs that can detect heart rate and respiration rate without the need for any contact-based sensors that are worn on the body. A WiFi access point, which employs the industry-standard 802.11 protocol, serves as the system's transmitter (or light source). The reference signal, which is sent directly from the source, and any reflected signals from the environment, including the one from the monitored individual, are captured using a Software-Defined Radio platform. The use of several signal processing methods allows for the extraction of the required vital indicators. There is a pressing demand in today's society for user-friendly, integrated, innovative, remote, omnipresent health monitoring systems, which is where the presented system comes in. Ambient RF sensing can improve people's quality of life, and the suggested system is a prime illustration of how that may work.

A multi-functional health monitoring remotely method is developed by combining several approaches of remote vital sign estimation (Bauder et al., 2023). Under ideal conditions, systems based on cameras may assess vital signs like temperature, blood pressure, SpO2, and heart rate. For the same reason, radar-based technologies are used to estimate the heart and respiration rates of patients in a more reliable manner. All of the important vital signs of human beings are recorded concurrently using these two approaches. The results demonstrate that the suggested system is capable of performing all of its functions with a high level of accuracy.

The article delves into the complex security issues that come with these systems, stresses the need for strong cybersecurity theories, and showcases successful security measures that have emerged from global cooperation initiatives. The document lays forth guidelines for creating, deploying, and overseeing safe systems, stressing the need for defense-in-depth tactics, least privilege, constant monitoring, and adaptive response systems (Alam, 2023) . Highlighting the ever-changing nature of threats to cybersecurity as well as the possibility of new technology to strengthen security measures, it also emphasizes current difficulties and areas where research could go next. The study stresses the need for ongoing research and cooperation to address the ever-changing security risks to water distribution networks and make them more resilient.

LeBaron (2022) emphasizes the important role that nurses may play in establishing and implementing RHM systems for older individuals with cancer care while also highlighting important obstacles and potential in that area. Personalized and tailored care, privacy and data security, interdisciplinary collaboration, addressing disparities in medical care and disparities, naturalistic data collection, caregiver perspectives, fast technological change, participant recruitment and burden, and user-centered design are some of the key topics. Developing RHM systems that are ideally helpful for patients, family members, physicians, and organizations requires nurses to be well-informed about the difficulties and possibilities in each of these areas.

The most recent developments in wearable sensor technologies that can assess vital signs with the same degree of precision as point-of-care testing are detailed in Mirjalali et al. (2022). That study primarily aims to concentrate on wearable sensors that can measure essential signals for the diagnosis and tracking of COVID-19, including respiratory behavior, body temperature, and blood oxygen level. An assortment of designs derived from diverse materials and operational systems are encapsulated (Khubrani & Alam, 2021). To wrap up their evaluation, they will look at the remaining obstacles and potential possibilities in that new area (A. Singh et al., 2022).

5. ARCHITECTURE AND DESIGN CONSIDERATIONS

Figure 2. Remote Monitoring System for IoT-based Healthcare

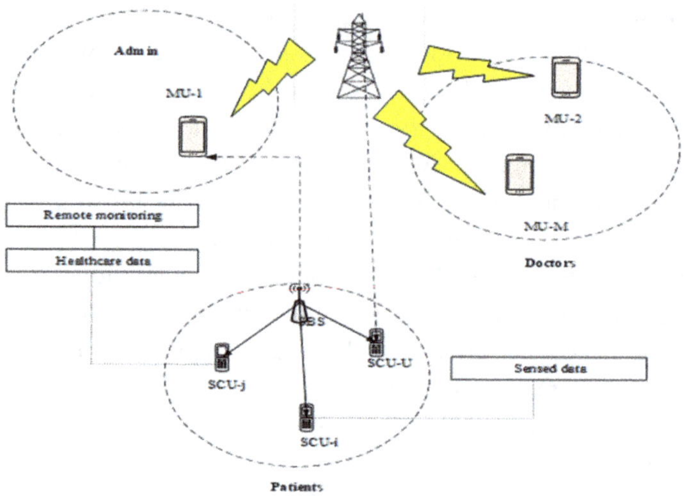

A new age in remote monitoring of patients and health data collecting has dawned with the integration of biosensors and multi-hop IoT systems in healthcare. To maintain smooth operation, transmit data in real-time, and make good use of data produced by biosensors, the design and architecture of such systems must be carefully considered (Karthik et al., 2025). To ensure the smooth incorporation of biosensors into healthcare-related multi-hop IoT systems, this section explores the critical architectural and design factors.

Adopting a scalable and flexible architecture is a fundamental part of creating multi-hop Internet of Things systems for biosensor integration. To meet the expanding needs of healthcare applications, scalability guarantees that the system can effectively manage a rising number of linked biosensors (Karthik et al., 2024). The ability to include different biosensors with different functions in a system without affecting its overall coherence is made possible by the modular architecture's adaptability.

5.1 Input Data Preparation

The use of convolutional neural networks (CNNs) for healthcare disease classification in machine diagnostics was motivated by their impressive feature learning and picture recognition capabilities, which are based on the image-processing idea. The usual 1D series of signals aren't always up to the task since they don't have the necessary 2D data structure or picture[27]. Image, matrix, time/frequency domain, wavelet, and short-time Fourier transformations are among the signal transformation methods used to get picture output from signal data. The measurement patterns that were created in this experiment were arranged in a matrix with the dimensions (N×M), where N is the number of samples and M is the number of measurement parameters[28]. In order to normalize the data to the range of -1 to 1, we used min-max normalization (Equation (4)). After that, the data was translated into a four-dimensional array with the dimensions (width, height, channel, sample size) as (rows, columns, routes, sample size) to represent the shape[29][30]. That is why the matrix data became (1, M, 1, " " N) in form. Each one was treated as an image with width=1, height=M, and channels=1 when the CNN model was fitted to the data.

$$\left(x_t^l\right)_{mar} = \frac{\left(x_{max}^l - x_{min}^l\right)\left(x_i^j - y'_{min}\right)}{y_{max} - y_{min}} + x_{min}$$

where $\left(x_i^f\right)_{nor}$ is the scaled value of the signal x_i^f, x_i^f is the novel i_{th} signal of the j_{th} sensor, x_{min}^f is the lowest value of the jth sensor, x_{max}^j is the supreme value of the jth sensor, $y_{min} = -1$, and $y_{max} = 1$.

5.2 CNN Architecture and Training

A training approach was used to ascertain the CNN model's architecture, which was utilized in this publication. Table 1 details its construction: two convolutional layers in quick succession, one pooling layer using the ReLU activation function, and a dropout layer sandwiched in the middle. ReLU is a piecewise linear function that returns zero for negative input values and keeps the input value unchanged for values greater than or equal to zero. Many convolutional neural networks (CNNs) use this activation function because it improves performance and avoids the vanishing gradient issue. There are 112 1×10 filters in the first convolutional layer with a stride of 1×1 and 212 1×2 filters in the second convolutional layer with a stride of 1×1. Both of these convolutional layers use input data to create output feature maps with representative signatures. For the downsampling process, an optimal pooling layer was used, which included filters measuring 1×2 and a stride of 1×1. A single fully connected layer came following the pooling layer, and immediately after that came a second dropout layer. The output layer, the last structural layer, uses probability distributions predicted by the softmax function to decide the class type. As an expansion of the standard stochastic gradient descent learning system, the

Adam optimization algorithm was chosen as the learning algorithm. High processing efficiency and low memory requirements are two of its advantages. All of the CNN models in the suggested hierarchy use the same hyperparameters.

5.2.1 Convolutional Layer

A CNN model is built upon convolutional layers. In order to create one or more feature maps that are reflective of the input data, they convolve groups of filters called kernels. Sliding the filter throughout the input data does the convolution. On each slide, the outcome is the result of multiplying the filter with the input data portion that underwent the convolution procedure. It has a corresponding mathematical expression:

$$y_l^k = f\left(w_l^k x_l^{k-1} + b_l^k\right)$$

where y_l^k is the output of the convolution for the filter k in layer I, x_l^{k-1} stands for the layer's input, f(·) for the activation function, and w and b for the weight (filter), along with bias values, respectively.

5.2.2 Pooling Layer

A few more names for the pooling layer include downsampling and subsampling. The pooling of the convolved features occurs in the subsequent layer of the convolutional layer. Most pooling algorithms employ either maximum or average pooling. While the latter takes the mean into account, the former filters an input feature map for the most valuable features inside a subset. This study made use of max pooling as it finds the most useful features in a convolved feature map and extracts them.

5.2.3 Fully-Connected Layer

The completely linked layer operates and is structured similarly to a standard multilayer perceptron. A feed-forward neural network based on backpropagation is essentially what it is. Common building blocks include an input layer, an output layer, and a concealed layer or levels in between. Producing meaningful outputs from the extracted features is the primary responsibility of this layer in the CNN process. It is necessary to flatten the feature outputs from the feature-learning part while the fully connected layer does not support multidimensional data input.

5.2.4 Output Layer

Finally, the CNN model's output layer executes the operation. A popular classification function is softmax, which may be found in Equation (3). To decide what category the incoming data falls into, it calculates probability values. All of the classes in the classification issue had their estimated probability values added up to one.

$$S\left(\vec{x}\right)_t = \frac{e^{xt}}{\sum_{j-1}^{c} e^{zj}} \text{ for } i = 1,2,\ldots,c$$

The input feature vector is denoted as $\vec{x}$, the typical exponential function for the input feature vector is e^xl, the total amount of classes in the classification problem is c, S is the softmax function, and e^{24} is the standard exponential function for the output.

Figure 3. Remote Healthcare Data Classification

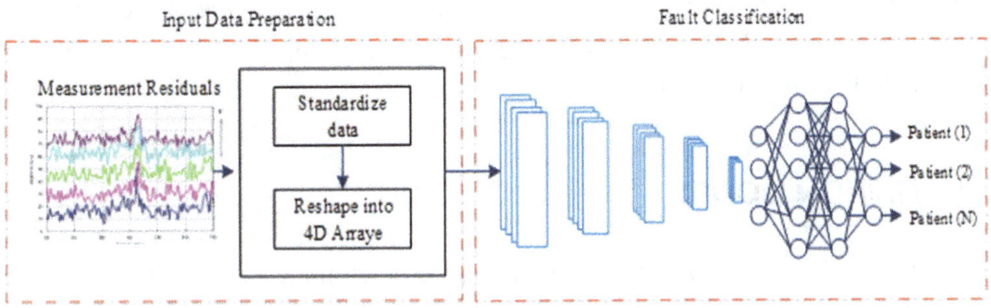

Figure 3 shows that there are two parts to the analysis process: transforming the input data and classifying the healthcare diseases. Improving classification performance and ensuring that each measurement is considered objectively requires first standardizing the input data. The next step is to reshape the input data so that the CNN algorithm built-in MATLAB can readily utilize it. Currently, the data is in a matrix format. Following this, the convolutional neural network (CNN) algorithm was taught to sift through the input data for characteristics that might be used to identify the various types of healthcare diseases. We will go over these stages in more detail later on.

Table 1. Details of the CNN architecture and learning hyperparameters

No.	Layers and Learning Hyperparameters	Description
1	Input layer	4D array input
2	Convolution Layer 1	Convolution with 112 filters of size [1·10] and stride [1·1]
3	Convolution Layer 2	Convolution with 212 filters of size [1·2] and stride [1·1]
4	Activation layer	ReLU
5	Dropout Layer 1	30% dropout
6	Pooling layer	Max pooling of size [1·2] with stride [1·1]
7	Dropout Layer 2	30% dropout
8	Fully connected layer	One fully connected layer
9	Output layer	Softmax
10	Optimizer	Adam
11	No. of epochs	20
12	Learning rate	0.01

Overfitting is a problem in deep learning that makes it hard to train excellent models. A more generic answer can only be achieved by controlling this phenomenon. The so-called "dropout" operation and cross-validation are two ways convolutional neural networks (CNNs) deal with overfitting. The trick is to temporarily and arbitrarily remove certain hidden neurons from the CNN architecture. The second one uses a dataset that wasn't utilized for training to apply a stopping condition for training. In this case, training the network should end whenever the validation error starts to rise and the training error goes down. As an additional strategy to combat overfitting and measure the degree of prediction uncertainty, deep ensemble approaches might be explored. Every dropout layer in the structure was subjected to the authors' 30% dropout notion in this study.

6. IMPLEMENTATION MODEL

PyTorch's built-in JIT compiler may be accessed via a special mode called TorchScript. It takes pre-existing Python code and turns it into serializable models. Without Python, a TorchScript application may be executed on its own. Without the need for Python packages, we can simulate any platform.

Table 2. Applications of sensors

Sensors	Applications
Accelerometer, Motion	Using motion and inactivity sensors, healthcare providers may identify whether a patient is moving or not.
Optical AFE, ECG	Industrial monitoring of heart rates, spo2 levels
Temperature	Environmental monitoring, HVAC, medical devices
Bio Impedance	Photoplethysmography and photodiode measurements
Capacitive sensors	When it comes to sensors that detect changes on touchscreens

Every patient's health state is unique, as we all know. Thus, we enable simple and efficient patient monitoring by using user input from the accompanying physician. Because every patient has a unique range for their heart rate and blood pressure, etc., this device notifies medical professionals and staff of any irregularities or decreases under the minimum range specified by the doctor, allowing for prompt treatment. By doing so, we can lessen the number of fatalities caused by physicians not keeping tabs on patients or communicating with one another. With further development, we may make it possible to track the healing process of shattered bones and display the patient's and doctor's percentage of recovery. It would also provide the patient with important medical appointment reminders. We can also store the tensors at bit widths smaller than the floating-point precision by using quantization. While working with tensors, the recently quantized model reduces the accuracy of some or all operations. Theoretically, this seems weak, but in practice, it has little effect on the accuracy. The reason is that most models are overparameterized, and this one was trained on floating point accuracy. We have a lot of space for mistakes because of this. The values in floating point are converted to integers using a mapping function. An equation (1) that provides a linear transformation is frequently employed as a mapping function.

$$Q(r) = \text{round}\left(\frac{r}{S} + Z\right)$$

In this case, the scaling factor (S) and zero-point (Z) are the quantization parameters. In quantized space, a 0 input translates to a 0 output, and the zero point works as a bias to achieve this. The scaling coefficient is just the ratio of the variety of inputs to the output range.

Evaluation Index

This research employed four popular performance metrics—Macro-precision, Macro-recall, accuracy, and F-Score—to confirm and assess the efficacy of the suggested approach. First, the arithmetic mean with all categories is computed, and then the precision for each class is represented by macro-precision. The recall for each class is represented by macrorecall, which is followed through the arithmetic mean for all categories. A measure of accuracy is the proportion of samples that were identified correctly relative to the overall amount of samples. Formulas (15)–(17) demonstrate how to get the precision, recall, and accuracy single category values from the confusion matrix:

$$\text{Precision} = \frac{TP}{TP + FP}$$

$$\text{Recall} = \frac{TP}{TP + FN}$$

$$\text{Accuracy} = \frac{TP + TN}{TP + TN + FP + FN}$$

True positives (TP), true negatives (TN), false positives (FP), and false negatives (FN) are the variables used here.

The F-Score is designed to take Macro-precision and Macro-recall into full consideration. As seen in Formula (18), it stands for the weighted harmonic mean of Macro-precision and Macro-recall:

$$\text{One- Score} = (1 + \beta^2)\frac{\text{Precision} \times \text{Recall}}{\beta^2 \times (\text{Precision} + \text{Recal})}$$

To get a suitable assessment measure and to balance the effects of recall and accuracy on the prediction outcomes, β is usually set to one, which is called F1 - Score.

7. CONCLUSIONS

The delivery of healthcare services to the constantly increasing older population is a significant problem for governments as well as healthcare authorities. It is not feasible for older people to visit hospitals every day to update physicians on their health and get recommendations. As a result, it provides a workable answer for both physicians and their senior patients. In this research, we surveyed the literature on the topic of effective RHMS development.

Current data sensing and gateway technologies, together with cutting-edge HAR systems, were examined. To get beyond cloud computing's drawbacks, including slow speeds, high latency, and excessive power consumption, our study delves into the advantages of Fog with mobile edge computing. A new computing architecture known as "fog computing" or "edge computing" has evolved for data processing analytics, with storage close to edge devices in real-time, as well as for sensors. Future research may benefit from the study's findings, which support the deployment of edge and fog computing to health applications for real-time actuator response.

To further emphasize their potential in healthcare, we also included promising current Remote Monitoring systems. Finally, we outlined and discussed the present obstacles to remote monitoring system development. Following this study, we want to tackle problems with idea drift in distributed fog health tracking models in our future work. Concept drift must be taken into account to guarantee the precision and dependability of health surveillance systems.

Finally, remote monitoring systems show great potential for meeting the healthcare requirements of older people. By using fog and edge computing, we can improve the quality of healthcare for older people and make health monitoring systems more efficient. This will allow for real-time reactions and improve the whole system.

REFERENCES

Ahmed, M., Hassan, H., Eldeeb, A., & Khattab, T. (2023). Towards Contactless Remote Health Monitoring using Ambient RF Sensing. *2023 21st Mediterranean Communication and Computer Networking Conference (MedComNet)*, 135–142.

Alam, S. (2023). Security concerns in smart agriculture and blockchain-based solution. *2022 OPJU International Technology Conference on Emerging Technologies for Sustainable Development (OTCON)*, 1–6. DOI: 10.1109/OTCON56053.2023.10113953

Alam, S., Bhatia, S., Shuaib, M., Khubrani, M. M., Alfayez, F., Malibari, A. A., & Ahmad, S. (2023). An overview of blockchain and IoT integration for secure and reliable health records monitoring. *Sustainability (Basel), 15*(7), 5660. DOI: 10.3390/su15075660

Bauder, C. J., Moadi, A.-K., Theilmann, P. T., & Fathy, A. E. (2023). Development of a multi-functional remote health monitoring system. *2023 International Microwave and Antenna Symposium (IMAS)*, 103–106. DOI: 10.1109/IMAS55807.2023.10066893

Bellino, F., Turvani, G., Garlando, U., & Riente, F. (2022). An integrated multi-sensor system for remote bee health monitoring. *2022 IEEE Workshop on Metrology for Agriculture and Forestry (MetroAgriFor)*, 334–338. DOI: 10.1109/MetroAgriFor55389.2022.9965130

Carter, D., Kolencik, J., & Cug, J. (2021). Smart internet of things-enabled mobile-based health monitoring systems and medical big data in COVID-19 telemedicine. *American Journal of Medical Research (New York, N.Y.), 8*(1), 20–29. DOI: 10.22381/ajmr8120212

Coman, L.-I., Ianculescu, M., Paraschiv, E.-A., Alexandru, A., & Bădărău, I.-A. (2024). Smart solutions for diet-related disease management: Connected care, remote health monitoring systems, and integrated insights for advanced evaluation. *Applied Sciences (Basel, Switzerland), 14*(6), 2351. DOI: 10.3390/app14062351

Dalloul, A. H., Miramirkhani, F., & Kouhalvandi, L. (2023). A review of recent innovations in remote health monitoring. *Micromachines, 14*(12), 2157. DOI: 10.3390/mi14122157 PMID: 38138326

Javed, H., Abaid, Z., Akbar, S., Ullah, K., Ahmad, A., Saeed, A., Ali, H., Ghadi, Y. Y., Alahmadi, T. J., Alkahtani, H. K., & Raza, A. (2023). Blockchain-based logging to defeat malicious insiders: The case of remote health monitoring systems. *IEEE Access : Practical Innovations, Open Solutions, 12*, 12062–12079. DOI: 10.1109/ACCESS.2023.3346432

Karmakar, K., Saif, S., Das, P., Neogy, S., & Biswas, S. (2022). FDRF: Fault detection and recovery framework for seamless data transmission in remote health monitoring using WBAN. *Wireless Personal Communications, 123*(1), 325–356. DOI: 10.1007/s11277-021-09134-3

Karthik, A., Hamatta, H. S. A., Patthi, S., Krubakaran, C., Pradhan, A. K., Rachapudi, V., Shuaib, M., & Rajaram, A. (2024). Ensemble-based multimodal medical imaging fusion for tumor segmentation. *Biomedical Signal Processing and Control, 96*, 106550. DOI: 10.1016/j.bspc.2024.106550

Karthik, A., Sahoo, S. K., Kumar, A., Patel, N., Chinnaraj, P., Maguluri, L. P., & Rajaram, A. (2025). Unified approach for accurate brain tumor Multi-Classification and segmentation through fusion of advanced methodologies. *Biomedical Signal Processing and Control*, *100*, 106872. DOI: 10.1016/j.bspc.2024.106872

Khubrani, M. M., & Alam, S. (2021). A detailed review of blockchain-based applications for protection against pandemic like COVID-19. *Telkomnika*, *19*(4), 1185–1196. DOI: 10.12928/telkomnika.v19i4.18465

LeBaron, V. (2022). Challenges and opportunities in designing and deploying remote health monitoring technology for older adults with cancer. *Innovation in Aging*, *6*(6), igac057. DOI: 10.1093/geroni/igac057 PMID: 36452048

Mirjalali, S., Peng, S., Fang, Z., Wang, C., & Wu, S. (2022). Wearable sensors for remote health monitoring: Potential applications for early diagnosis of Covid-19. *Advanced Materials Technologies*, *7*(1), 2100545. DOI: 10.1002/admt.202100545 PMID: 34901382

Peyroteo, M., Ferreira, I. A., Elvas, L. B., Ferreira, J. C., & Lapão, L. V. (2021). Remote monitoring systems for patients with chronic diseases in primary health care: Systematic review. *JMIR mHealth and uHealth*, *9*(12), e28285. DOI: 10.2196/28285 PMID: 34932000

Rehman, S. U., Usman, M., Toor, M. H. Y., & Hussaini, Q. A. (2024). Advancing structural health monitoring: A vibration-based IoT approach for remote real-time systems. *Sensors and Actuators. A, Physical*, *365*, 114863. DOI: 10.1016/j.sna.2023.114863

Schütz, N., Knobel, S. E. J., Botros, A., Single, M., Pais, B., Santschi, V., Gatica-Perez, D., Buluschek, P., Urwyler, P., Gerber, S. M., Müri, R. M., Mosimann, U. P., Saner, H., & Nef, T. (2022). A systems approach towards remote health-monitoring in older adults: Introducing a zero-interaction digital exhaust. *NPJ Digital Medicine*, *5*(1), 116. DOI: 10.1038/s41746-022-00657-y PMID: 35974156

Sharma, S. K., Rao, R. S., Singh, P., & Khan, S. A. (2022). Evaluation of VANETs routing protocols for data-based smart health monitoring in intelligent transportation systems. *International Journal of Mathematical. Engineering and Management Sciences*, *7*(2), 211.

Shuaib, M., Alam, S., & Reegu, F. A. (2023). Blockchain-based self-sovereign identity for COVID-19 medical passports and immunity certificates. *AIP Conference Proceedings*, *2587*(1), 070003. DOI: 10.1063/5.0150394

Singh, A., Joshi, K., Alam, S., Bharany, S., Shuaib, M., & Ahmad, S. (2022). Internet of Things-Based Integrated Remote Electronic Health Surveillance and Alert System: A Review. *2022 IEEE International Conference on Current Development in Engineering and Technology (CCET)*, 1–6. DOI: 10.1109/CCET56606.2022.10080629

Singh, B., & Kaunert, C. (2024). Integration of cutting-edge technologies such as internet of things (IoT) and 5G in health monitoring systems: A comprehensive legal analysis and futuristic outcomes. *GLS Law Journal*, *6*(1), 13–20. DOI: 10.69974/glslawjournal.v6i1.123

Singh, V. K., Bangari, N., Ali, Z., Vyas, A., Verma, R. K., & Saxena, A. (2023). Parachute shape ultra-wideband wearable antenna for remote health care monitoring. *International Journal of Communication Systems*, *36*(10), e5488. DOI: 10.1002/dac.5488

Chapter 7
The Role of Personalized Medicine and Internet of Things in Shaping Precision Healthcare

N. Mahesh Kumar
https://orcid.org/0009-0008-9509-245X
Dayanandasagar College of Engineering, India

T. R. Chenthil
https://orcid.org/0000-0001-9692-5195
Jeppiaar Engineering College, India

Nirmalkumar S. Benni
RNS Institute of Technology, India

S. Ramesh
SRM Institute of Science and Technology, India

G. Deepak
Global Academy of Technology, India

A. Rajaram
E.G.S. Pillay Engineering College, India

Mustafa Ali Khan
Compunnel Software Group Inc., USA

ABSTRACT

In order to encourage a healthy lifestyle, people should eat a balanced diet and work out in a way that is relevant to their needs and concerns. To help consumers easily gauge their health status without seeing a doctor, we provide a framework in this research that takes into account preexisting medical issues. The data set includes vitals measured by an Internet of Things (IoT) device, including heart rate (BPM), blood oxygen saturation (SpO2), body mass index (BMI), and core temperature. The data was cleaned and corrected using ML methods before analysis. Based on the data analysis, our framework proposes a healthy diet and regular exercise using a two-stage classifier method. This study use machine learning algorithms to examine datasets tailored to healthcare systems for adults. This investigation employs a variety of approaches, such as Random Forest, CatBoost classifier, Logistic Regression, and MLP classifier. We have also built an interactive online platform that makes it easier to engage using the framework that is in place, which improves accessibility and user experience.

DOI: 10.4018/979-8-3373-1022-0.ch007

1. INTRODUCTION

The term "Internet of Things" (IoT) refers to the network of interconnected computing devices that allow for various types of data transfer and interaction via multiple forms of network infrastructure. Many parts of our everyday lives now make use of IoT. One of the most popular uses of the IoT is in healthcare, where it enables the remote and ongoing surveillance of patients in hospitals or at home, allowing for the prompt provision of medical aid in an emergency. Data gathered from various health sensors and sent over wireless networks poses significant privacy and security risks for healthcare IoT applications (Alqahtani et al., 2023). Because medical sensor nodes have low computational capabilities, traditional security methods do not apply to healthcare IoT applications. Using cryptographic keys is essential for secure end-to-end communication. Additionally, before exchanging keys, make sure both parties have authenticated each other. For healthcare IoT networks to provide secured broadcast or multicast communication, a crucial feature is secure group key distribution (Reddy et al., 2024). There is little focus on group key negotiation in most existing protocols, but most do include pairwise key exchange for unicast communication (Singh et al., 2022).

Healthcare management is in charge of running a healthcare facility, whether it is a hospital, clinic, or other similar establishment (Bharany et al., 2023). A healthcare manager is someone who keeps an eye on the institute's finances, oversees the facility's people and material resources, and makes sure everything runs according to plan, all while keeping the facility's goal and vision in mind (Obijuru et al., 2024). On a daily basis, several healthcare institutions throughout the globe produce massive amounts of data. With the use of this medical facility data, valuable insights may be drawn, allowing the institution to thrive in terms of income, human relations, and technology. A potential goal of this research is to collect all of this information logically so that we can build process models that will lead us to a better understanding of how the medical staff and other stakeholders in the healthcare institution operate together.

Figure 1. Strategy for IoT Healthcare Systems

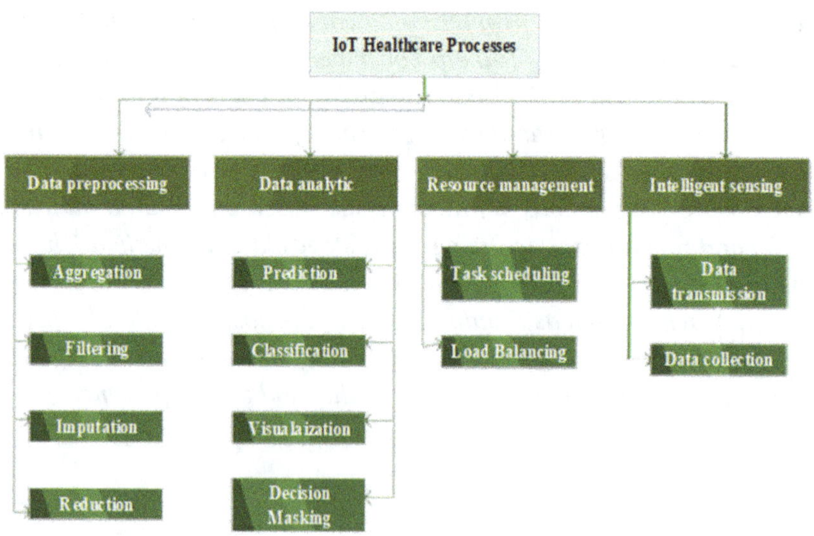

One of the primary goals of the Internet of Things (IoT)-based Framework for Personalised Health Evaluation and Recommendation utilizing Machine Learning techniques is to develop a system that can evaluate a person's health condition and deliver tailored suggestions based on that evaluation (Alam et al., 2023). Wearable sensors and health monitoring devices are only two examples of the Internet of Things (IoT) gadgets that this framework intends to use machine learning algorithms to examine (Matthews & Rhodes-Maquaire, 2024). This information allows the framework to determine a person's health status and provide tailored suggestions for how to improve it. The end objective is to make it possible to use real-time monitoring and analysis of data produced by the IoT to allow individualized healthcare actions. Utilizing machine learning algorithms, the IoT-based framework for customized health evaluation and recommendations analyzes data from IoT devices and provides individualized health recommendations. By using machine learning approaches, the system is able to extract pertinent characteristics from data collected from health monitoring devices and wearable sensors and then detect trends or abnormalities. This study is the basis for the framework's evaluation of an individual's health state, risk detection, and general well-being. In order to provide tailored suggestions, machine learning takes into account the outcomes of health assessments, as well as the patient's medical history, lifestyle choices, and personal preferences. In order to improve individual health outcomes, the framework learns and adapts continually, adjusting the suggestions according to user input.

Personalized health management, early disease detection and prevention, continuous condition monitoring, data-driven insights into individual health patterns, and improved efficiency and convenience in accessing personalized care are some of the potential benefits of an IoT-based framework (Kishor Kumar Reddy et al., 2025). The system gives personalized health evaluations and suggestions by combining machine learning with real-time data from the Internet of Things devices. This foresightful method allows for prompt intervention, encourages preventative actions, and gives people agency over their own health.

In order to sort and rank pertinent data, the recommendation system makes use of a number of criteria, some of which are user-supplied. The algorithm finds suitable matches between users and resources by looking at demographic information like age, gender, height, weight, body fat percentage, and personal preferences like whether they want to lose or gain weight. In order to provide tailored suggestions, the system also considers physiological parameters like core temperature, saturation of oxygen, and heart rate. Sensors are deployed to capture this data, which is subsequently compared with a vast database of information. Based on the data, the system proposes suitable food choices and diet regimens for the user.

The key contributions made in the article are as follows:

- Constructing an all-encompassing system that can analyze a person's current health status and then provide individualized suggestions for exercise and nutrition.
- Data is enhanced and balanced using machine learning algorithms before analysis of health parameters relating to different health indicators is performed.
- Two-stage classifiers trained using machine learning algorithms to assess health metrics and give dietary and activity recommendations.
- Building an engaging online environment that makes working with the framework a breeze.
- A focus on helping people lead healthier lives by recommending certain foods and exercise routines.

2 IMPORTANCE OF HEALTHCARE MANAGEMENT

Healthcare data management is the act of collecting, organizing, analyzing, and making sense of medical records from a wide variety of sources. Medical records provide a wealth of information that may be analyzed for summary purposes, such as patient diagnosis, therapy, and healthcare administration, using a systematic method. The subject matter of medical information presents several obstacles, even if the work seems straightforward at first. For many reasons, healthcare management of data is crucial:

- It facilitates directed engagement with patients and caregivers and helps model several stakeholders, including consumers, caretakers, and patients.
- It aids the medical facility in making crucial business choices that enhance the interaction with the many stakeholders associated with the medical facility.
- It's useful for hospitals and other medical centers to track and evaluate doctor, patient, and staff actions and then compare them to the institute's stated goals and objectives.
- We need a thorough understanding of the healthcare data in order to make larger-scale use of the healthcare system successfully. Here, we'll have a look at the characteristics of the healthcare data.

3 COMMON DATA SOURCES IN HEALTH CARE

In almost any healthcare system, you may find the following data sources (Heart et al., 2017).

- EMRs, or electronic medical records, are a computerized representation of a patient's paper medical record. Medical staff utilize it to document patient history, current status, planned treatments, etc. It is common practice for healthcare organizations to preserve electronic medical records digitally.
- EHRs, or electronic health records, are a trove of digital data pertaining to a patient's overall health. This data contains not just medical records but also information about the patient's treatment history from other healthcare providers, test results, etc. EHR essentially follows clients and is used among various healthcare practitioners as needed.
- This data is specific to information gathered by a subset of healthcare organizations' internal departments. While some departments do not need this data, it is essential for the operation of others.
- Administrative information—Healthcare management systems collect this data as they oversee the overall functioning of the healthcare setting. It provides valuable information for the upper administration of the institution. Optimization and use of data (human and non-human) is also part of it (Yadav et al., 2025).
- Financial data is usually kept in financial database systems in major firms, and this is confidential information.

Figure 2. Personalized Model for IoT Networks

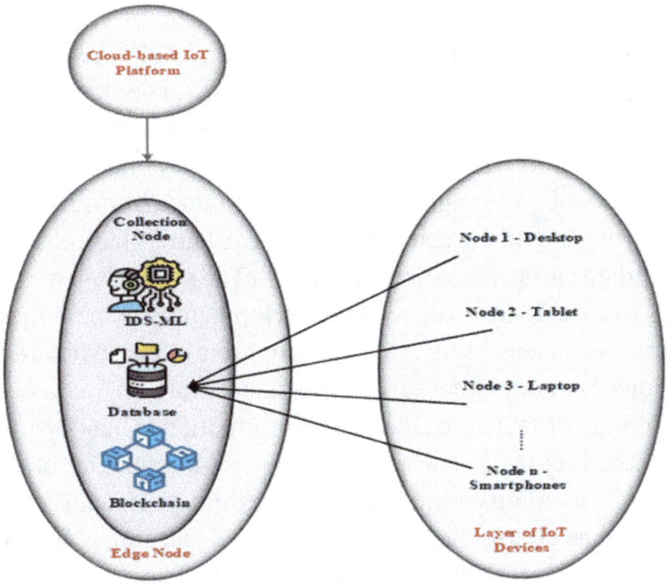

4. CURRENT METHODS FOR PERSONALIZED MEDICINE USING IOT

In order to conduct a comprehensive analysis of the prediction of liver disease stages, investigators used a dataset from Siksha 'O' Anusandhan University Medical Laboratory. That dataset had 6,780 samples obtained from 6,780 individuals, both manually and via IoT sensor sources. A thorough cleaning of the dataset was performed prior to its transmission to the machine learning process. To forecast the phases of liver illness, they used several machine learning models in Python, including Naïve Bayes, sequential minimum optimization, random forest, K-STAR, and multi-class classification. Their simulation results showed that the SMO model outperformed the competition. They continued by including more machine learning boosting techniques into their research, using SMO as the foundational model: AdaBoost, gradient boost, XGBoost, CatBoost, and LightGBM. Gradient boost surprised everyone by achieving an incredible 96% accuracy.

Reviewing the literature on the IoT and its healthcare applications and evaluating data from cases of IoT technology's deployment in personal healthcare are both qualitative and quantitative techniques used in the study (Erlinawati et al., 2024). Remote patient condition monitoring, data-driven illness prediction, personalized treatment modification, and healthcare system cost efficiency are just a few of the ways that the study's findings highlight the enormous potential of IoT applications to enhance personal healthcare. System security, security of information, and cross-platform integration are some of the obstacles that must be addressed in order to fully realize the advantages of using IoT technology (Kaza et al., 2024). That research found that the use of IoT in healthcare will lead to future-tailored healthcare that is more effective and efficient. To be effective, these apps must overcome technological, ethical, and security problems. In order to guarantee better individualized healthcare in the future, it is important to have a deeper grasp of the pros and cons of using the IoT in healthcare.

Personalized healthcare is made possible by technology, which improves health outcomes and provides tailored treatment and intervention measures (Ramalingam et al., 2024). Predicting future health problems and constantly monitoring people's health statuses is a challenge for contemporary healthcare. Checkups and manual data entry are commonplace in traditional medicine, but they may not be adequate to catch minor health problems or respond to crises. In order to significantly enhance patient care, it is necessary to review the massive amounts of patient-generated medical information in a trustworthy and efficient manner. Together, ML algorithms and the Internet of Medical Things have the potential to revolutionize healthcare and set new standards for personalized treatment. The system's goal is to unite healthcare, ML, and the Internet of Things in order to investigate new developments in illness monitoring and prediction. Metrics such as recall, error rate, sensitivity, and F-score are used to evaluate the efficacy of the ML model that is integrated into the model; these parameters constitute the main outcome parameter of the research (Khan et al., 2024b). In order to provide useful information to healthcare practitioners, they may use these factors to assess the accuracy, efficacy, and temporal complexity of the model's predictions.

Research conducted in a developing nation found that 56 third-year medical students were enrolled in a preclinical Doctor of Medicine course that used an IoT-based learning platform. Students participated in dynamic, experiential learning activities that mimicked clinical practice in an IoT-enabled classroom. In sum, medical education has been transformed into something far more successful, interesting, and student-centered via the implementation of IoT. Sharing that technique early on in the development process is a novel endeavor that might generate interest in using that strategy and pave the way for more development (Mastour et al., 2025).

Using an altered capsule neural network with multicenter mammography, the authors of that paper provide a new framework they name MLT-UniCaps (Wang et al., 2022). In order to achieve an intelligent remote assistant diagnosis, the suggested MLT-UniCaps combines Attentional Pose Embedding, Dynamic Source Capsule Traversal with Adaptive Target Capsule Fusion. By using an adversarial convolutional neural network along with an attention-based layer, Attentional Pose Embedding recovers feature vectors from postures that vary in location, orientation, size, and illumination. In order to construct source cancer classifiers for single-center mammography screening, Dynamic Source Capsule Traversal uses a dynamic routing method between neurons based on the posture presentation. Adaptive Target Capsule Fusion maximizes the transformation-likelihood of the heterogeneous distribution across the mammography centers and uses the source cancer classifier to integrate them as universal cancer detectors. Because of these three factors, MLT-UniCaps is able to enhance the outcomes of breast cancer screenings conducted at single centers and to contribute to the detection of breast cancers conducted at several centers. The suggested MLT-UniCaps achieves 90.1% overall classification precision on single-center trials with 73.8% overall F1 ranking on multicenter trials, according to thorough studies conducted on 58,965 samples.

The use and use of AI methodology in several healthcare domains is covered in the study of AI for IoT with medical systems (Oniani et al., 2020). Research into medical applications of artificial intelligence has uncovered four primary domains: the detection of cardiovascular illness, prediction approaches, robotic surgery, and individualized treatment plans. We can see from the findings that the top artificial intelligence techniques are k-nearest neighbors, SVM, SVR, linear regression, regression tree, Naïve Bayes, classification tree, and random forest. In order to better patients' health, these approaches are mostly used to analyze their data. There are a number of benefits to using robotic surgery systems like the Automated Endoscopic System for Optimal Positioning and Transoral Robotic Surgery. These approaches provide less invasive treatments with better outcomes in terms of blood loss and speedier recovery. Diabetes, critical biophysical parameter monitoring, and medical decision-making support systems are just a few of the many health issues that the Internet of Medical Things aims to solve.

An examination of the IoT in healthcare has been conducted in (Veeraiah et al., 2022), with a particular emphasis on its application to the dynamic field of customized medicine. It addresses both everyday medical situations and state-of-the-art, complex approaches derived from the IoT. It brings to light the ethical, scientific, and financial obstacles to creating a more effective healthcare system for early disease diagnosis. Finally, the IoT is enabling modern medicine to respond quickly to current needs by establishing a communication platform across many health sectors, offering digital assistance at every level, etc.

Patients with Parkinson's disease can now benefit from personalized medicine in addition to symptomatic treatment through the use of passive (through IoT devices) and active (through mobile app) patient monitoring and evaluation, as outlined in the design of an EHR-agnostic clinical decision support system (Gatsios et al., 2021). The most important design principles include well-defined shared decision-making, flexibility to address variations among clinicians, and integration of knowledge and data from various sources. These principles rely on current research on CDSS, the results of recent studies monitoring m-health for PD, and an evaluation of user needs. An outline of the platform's components and a presentation of the functional and dashboard requirements for the CDSS are included.

Article (Aileni et al., 2020)discusses several facets of the IoT and communication technology synergy for healthcare remote services, particularly for patients with greater risks who need remote monitoring. Study after study by STATISTICA predicts that the number of IoT devices will increase from 26.66 billion in 2018 to around 75.44 billion in 2025, with a quarter of all cyberattacks aimed at these devices. Considering the potential dangers to data security posed by these applications, a number of scenarios regarding the use of 5G and IoT-based communications services are taking shape inside the new framework of customized medicine. Because of the strong direct association between securities and high-power computing, low-power computing may introduce new cybersecurity vulnerabilities.

A unique integration of the IoT along with big data analytics technologies, the intelligent, interconnected healthcare system, is introduced in (Abatal et al., 2024). Its purpose is to transform proactive and customized healthcare. With the help of IIHS, a steady flow of complete healthcare data may be created by integrating real-time data from a variety of devices, environmental sensors, and hospital equipment. Using cutting-edge data analysis, IIHS provides practical insights for continuous patient health surveillance, trend prediction with machine learning, and easy access to information with a user-friendly interface (Singh et al., 2025). That system's design improves data management efficiency and security by combining centralized cloud storage with edge storage at healthcare institutions. Two hospitals have shown that IIHS is beneficial by reporting a considerable decrease in patient readmission rates and duration of stay. That indicates that the technology can work well with current healthcare systems and can enhance patient care. As a scalable, patient-centric system that bolsters the continuous shift towards data-driven healthcare, IIHS embodies the future of digital and customized medicine (Khubrani & Alam, 2021).

5. METHODOLOGY

The study's methodology, including its design, data gathering processes, algorithms, and statistical analysis methods, are described in depth in this part. To help other researchers confirm the results and conduct their studies, we also provide a detailed account of the steps used to accomplish the research goals.

Figure 3. Healthcare Parameters Using IoT

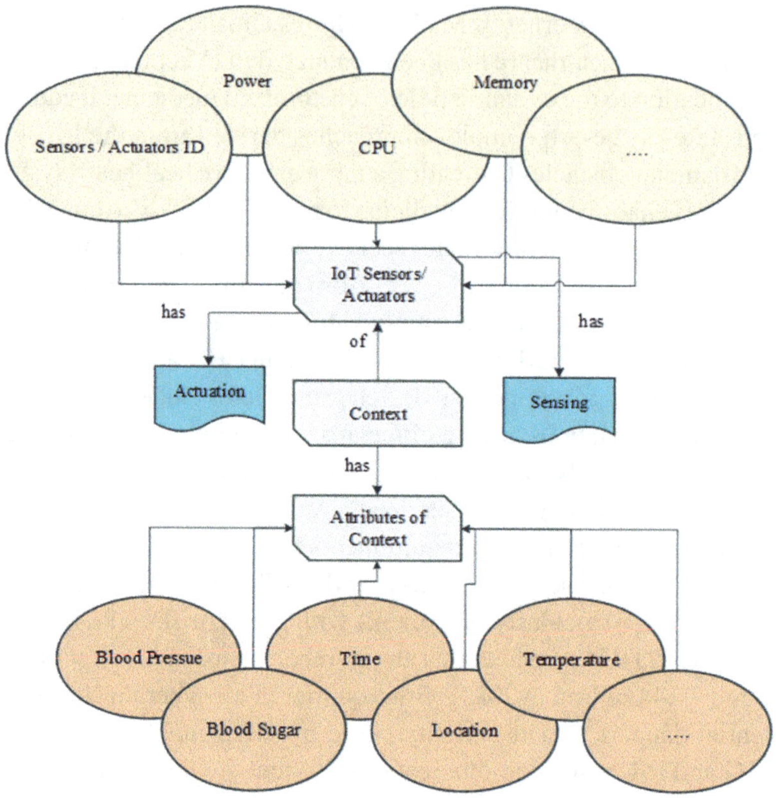

5.1. IoT Sensor Parameters

It is crucial to always keep an eye on adults' vital signs. It is more important than ever to monitor our physical health and make the required changes to our routines in light of the rising prevalence of chronic illnesses and sedentary lifestyles (Karthik et al., 2025). When evaluating health problems, it is essential to take the following into account.

5.1.1. Heart Rate

The frequency at which the heart contracts and relaxes is called the pulse rate or heart rate. The average adult heart rate, as reported by the American Heart Association (AHA), is 60 to 100 beats per minute (bpm). However, a person's pulse rate may be affected by several things, including their age, smoking habits, level of physical fitness, ambient temperature, mental state, medications they take, body size, and dimensions (Maguluri et al., 2024). Standard heart rates may also vary across sexes. Tachycardia, in which the heart rate is faster than 100 beats per minute, may be brought on by a number of things, such as being under a lot of stress, drinking too much alcohol, having high blood pressure, having hyperthyroidism, having poor blood flow, or having an electrolyte imbalance. In the framework of the Internet of Health

Things, a study delves into the most recent findings about online monitoring, detection, and diagnostic assistance for cardiovascular disorders using heart rate data (Kalaivani et al., 2023).

5.1.2. Oxygen Level

Using an oximeter, one may measure the blood oxygen level, which is also called SpO2. In adults, a normal range is usually between 95% and 100% saturation, or 80 and 100 mm Hg. Heart disease, COPD, and bronchial asthma are among the underlying diseases that abnormal oxygen levels might indicate. To control chronic illnesses and enhance general health, a healthy diet, and regular exercise are essential. Symptoms of hypoxemia, in which the blood oxygen level drops below normal, include difficulty breathing, chest discomfort, disorientation, headache, and irregular pulse.

5.1.3. Temperature

While a temperature of 98.6 degrees Fahrenheit (37 degrees Celsius) is generally thought to be the normal range, little deviations from this mark do not always point to disease. Body temperature is affected by a number of things, such as gender, age, activity level, and the time of day. Even among healthy people, there may be noticeable temperature variation, with daily averages ranging from 0.25 to 0.5 °C. The American College of Critical Care Medicine defines fever as a temperature of 100.9 °F (38.3 °C) or above.

5.1.4. Body Mass Index (BMI)

A person's body mass index (BMI) is a measure of their fat mass that is calculated by dividing their weight (in kilograms or pounds) by their height (in meters squared or feet). It is not possible to determine a person's health or body fat using their BMI alone; however, a high BMI may suggest a high level of body fat. But it may show you which weight groups are most likely to cause health issues. Cut down on calories, but that's not all you need to lose weight.

5.2 Machine Learning

Building a machine learning algorithm into the thermal therapy framework opens up new possibilities for health parameter prediction analysis. Algorithms like this may analyze both past and present data to deduce patterns and predict future health hazards, including cardiac issues detected by heart rate monitors or exercise.

Figure 4. AI Method and Algorithms (Machine learning and Deep learning)

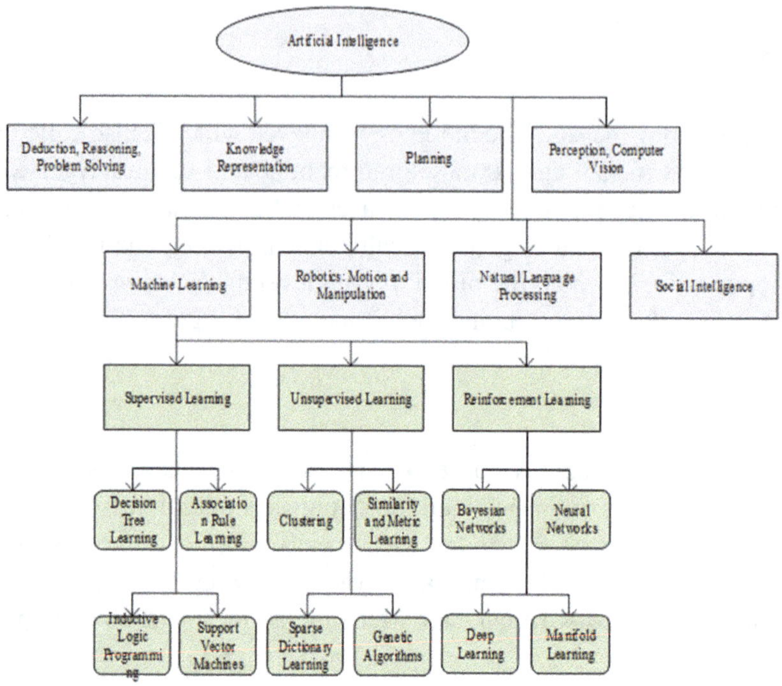

Customizing thermal treatment courses also benefits significantly from artificial intelligence (AI), which may maximize therapeutic results by suggesting alterations based on patient variables. Artificial intelligence may detect the first signs of emerging ailments, including musculoskeletal or neurological disorders, by evaluating data pertaining to rest and physical activity (Chinthala et al., 2022). When it comes to addressing any unfavorable consequences and implementing preventative measures, this competence is crucial. This feature's incorporation into our system allows it to aid healthcare practitioners in their daily operations by recommending the best course of patient management and classifying patients according to their level of medical need. Critical to their success is AI and ML's capacity to learn from the data they acquire and enhance their performance thereafter. This technology streamlines the supply of thermal services to patients' homes and improves The communication of our solution inside telemedicine infrastructures. It also helps patients and doctors work together more effectively. Through the detection and countermeasure of illegal access or aberrant data consultation paths, AI helps to improve security and privacy assurances, which are important elements. Another advantage of AI systems is their ability to react to patients' requirements via mobile apps. These apps may guide good living choices and autonomously handle health concerns depending on discovered data. As a whole, medicinal procedures are enhanced when AI and ML are integrated into these fields. The healthcare system becomes increasingly more connected, coordinated, and responsive to each patient's demands as a result of the patient's perspective and support of their providers expanding.

- *CatBoost:* The CatBoost method is an ML framework based on gradient-boosted decision trees. The method trains by constructing a succession of decision trees sequentially, with the goal of minimizing loss as built. The default values dictate how many trees are to be built. Among CatBoost's many healthcare applications are the prediction of illness outcomes and the identification of people at high risk for specific disorders. Furthermore, it may be used in combination with data on food and physical activity to provide tailored suggestions to persons seeking to enhance their well-being. With the use of a patient's health metrics and lifestyle variables, CatBoost may recommend dietary and activity adjustments that can significantly improve their health and well-being. The capacity of the CatBoost algorithm to streamline and make the process of constructing models is one of its most striking features. It is very uncommon for categorical feature conversion into a numerical format to be a challenging undertaking when working with datasets. Using CatBoost in these cases may make building the learning model much easier. Furthermore, compared to other machine learning algorithms, CatBoost's speed is unmatched. In addition, it should provide operations that are both efficient and speedier, regardless of whether they are run on a CPU or GPU.

- *Logistic Regression:* Forecasting the likelihood of binary outcomes, such as a patient's likelihood of developing a certain ailment, is a common use case for Logistic Regression in healthcare applications. The method is straightforward to understand and use, but it packs a significant punch. It is simple to make decisions based on the anticipated probability since this method uses the logistic function, which transfers every input value to a value of probability between 0 and 1. Diet recommendation systems may employ logistic regression to help patients get the most out of their food and exercise regimens by estimating the probability that they will be overweight or obese.
- *Random Forest:* To improve the accuracy of its predictions, the potent machine-learning program RF employs a network of decision trees. The total accuracy of the model may be improved by combining the predictions of many decision trees. Several healthcare applications have found success with this technology, including illness diagnostic prediction and the identification of risk factors for specific health disorders. Medical practitioners are able to assess each patient's individual needs better and develop individualized treatment programs with the use of RF. RF has also used individuals' health data to provide food suggestions. With the use of RF, people may keep up a healthy lifestyle by assessing their body temperature and body mass index (BMI) and then getting personalized recommendations for food and exercise (Khan et al., 2024a).
- *MLP:* Multi-layer perceptrons (MLPs) are a kind of feed-forward artificial neural network that takes in data in a variety of forms and outputs a predetermined set of results. What sets multi-layer perforation (MLP) models apart from others is the directed network that links the input nodes of the previous layers to the ones that contain the outputs.

5.3 Mobile APP Integration

An important step in providing better, more comfortable treatment for patients has been creating a mobile app that works in tandem with the state-of-the-art thermal monitoring system. Consciously and interactively empowering patients to take charge of their health care, this new app is a natural progression from our diagnostic tools and has an intuitive and engaging user experience. By using the app, our patients may get personalized consultations that are crafted using data gathered from their sensors, as well as information about their interactions and lifestyle habits. So, for instance, if the patient has mentioned feeling more stressed, they may provide tailored advice on how to relax and improve their overall health. Users are also given the chance to accomplish and manage their own health objectives inside the software, such as enhancing their sleep environment or decreasing stress levels. A system-based feedback approach that motivates patients to adhere to or make necessary adjustments to their regimens may bolster these objectives. Mood, discomfort, dietary choices, and hydration status are some of the other data that may be entered into the app. Going beyond the basic characteristics obtained separately by the sensing devices, this gives a far better and more comprehensive picture of the subject's health status. The app's reporting and notification features are also crucial, as they allow for the prompt transmission of notifications in the event that the patient's safety parameters exhibit any irregularities or in order to remind the patient of upcoming treatments and medical tests. The interface has been thoughtfully designed to be user-friendly for all types of users. It includes both visual and grammatical explanations to make the program easy to understand and use. You can see the subject's current schedule as well as their forthcoming treatments for the current month in a portion of the app that is connected to their therapy program. Other screens in the app let you integrate the subject's data with information about the medical course they are going to pursue. With the thermal management system and this app working in tandem, data may flow directly and continuously between the wearables and the app. In order to provide real-time insights and comments, the gathered data is readily available in a dedicated area of the app. Not only are all the monitoring system's metrics shown and reported in the real-time and day-by-day format in that part, but users can also see the trend discovered in terms of frequency from the last week or months.

5.4 Diet and Fitness Recommendation

Using HTML and the Flask web framework, we built a fitness and nutrition app that can track your progress in real-time. When hit, the app's front-end request button will trigger the sensor to provide the app with real-time data 10 seconds later. According to the app's interpretation of the sensor's digital output, users are categorized as fit, medium-risk, or high-risk and then given dietary and activity recommendations. In a Jupyter Notebook, the Flask web framework generates a local host by storing the sensor data as a list and using pickle files. In this procedure, we use the Catboost classifier, which is known for its greatest accuracy, to create a tailored workout and nutrition plan.

6. PERFORMANCE STANDARDS

When it comes to healthcare applications of machine learning, performance metrics like recall, accuracy, precision, and F1 score are essential. A model's ability to forecast outcomes, diagnose illnesses, and suggest treatments may be assessed using these metrics. Accurate forecasts and diagnoses are of the utmost importance in healthcare, where mistakes may have devastating effects.

- Accuracy: the ratio of correct positive results to the sum of all possible results, including both true and false negatives
- Recall: We recall this as the percentage of correct guesses to total predictions.
- F1 score: This statistic takes Precision and Recall into consideration and combines them into a single number between zero and one.
- Precision: Fourth, precision, or the ratio of correct forecasts to total predictions.

7. CONCLUSION

To guarantee excellent medical care at a fraction of the cost that hospitals or assisted living facilities presently pay, smart healthcare offers a safe, effective, and simply deployable health monitoring system. Modern wearables and cellphones for vitals monitoring, AI for the diagnosis of three major illnesses (COVID-19, cardiovascular disease, and diabetes), and frameworks created to support individuals in ambient assisted living settings were briefly covered in this study. Briefly, this evaluation demonstrates the software integration platforms that are quite important for developing smart healthcare. We have weighed the pros and cons of several methods. We also covered the key issues with newly created smart healthcare frameworks, which are the biggest roadblocks to creating helpful prototypes. To further enhance the current healthcare system, several possible avenues for future study are suggested. Tech couldn't possibly take over healthcare as a whole, but it may ease the workload of doctors and nurses by implementing new systems. When researchers and medical professionals collaborate on a platform, the creation of such assistive devices becomes a realistic possibility.

REFERENCES

Abatal, A., Mzili, M., Mzili, T., Cherrat, K., Yassine, A., & Abualigah, L. (2024). Intelligent Interconnected Healthcare System: Integrating IoT and Big Data for Personalized Patient Care. *International Journal of Online & Biomedical Engineering*, *20*(11), 46–65. DOI: 10.3991/ijoe.v20i11.49893

Aileni, R. M., Suciu, G., Valderrama Sukuyama, C. A., & Pasca, S. (2020). Internet of Things and communication technology synergy for remote services in healthcare. *IoT and ICT for Healthcare Applications*, 59–82.

Alam, S., Jasim Mohammad, O. K., Alfurhood, B. S., Saxena, K. K., Anand, M., Mahaveerakannan, R., & Savitha, V. (2023). Effective sound detection system in commercial car vehicles using Msp430 launchpad development. *Multimedia Tools and Applications*. Advance online publication. DOI: 10.1007/s11042-023-15373-2

Alqahtani, N., Alam, S., Aqeel, I., Shuaib, M., Mohsen Khormi, I., Khan, S. B., & Malibari, A. A. (2023). Deep belief networks (DBN) with IoT-based Alzheimer's disease detection and classification. *Applied Sciences (Basel, Switzerland)*, *13*(13), 7833. DOI: 10.3390/app13137833

Bharany, S., Alam, S., Shuaib, M., & Talwar, B. (2023). *Sentiment Analysis of Twitter Data for COVID-19 Posts BT - Data Intelligence and Cognitive Informatics* (I. J. Jacob, S. Kolandapalayam Shanmugam, & I. Izonin, Eds.; pp. 457–466). Springer Nature Singapore.

Chinthala, K. K. R., Thakur, M. S., Shuaib, M., & Alam, S. (2022). Prospects of Computational Intelligence in Society: Human-Centric Solutions, Challenges, and Research Areas. *Journal of Computational and Cognitive Engineering*.

Erlinawati, N. D., Anurogo, D., Hasyim, D. M., & Ardi, A. (2024). Application of the Internet of Things (IoT) in Health: The Future of Personal Care. *Journal of World Future Medicine. Health and Nursing*, *2*(1), 79–92. PMID: 38291421

Gatsios, D., Rigas, G., & Konitsiotis, S. (2021). Design of a clinical decision support system powered by mhealth for the management of Parkinson's disease. *2021 6th South-East Europe Design Automation, Computer Engineering,Computer Networks and Social Media Conference (SEEDA-CECNSM)*, 1–4.

Heart, T., Ben-Assuli, O., & Shabtai, I. (2017). A review of PHR, EMR and EHR integration: A more personalized healthcare and public health policy. *Health Policy and Technology*, *6*(1), 20–25. DOI: 10.1016/j.hlpt.2016.08.002

Kalaivani, K., Kshirsagarr, P. R., Sirisha Devi, J., Bandela, S. R., Colak, I., Nageswara Rao, J., & Rajaram, A. (2023). Prediction of biomedical signals using deep learning techniques. *Journal of Intelligent & Fuzzy Systems*, *44*(6), 9769–9782. DOI: 10.3233/JIFS-230399

Karthik, A., Sahoo, S. K., Kumar, A., Patel, N., Chinnaraj, P., Maguluri, L. P., & Rajaram, A. (2025). Unified approach for accurate brain tumor Multi-Classification and segmentation through fusion of advanced methodologies. *Biomedical Signal Processing and Control*, *100*, 106872. DOI: 10.1016/j.bspc.2024.106872

Kaza, V. S., Alamer, A., Alam, S., Shuaib, M., Basudan, S., & Sheneamer, A. (2024). Detecting and forecasting cryptojacking attack trends in Internet of Things and wireless sensor networks devices. *PeerJ. Computer Science, 10*, e2491. DOI: 10.7717/peerj-cs.2491 PMID: 39650421

Khan, A., Zubair, S., Shuaib, M., Sheneamer, A., Alam, S., & Assiri, B. (2024a). Development of a robust parallel and multi-composite machine learning model for improved diagnosis of Alzheimer's disease: Correlation with dementia-associated drug usage and AT (N) protein biomarkers. *Frontiers in Neuroscience, 18*, 1391465. DOI: 10.3389/fnins.2024.1391465 PMID: 39308946

Khan, A., Zubair, S., Shuaib, M., Sheneamer, A. A. M., Alam, S., & Assiri, B. (2024b). Development of a robust parallel and multi-composite machine learning model for improved diagnosis of Alzheimer's disease: Correlation with dementia-associated drug usage and AT (N) protein biomarkers. *Frontiers in Neuroscience, 18*, 1391465. DOI: 10.3389/fnins.2024.1391465 PMID: 39308946

Khubrani, M. M., & Alam, S. (2021). A detailed review of blockchain-based applications for protection against pandemic like COVID-19. *Telkomnika, 19*(4), 1185–1196. DOI: 10.12928/telkomnika.v19i4.18465

Kishor Kumar Reddy, C., Kaza, V. S., Madana Mohana, R., Alhameed, M., Jeribi, F., Alam, S., & Shuaib, M. (2025). Detecting anomalies in smart wearables for hypertension: A deep learning mechanism. *Frontiers in Public Health, 12*, 1426168. DOI: 10.3389/fpubh.2024.1426168 PMID: 39850864

Maguluri, L. P., Chouhan, K., Balamurali, R., Rani, R., Hashmi, A., Kiran, A., & Rajaram, A. (2024). Adversarial deep learning for improved abdominal organ segmentation in CT scans. *Multimedia Tools and Applications, 83*(35), 82107–82129. DOI: 10.1007/s11042-024-18578-1

Mastour, H., Khoshgoftar, Z., Ahmady, S., & Sohrabi, S. (2025). Implementing an Internet of Things-based learning platform into medical education: Addressing educational challenges with innovative solutions. *Medical Teacher*, •••, 1–4. DOI: 10.1080/0142159X.2024.2445036 PMID: 39773016

Matthews, P., & Rhodes-Maquaire, C. (2024). Personalisation and Recommendation for Mental Health Apps: A Scoping Review. *Behaviour & Information Technology*, •••, 1–16. DOI: 10.1080/0144929X.2024.2356630

Obijuru, A., Arowoogun, J. O., Onwumere, C., Odilibe, I. P., Anyanwu, E. C., & Daraojimba, A. I. (2024). Big data analytics in healthcare: A review of recent advances and potential for personalized medicine. *International Medical Science Research Journal, 4*(2), 170–182. DOI: 10.51594/imsrj.v4i2.810

Oniani, S., Marques, G., Barnovi, S., Pires, I. M., & Bhoi, A. K. (2020). Artificial intelligence for internet of things and enhanced medical systems. In *Bio-inspired neurocomputing* (pp. 43–59). Springer.

Ramalingam, S., Dharani, S. P., Priya, R., Devi, E. P., & Pavithra, S. (2024). Machine Learning Based Remote Health Care Data Monitoring and Prediction System Using IoMT. *2024 10th International Conference on Advanced Computing and Communication Systems (ICACCS), 1*, 2113–2118.

Reddy, K. K., Badam, R., Alam, S., & Shuaib, M. (2024). IoT-driven accessibility: A refreshable OCR-Braille solution for visually impaired and deaf-blind users through WSN. *Journal of Economy and Technology, 2*, 128–137. DOI: 10.1016/j.ject.2024.04.007

Singh, A., Joshi, K., Alam, S., Bharany, S., Shuaib, M., & Ahmad, S. (2022). Internet of Things-Based Integrated Remote Electronic Health Surveillance and Alert System: A Review. *2022 IEEE International Conference on Current Development in Engineering and Technology (CCET)*, 1–6. DOI: 10.1109/CCET56606.2022.10080629

Singh, A., Nagabhooshanam, N., Kumar, R., Verma, R., Mohanasundaram, S., Manjith, R., & Rajaram, A. (2025). Deep learning based coronary artery disease detection and segmentation using ultrasound imaging with adaptive gated SCNN models. *Biomedical Signal Processing and Control*, *105*, 107637. DOI: 10.1016/j.bspc.2025.107637

Veeraiah, V., Kumar, G. K. R., Singh, D. P., Chaudhary, A., Elkady, G., & Ross, D. S. (2022). A Descriptive Research on Internet of Things Implementation in Healthcare Sector. *2022 5th International Conference on Contemporary Computing and Informatics (IC3I)*, 308–312.

Wang, B., Hu, X., Zhang, J., Xu, C., & Gao, Z. (2022). Intelligent Internet of Things in mammography screening using multicenter transformation between unified capsules. *IEEE Internet of Things Journal*, *10*(2), 1536–1545. DOI: 10.1109/JIOT.2022.3209895

Yadav, G., Ubaidullah Bokhari, M., Alzahrani, S. I. I., Alam, S., Shuaib, M., Bokhari, M. U., Alzahrani, S. I. I., Alam, S., Shuaib, M., Ubaidullah Bokhari, M., Alzahrani, S. I. I., Alam, S., & Shuaib, M. (2025). Emotion-Aware Ensemble Learning (EAEL): Revolutionizing Mental Health Diagnosis of Corporate Professionals via Intelligent Integration of Multi-Modal Data Sources and Ensemble Techniques. *IEEE Access : Practical Innovations, Open Solutions*, *13*, 11494–11516. DOI: 10.1109/ACCESS.2025.3529032

Chapter 8
AI-Driven Operational Improvements in Healthcare

Ushaa Eswaran
https://orcid.org/0000-0002-5116-3403
Mahalakshmi Tech Campus, India

Vivek Eswaran
https://orcid.org/0009-0002-7475-2398
Medallia, India

Vishal Eswaran
https://orcid.org/0009-0000-2187-3108
CVS Health Centre, USA

Keerthna Murali
https://orcid.org/0009-0009-1419-4268
Dell, USA

ABSTRACT

Artificial Intelligence (AI) is transforming healthcare by improving clinical outcomes and enhancing operational efficiencies. AI technologies like machine learning (ML), natural language processing (NLP), and predictive analytics streamline processes, optimize resource management, and improve decision-making. These advancements impact areas such as patient scheduling, resource allocation, supply chain management, and clinical workflows, reducing human error and costs. This chapter explores AI's role in operational improvements, the challenges in adoption, and its potential to reshape healthcare systems, with a focus on ethical standards, data security, and workforce adaptability.

DOI: 10.4018/979-8-3373-1022-0.ch008

1. INTRODUCTION

1.1.Overview of AI in Healthcare

Artificial Intelligence (AI) has dramatically transformed the healthcare industry by enhancing both clinical outcomes and operational efficiency. Techniques such as machine learning (ML), natural language processing (NLP), and robotics are now being widely used across healthcare processes, from diagnostics to resource management. AI enables healthcare systems to analyze vast amounts of data, make data-driven decisions, and automate routine tasks, contributing to more accurate diagnoses, optimized resource use, and improved patient care.

1.2.The Role of AI in Operational Improvements within Healthcare Settings

AI is crucial in optimizing healthcare operations, particularly by automating administrative tasks, improving resource allocation, enhancing decision-making, and streamlining clinical workflows (Maleki Varnosfaderani, S,et.al,2024). By integrating AI into healthcare systems, organizations can address operational inefficiencies such as scheduling delays, supply chain disruptions, and inefficient clinical workflows. For example, AI systems can predict patient admissions, optimize bed and staff allocation, and assist in reducing administrative burdens, allowing healthcare providers to focus more on patient care.

1.3.Objectives and Scope of the Chapter

The primary aim of this chapter is to explore how AI-driven technologies are being used to improve operational efficiencies in healthcare settings. The chapter will address the various ways in which AI is implemented, such as in patient scheduling, resource management, supply chain optimization, and clinical workflow improvements. It will also delve into the challenges of AI adoption, including concerns about data privacy, workforce adaptation, and system integration. Additionally, the chapter will discuss the future potential of AI in healthcare and the ethical considerations that must be taken into account when integrating AI into healthcare operations. Table 1 discusses the AI Technologies in Healthcare Operations

Table 1. AI Technologies in Healthcare Operations

AI Technology	Application in Healthcare	Operational Benefits
Machine Learning (ML)	Predictive analytics for patient outcomes, diagnostics, and resource allocation	- Improved accuracy in patient diagnosis and treatment planning
	Real-time predictions for hospital admissions, equipment needs, and staffing	- More effective use of hospital resources
Natural Language Processing (NLP)	Automating clinical note-taking, patient documentation, and communication	- Faster and more accurate documentation
	Analyzing medical texts for clinical insights and automated reporting	- Reduced clinician workload and faster data retrieval for decision-making
Robotics (AI-powered)	Surgical assistance, hospital logistics, and automating administrative tasks	- Increased precision in surgeries; more efficient hospital operations

continued on following page

Table 1. Continued

AI Technology	Application in Healthcare	Operational Benefits
Predictive Analytics	Predicting disease outbreaks, patient readmission, and staffing needs	- Proactive management of patient care and resource allocation
Robotic Process Automation (RPA)	Automating routine administrative processes like billing and claims processing	- Reduced administrative overhead and minimized human errors
AI in Clinical Decision Support (CDS)	Assisting clinicians with diagnostic and treatment recommendations	- More timely, accurate, and personalized clinical decisions
AI-powered Chatbots/Virtual Assistants	Enhancing patient engagement, appointment reminders, and follow-up care	- Improved patient satisfaction through efficient communication and personalized care
AI in Supply Chain Management	Predicting inventory needs and managing medical supplies	- Reduced waste, stockouts, and overstocking, leading to cost savings and better resource management

AI-driven technologies are revolutionizing operational processes in healthcare, making systems more efficient and responsive. From predictive analytics to resource management, AI is enabling hospitals and healthcare providers to optimize operations, enhance clinical decision-making, and improve patient care. However, the successful integration of AI requires addressing challenges such as data privacy, ethical concerns, and workforce readiness. As AI adoption in healthcare grows, it is important to ensure that these technologies are implemented responsibly, with an emphasis on equity, transparency, and accountability.

2. UNDERSTANDING AI TECHNOLOGIES IN HEALTHCARE OPERATIONS

2.1.Machine Learning (ML)

Machine Learning (ML) is one of the most powerful AI technologies utilized in healthcare for optimizing various processes, such as resource management, predicting patient outcomes, and improving patient care coordination. ML models are designed to learn from large datasets by identifying complex patterns and generating insights that can aid in decision-making. These models use historical and real-time data to predict patient health trends, anticipate demand for healthcare services, and optimize staffing levels based on predicted patient volumes. ML can also enhance clinical workflows by recommending personalized treatment plans based on a patient's medical history, current conditions, and genetic information.

For example, in a hospital setting, ML can be used to predict patient admissions, discharge times, and the need for ICU beds, enabling better resource allocation (Awasthy, R., Malhotra, M., Seavers, M. L., & Newman, M. 2024). In diagnostics, ML algorithms have been successfully employed to analyze medical imaging (e.g., radiology scans) for signs of diseases like cancer, thus improving diagnostic accuracy and reducing the time taken to identify critical conditions. Additionally, ML can be used to streamline the patient journey by identifying bottlenecks in care processes and recommending interventions to reduce waiting times, improve patient flow, and enhance overall healthcare delivery.

2.2.Natural Language Processing (NLP)

Natural Language Processing (NLP) is a subfield of AI that focuses on the interaction between computers and human language, enabling computers to process and understand vast amounts of unstructured textual data in healthcare. The data often comes in the form of clinical notes, medical literature, patient feedback, and electronic health records (EHR). NLP plays a crucial role in improving documentation efficiency, enhancing communication, and supporting clinical decision-making by extracting valuable information from unstructured text.

NLP applications in healthcare include automatically converting physician's notes into structured formats for easy integration with EHRs, which reduces the need for manual data entry and streamlines clinical documentation processes. NLP is also used to analyze patient feedback from surveys, online reviews, and other sources to gain insights into patient satisfaction, allowing healthcare providers to improve service delivery. Additionally, NLP can assist in clinical decision-making by scanning medical literature and research papers to provide clinicians with up-to-date evidence and best practices for treating patients, ultimately supporting evidence-based care.

Furthermore, NLP systems can be used to identify key terms in clinical records that may indicate serious medical conditions such as infections, allergic reactions, or potential drug interactions, facilitating early intervention and improving patient safety.

2.3.Predictive Analytics

Predictive analytics in healthcare involves using statistical algorithms and machine learning models to analyze historical data and forecast future outcomes (B. Nithya and V. Ilango,2017). These predictive models are designed to identify patterns and trends that can help healthcare organizations optimize operational workflows, predict patient outcomes, and improve resource management. By leveraging large datasets, predictive analytics can anticipate patient needs, prevent complications, and minimize operational inefficiencies.

For example, predictive models can identify high-risk patients who are more likely to require emergency care or readmission, allowing healthcare providers to take proactive steps to prevent these outcomes. Predictive analytics can also help hospitals forecast demand for services, such as surgeries, diagnostic tests, and emergency care, ensuring that resources such as staff, equipment, and facilities are appropriately allocated. In terms of operational efficiency, predictive models can help predict staffing requirements, patient discharge times, and even anticipate supply chain needs, thus preventing overstocking or shortages of critical medical supplies.

Moreover, predictive analytics tools can help in the identification and management of chronic diseases by forecasting exacerbations and complications in patients with conditions like diabetes, heart disease, or chronic respiratory issues. This enables healthcare providers to deliver more personalized and timely interventions, improving patient outcomes while reducing healthcare costs.

2.4.Robotic Process Automation (RPA)

Robotic Process Automation (RPA) is a technology used to automate repetitive and rule-based administrative tasks within healthcare settings, such as data entry, claims processing, appointment scheduling, and billing (Dhatterwal, J.S, 2023). RPA is essentially the application of software robots or "bots" that can mimic human interactions with digital systems to carry out tasks with greater accuracy, speed, and efficiency than humans. The integration of RPA in healthcare operations has been transformative, especially in reducing the administrative burden on healthcare providers and staff.

RPA can be used to automate routine tasks, such as processing insurance claims, handling patient referrals, and managing appointments. By eliminating manual processes, RPA frees up human resources to focus on more complex tasks, such as patient care, decision-making, and strategy development. It also reduces human errors, ensuring that administrative tasks are carried out accurately and consistently. Additionally, RPA systems can operate around the clock, providing greater operational efficiency and faster turnaround times for administrative processes.

RPA can also enhance data management by automating the extraction of patient information from various systems, consolidating it into centralized databases for easier access and analysis. This improves operational efficiency, facilitates data-driven decision-making, and ensures compliance with regulatory requirements, particularly in billing and coding.

2.5. AI in Clinical Decision Support (CDS)

AI-powered Clinical Decision Support (CDS) systems assist healthcare providers in making evidence-based decisions by offering insights based on a vast amount of data, including clinical records, patient history, medical literature, and research findings. CDS tools can process and analyze this data to provide recommendations for diagnosis, treatment, and patient management. These systems help clinicians by presenting relevant clinical information at the point of care, reducing cognitive overload and aiding in the decision-making process(C. Comito, 2022).

CDS systems leverage AI technologies such as machine learning, natural language processing, and predictive analytics to provide real-time, context-sensitive recommendations. For instance, AI-driven CDS tools can alert clinicians to potential drug interactions, allergies, or deviations from clinical guidelines. They can also assist in predicting the likelihood of certain outcomes, such as readmissions, based on the patient's medical history and current conditions, helping clinicians prioritize interventions.

Furthermore, AI can support personalized treatment plans by analyzing large datasets from multiple sources, including genomics, medical imaging, and clinical trials. This allows for more tailored and precise treatment strategies that are aligned with individual patient needs, ultimately improving patient outcomes. By assisting with routine clinical decisions, AI in CDS helps reduce diagnostic errors, optimize treatment paths, and enhance the quality of care provided to patients.

In summary, AI technologies such as machine learning, natural language processing, predictive analytics, robotic process automation, and clinical decision support are transforming healthcare operations by enhancing clinical outcomes and improving operational efficiency. These technologies streamline administrative tasks, optimize resource allocation, and enable data-driven decision-making. However, the successful integration of AI in healthcare requires overcoming challenges like data privacy, algorithmic fairness, and workforce adaptability. Despite these hurdles, the potential benefits, including reduced operational costs and improved patient care, are substantial. As AI continues to evolve, its role in healthcare operations will expand, driving further advancements in quality, accessibility, and sustainability in healthcare delivery (Eswaran et al., 2024a).

3. AI-DRIVEN OPERATIONAL IMPROVEMENTS IN HEALTHCARE

3.1. Patient Scheduling and Flow Management

AI systems are increasingly being deployed in healthcare settings to enhance patient scheduling, reduce wait times, and streamline patient flow management. Patient scheduling is a complex task involving numerous variables, such as physician availability, patient preferences, medical urgency, and hospital capacity. AI-driven scheduling tools leverage machine learning algorithms to analyze historical appointment data and predict optimal time slots for patients, considering all these variables. This reduces administrative burden, enhances patient satisfaction, and prevents scheduling conflicts.

Moreover, AI tools can predict patient no-shows, cancellations, and appointment delays, allowing healthcare providers to proactively adjust schedules and allocate time slots accordingly. This is particularly valuable in busy healthcare environments like hospitals and outpatient clinics, where maximizing resource utilization is critical. By anticipating patient cancellations or delays, AI enables healthcare administrators to adjust workflows in real-time, ensuring more efficient operations and reducing downtime.

Figure 1 illustrates the interconnected components of AI-driven patient scheduling and flow management within a healthcare system. It highlights how AI tools predict optimal appointment times, manage patient flow through hospital departments, and allocate resources effectively, ultimately enhancing operational efficiency and patient satisfaction.

Figure 1.AI-Driven Patient Scheduling and Flow Management Component Diagram

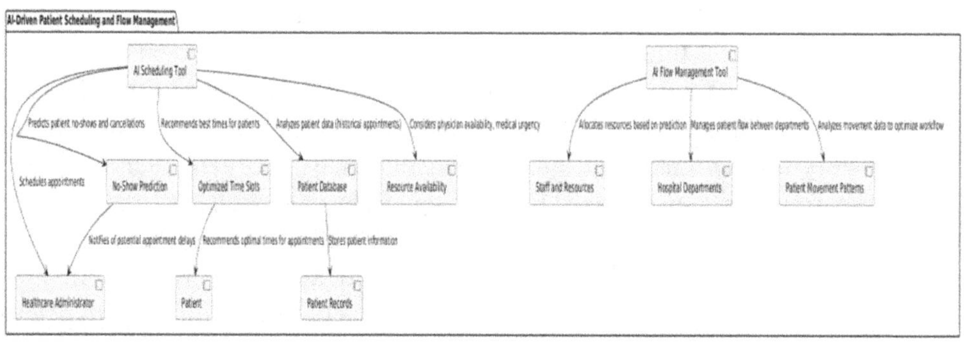

AI-based flow management tools also help optimize patient movement through different departments within the hospital, reducing bottlenecks in areas such as emergency departments, imaging, or outpatient clinics (Pierre, K,et.al,2023). Predictive algorithms can analyze historical data to forecast patient volume and patient movement patterns, ensuring that staff and resources are appropriately allocated to reduce waiting times and enhance the overall patient experience.

3.2.Resource Management and Allocation

AI plays a pivotal role in managing hospital resources, such as beds, medical equipment, and healthcare staff. Resource allocation is a dynamic and multifaceted challenge, with hospitals needing to efficiently distribute limited resources based on real-time patient needs, hospital capacity, and operational constraints. AI-powered systems address this by using predictive analytics and real-time data to optimize resource distribution.

For example, AI models can predict the number of beds required in different hospital departments based on patient admission trends, reducing overcrowding and ensuring that resources are available where they are most needed. Furthermore, AI-driven dynamic scheduling systems can adjust the deployment of healthcare staff in real-time, ensuring that adequate personnel are available for high-demand areas, such as emergency rooms or critical care units.

Another critical application of AI in resource management is in the allocation of medical equipment such as ventilators, imaging machines, and diagnostic tools. AI systems can monitor equipment usage, predict future demand, and suggest optimal allocation based on patient needs (Al-Anazi,,et.al,2024). This minimizes downtime and ensures that expensive medical equipment is used effectively, enhancing patient care while reducing costs.

3.3.Supply Chain Management

AI technologies are increasingly being used to optimize supply chain operations in healthcare settings, helping hospitals and healthcare providers manage inventory, reduce waste, and ensure that medical supplies are readily available when needed. The healthcare supply chain is complex, involving the procurement, storage, and distribution of a wide range of products, from pharmaceuticals to surgical instruments. AI-based tools help improve forecasting accuracy and streamline procurement processes.

AI can predict future inventory needs by analyzing historical data, seasonal trends, and current supply chain conditions, helping healthcare providers maintain optimal stock levels. This ensures that essential supplies are always available while minimizing the risk of overstocking, which can lead to waste. AI systems can also detect potential stockouts in real-time, allowing hospitals to take proactive steps to restock supplies before shortages occur. Additionally, AI algorithms optimize procurement strategies by evaluating suppliers based on price, reliability, and delivery times, leading to cost savings and more efficient supply chain operations (Eswaran.U,et.al, 2024b)

In terms of logistics, AI-driven technologies can optimize the movement of goods within hospitals and healthcare facilities. For example, AI can track the location and movement of medical supplies and equipment in real-time, ensuring that critical materials are always available where they are needed most, such as in operating rooms or emergency departments.

3.4.Clinical Workflows and Efficiency

AI has a transformative impact on clinical workflows by enhancing diagnostic accuracy, improving treatment planning, and optimizing patient care coordination. AI tools help healthcare providers analyze patient data more quickly and accurately, facilitating better decision-making and more efficient care delivery. For instance, AI-powered diagnostic systems can analyze medical images, such as X-rays, MRIs, and CT scans, to detect abnormalities or signs of diseases like cancer or fractures. These systems help radiologists and clinicians identify conditions more quickly and accurately, leading to earlier interventions and better patient outcomes.

In treatment planning, AI can assist in generating personalized treatment options by analyzing patient data, including genetic information, medical history, and current health status. This enables clinicians to make more informed, individualized decisions, which can improve the effectiveness of treatments and reduce adverse reactions.

AI also plays a key role in improving patient care coordination by automatically managing and tracking patient data across different departments, facilitating communication between healthcare providers, and ensuring that no critical information is missed. This leads to fewer errors in care delivery, improved patient outcomes, and enhanced collaboration among clinical teams.

In addition, AI can automate routine administrative tasks within clinical workflows, such as updating electronic health records (EHR), processing test results, and preparing discharge summaries. This reduces the administrative burden on healthcare providers, allowing them to spend more time with patients and focus on clinical care rather than paperwork.

3.5.Patient Engagement and Communication

AI-powered tools are significantly enhancing patient engagement and communication by offering personalized interactions, improving patient education, and enabling more timely and effective communication between patients and healthcare providers (Thorat V,et.al, 2024). One of the most popular applications of AI in patient engagement is the use of chatbots and virtual assistants. These systems are capable of interacting with patients in natural language, answering questions, providing appointment reminders, and offering basic medical advice.

AI-driven chatbots can be integrated into healthcare websites, mobile apps, or patient portals to provide immediate responses to patient queries. They can handle routine questions related to appointments, medications, and general health concerns, ensuring that patients have quick access to information. Additionally, these chatbots can be used to collect patient data, such as symptoms or medical history, before the patient sees a doctor, which helps streamline the intake process.

In terms of patient education, AI systems can analyze patient preferences and medical history to deliver personalized educational content, such as articles, videos, or recommendations for lifestyle changes. These tailored resources can help patients better understand their conditions, treatment options, and ways to improve their health, leading to better adherence to treatment plans and healthier outcomes.

Furthermore, AI-powered communication tools enhance collaboration between patients and healthcare providers. Virtual assistants can facilitate follow-up appointments, send reminders for medication refills, and provide post-discharge care instructions. This ensures continuous communication and reduces the likelihood of patients missing critical steps in their care journey. Table 2 discusses the Key AI-Driven Operational Improvements in Healthcare

Table 2. Key AI-Driven Operational Improvements in Healthcare

Operational Area	AI Technology/Method	Operational Impact
Patient Scheduling & Flow Management	Machine Learning (ML), Predictive Analytics	Optimizes patient appointments, reduces wait times, and predicts no-shows/cancellations, improving overall patient flow.
Resource Management & Allocation	Machine Learning, Predictive Analytics	Optimizes resource allocation (beds, equipment, staff), ensuring efficient use of resources and reducing downtime.
Supply Chain Management	Predictive Analytics, Machine Learning, IoT	Forecasts inventory needs, reduces waste, prevents stockouts, and optimizes procurement, ensuring medical supplies are available when needed.
Clinical Workflows & Efficiency	AI in Diagnostics, Treatment Planning, Automation	Enhances diagnostic accuracy, improves treatment planning, automates administrative tasks, and ensures efficient care coordination among healthcare providers.
Patient Engagement & Communication	AI Chatbots, Virtual Assistants, Natural Language Processing (NLP)	Improves patient communication through appointment reminders, queries, personalized education, and follow-ups, fostering better patient engagement.

In conclusion, AI-driven operational improvements in healthcare extend across various domains, from patient scheduling to resource management and patient communication. By optimizing workflows, improving resource allocation, enhancing decision-making, and automating administrative tasks, AI technologies contribute to more efficient, cost-effective, and patient-centered healthcare operations (Knight, D. R. T.,,et.al,2023). The continued integration of AI will drive further advancements in operational efficiency and clinical outcomes, ultimately transforming the healthcare landscape for the better.

4. CHALLENGES IN AI ADOPTION IN HEALTHCARE OPERATIONS

4.1.Data Privacy and Security Concerns

One of the most significant challenges in the adoption of Artificial Intelligence (AI) in healthcare operations is ensuring the privacy and security of sensitive patient data(Lee, D,et.al,2021). Healthcare organizations deal with vast amounts of personally identifiable health information (PHI), making them prime targets for data breaches and cyberattacks. AI systems often require large datasets to function effectively, and these datasets are often composed of sensitive medical data, including patients' medical histories, test results, and personal information. Protecting this data from unauthorized access and ensuring that it is securely stored and transmitted is paramount.

Regulatory frameworks such as the Health Insurance Portability and Accountability Act **(HIPAA)** in the United States and the General Data Protection Regulation **(GDPR)** in the European Union provide guidelines on the secure handling of patient data. These regulations mandate strict rules on consent, access control, and data anonymization, all of which must be incorporated into AI systems deployed in healthcare. Compliance with these regulations is essential for healthcare organizations to avoid legal and financial penalties, as well as to maintain patient trust. Additionally, healthcare organizations must consider the ethical implications of data use, ensuring that AI systems are designed with robust privacy protections.

4.2.Integration with Existing Systems

The integration of AI into legacy healthcare IT systems presents another major challenge. Many healthcare organizations still rely on outdated IT systems that are not designed to work with modern AI technologies. These systems often lack interoperability, which is the ability of different software applications to communicate and share data seamlessly. For AI tools to be effective in healthcare settings, they must be able to access and process data from a variety of existing platforms, such as Electronic Health Records (EHR), Picture Archiving and Communication Systems (PACS), and other legacy databases.

Integrating AI solutions with legacy systems often requires significant investment in infrastructure upgrades, including data standardization and the implementation of Application Programming Interfaces (APIs) to enable communication between platforms. Moreover, the complexity of healthcare IT environments, with various departments using different software and systems, adds another layer of difficulty. Ensuring that AI solutions can interact smoothly across these disparate systems is crucial for achieving operational improvements and maximizing the benefits of AI adoption in healthcare.

4.3.Bias and Fairness in AI Algorithms

AI algorithms, particularly those driven by machine learning (ML), can inadvertently inherit biases present in the data used to train them. Healthcare data is often collected from a variety of sources, and these datasets may reflect historical inequalities or imbalances in healthcare access. For instance, if an AI model is trained on data that predominantly comes from a certain demographic group, it may not perform well for underrepresented groups. This can lead to biased or discriminatory outcomes, such as incorrect diagnoses, unequal resource allocation, or unfair treatment recommendations, which could exacerbate existing healthcare disparities.

Addressing bias in AI algorithms is a critical challenge to ensure equity and fairness in healthcare decision-making. It is essential for healthcare providers to be aware of the potential for bias in AI systems and to take steps to mitigate it. This includes using diverse and representative datasets, continuously auditing AI models for fairness, and incorporating input from diverse stakeholders to ensure that AI systems reflect the needs of all populations. By fostering transparency in AI development and deployment, healthcare organizations can build trust in AI-driven tools and ensure that these technologies contribute to more equitable and just healthcare outcomes.

The diagram illustrates the flow of data and processes involved in AI-driven decision-making in healthcare, highlighting how AI models are trained using diverse datasets and the importance of bias detection and mitigation. It emphasizes the need for continuous auditing and modification of AI algorithms to ensure fairness in healthcare decisions, thereby addressing potential biases that could impact diagnosis, treatment recommendations, and resource allocation.

The integration of bias mitigation strategies in AI systems is essential for promoting equitable healthcare outcomes and ensuring AI tools serve diverse populations effectively. Figure 2 shows the Bias and Fairness in AI Algorithms for Healthcare

Figure 2. **Bias and Fairness in AI Algorithms for Healthcare**

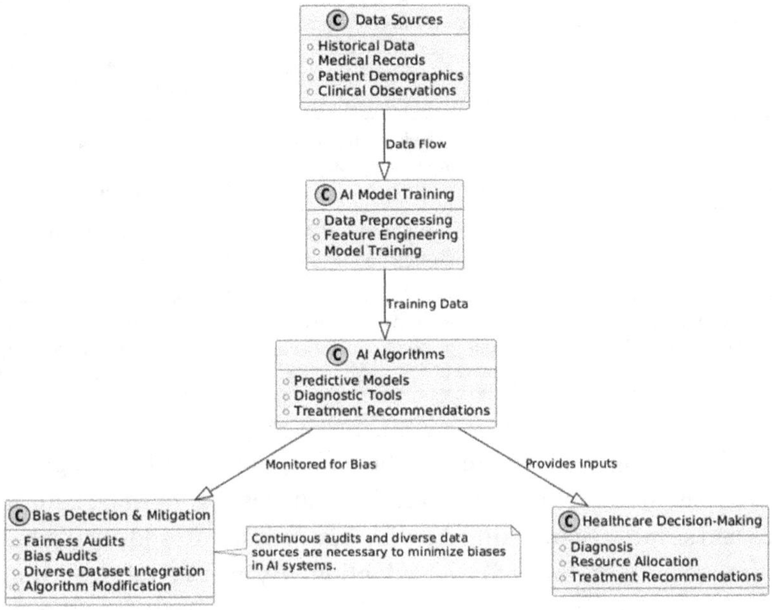
Data Sources
Historical Data
Medical Records
Patient Demographics
Clinical Observations
Data Flow
AI Model Training
Data Preprocessing
Feature Engineering
Model Training
Training Data
AI Algorithms
Predictive Models
Diagnostic Tools
Treatment Recommendations
Monitored for Bias
Provides Inputs
Bias Detection & Mitigation
Fairness Audits
Bias Audits
Diverse Dataset Integration
Algorithm Modification
Continuous audits and diverse data sources are necessary to minimize biases in AI systems.
Healthcare Decision-Making
Diagnosis
Resource Allocation
Treatment Recommendations

4.4.Workforce Readiness and Adaptability

The integration of AI into healthcare operations requires a workforce that is not only ready to use new technologies but also adaptable to the ongoing changes AI introduces. Healthcare professionals, including doctors, nurses, and administrative staff, may initially resist AI adoption due to concerns about its impact on their roles (Nasrullah Abbasi, 2023). Some may fear job displacement, while others may be apprehensive about the need to learn new skills and technologies. It is essential to recognize that AI is not meant to replace human workers but to enhance their capabilities and improve operational efficiency.

To facilitate AI adoption, healthcare organizations must invest in training programs that equip staff with the skills necessary to effectively use AI tools. This includes training on how to interact with AI systems, interpret AI-generated insights, and apply these insights in clinical and operational decision-making. Additionally, fostering a culture of adaptability and continuous learning is crucial to ensuring that healthcare professionals remain engaged with AI technologies as they evolve. Providing clear communication about how AI will improve workflow and patient outcomes, rather than replace jobs, is essential to overcoming resistance and encouraging acceptance among healthcare workers. Table 3 discuses the Key Challenges in AI Adoption in Healthcare

Table 3. Key Challenges in AI Adoption in Healthcare

Challenge	Description	Potential Solutions
Data Privacy and Security Concerns	AI systems require access to large volumes of sensitive patient data, raising concerns about data breaches and compliance with privacy regulations like HIPAA and GDPR.	Implement robust data encryption, anonymization, and access control measures; ensure compliance with legal frameworks.
Integration with Existing Systems	Legacy healthcare IT systems often lack interoperability with modern AI technologies, making integration complex and costly.	Invest in infrastructure upgrades; implement APIs for seamless communication between different systems and platforms.
Bias and Fairness in AI Algorithms	AI algorithms can inherit biases from historical data, potentially leading to unfair or discriminatory healthcare outcomes.	Use diverse and representative datasets; audit AI models for fairness; incorporate stakeholder input to ensure equity.
Workforce Readiness and Adaptability	Healthcare professionals must adapt to AI technologies, which may lead to concerns about job displacement and the need for new skills.	Invest in training programs, create a culture of continuous learning, and communicate the benefits of AI-enhanced workflows.

In conclusion, while the adoption of AI in healthcare has the potential to significantly improve operational efficiency and patient care, there are several challenges that must be addressed. These include ensuring data privacy and security, integrating AI with legacy systems, addressing bias in AI algorithms, and preparing the healthcare workforce for AI adoption. By proactively tackling these challenges, healthcare organizations can harness the full potential of AI while ensuring ethical, fair, and effective implementation.

5. CASE STUDIES AND EXAMPLES OF AI-DRIVEN OPERATIONAL IMPROVEMENTS

5.1.Hospital and Healthcare System Case Studies

Hospitals and healthcare systems around the world are increasingly leveraging AI to optimize operational efficiency and improve patient care outcomes (Mitchell MD, 2010). For instance, AI-driven patient flow management systems have been implemented to predict patient admissions, discharge patterns, and resource needs. By analyzing historical data, these systems can forecast the number of patients expected on a given day, allowing hospitals to prepare adequate staffing levels and manage beds more effectively. In some cases, AI tools have been employed to optimize surgical workflows, from scheduling surgeries to managing the availability of operating rooms and personnel, resulting in fewer delays and better utilization of resources.

A key example comes from the implementation of AI-based bed management systems in a large hospital in the UK. These systems use predictive models to forecast patient discharges and optimize the allocation of beds. By doing so, hospitals can reduce bottlenecks in patient admission, improve patient flow, and enhance overall operational efficiency. Additionally, AI algorithms have been used to predict patient outcomes based on clinical data, helping clinicians make more informed decisions regarding treatment plans and interventions.

5.2.AI in Supply Chain Optimization

AI has also made significant strides in optimizing healthcare supply chains, leading to more efficient management of inventory and reducing waste. Hospitals often face challenges in maintaining the right balance of medical supplies—too little can result in stockouts, while overstocking leads to increased costs and waste. AI-powered supply chain management systems help address these issues by forecasting demand for medical supplies, predicting shortages, and automating procurement processes.

For example, **AI tools** have been used by major hospitals to predict the demand for critical supplies such as personal protective equipment (PPE) and medications. In one such case study, AI was integrated with hospital management systems to track real-time inventory levels, analyze historical consumption patterns, and anticipate future needs. This allowed the hospital to order supplies proactively, reducing both stockouts and excess inventory. Furthermore, AI-enabled systems have helped optimize **logistics**, ensuring that supplies are delivered at the right time and reducing operational delays.

5.3.Predictive Analytics in Patient Care

Predictive analytics has become a vital tool in patient care by allowing healthcare providers to monitor patient conditions in real-time and take proactive steps. Predictive models leverage patient data, such as vital signs, lab results, and medical history, to forecast health outcomes, detect potential complications, and inform personalized treatment plans. By analyzing this data, predictive analytics tools assist clinicians in identifying early signs of deterioration, enabling timely interventions that can enhance patient outcomes (Eswaran.U,et.al, 2024c).

One notable example comes from the use of predictive analytics in managing patients with chronic conditions, such as diabetes or heart disease. AI tools have been used to monitor patients remotely through wearable devices, providing real-time data on their health status. By analyzing trends and patterns in this data, AI models can predict when a patient's condition is likely to worsen, alerting healthcare providers to intervene before a crisis occurs. In this way, predictive analytics not only improves the quality of care but also reduces hospital readmissions and healthcare costs.

5.4.AI in Administrative and Billing Tasks

Administrative tasks, including medical coding, billing, and claims processing, have traditionally been time-consuming and prone to human error. However, AI systems have successfully automated many of these functions, leading to significant reductions in administrative costs and errors. AI-driven tools use natural language processing (NLP) and machine learning algorithms to extract information from clinical notes, medical records, and billing documents to generate accurate codes and process claims more efficiently.

For instance, AI has been applied in the medical coding process, where it can automatically assign the correct diagnosis and procedure codes based on patient records. This reduces the workload of medical coders, improves accuracy, and speeds up the reimbursement process. Similarly, AI has been used to automate claims processing by verifying patient eligibility, checking for billing errors, and reducing the time spent manually handling insurance claims. By streamlining these administrative tasks, AI allows healthcare providers to focus more on patient care and less on back-office operations. Table 4 discusses the Case Studies and Examples of AI-Driven Operational Improvements

Table 4. Case Studies and Examples of AI-Driven Operational Improvements

AI-Driven Improvement	Description	Real-World Example	Impact
Patient Flow Management	AI tools optimize patient admissions, discharges, and bed management to enhance hospital operations and improve patient care.	AI-based bed management system in the UK hospital.	Reduced bottlenecks in patient admission, improved bed utilization, and smoother patient flow.
AI in Surgical Workflows	AI optimizes surgical scheduling, resource allocation, and operating room utilization, ensuring efficient use of hospital resources.	Surgical workflow optimization system in a hospital.	Reduced surgical delays, better resource utilization, and improved patient outcomes.
Supply Chain Management	AI forecasts demand, optimizes procurement, and manages inventory, reducing waste and ensuring timely availability of supplies.	AI-powered inventory and supply chain management in hospitals for critical supplies.	Minimized stockouts and excess inventory, reduced procurement costs.
Predictive Analytics in Patient Care	AI models analyze patient data to predict outcomes, identify complications, and guide personalized care.	AI-powered predictive tools for chronic disease management, such as diabetes and heart disease.	Early detection of complications, proactive care, reduced hospital readmissions.
AI in Medical Coding and Billing	AI automates administrative tasks like coding, claims processing, and billing, improving efficiency and reducing errors.	AI-driven medical coding and claims processing systems in healthcare organizations.	Reduced administrative costs, faster reimbursement, improved accuracy in coding.

AI-driven operational improvements are transforming healthcare by making processes more efficient, reducing costs, and improving patient outcomes. Case studies from healthcare systems around the world demonstrate the tangible benefits of AI in areas such as patient flow management, supply chain optimization, predictive analytics, and administrative automation. By incorporating AI into these critical areas, healthcare organizations are not only enhancing operational efficiencies but also ensuring that patients receive more personalized, timely, and effective care. These advancements are setting the stage for a more sustainable and efficient future for healthcare operations globally.

6. ETHICAL CONSIDERATIONS IN AI-DRIVEN OPERATIONAL IMPROVEMENTS

6.1. Transparency and Explainability of AI Models

Transparency and explainability are fundamental principles in ensuring the ethical application of Artificial Intelligence (AI) in healthcare. As AI models become more involved in decision-making, healthcare providers and patients must understand how AI systems arrive at their conclusions. This understanding builds trust and confidence in AI technologies and ensures that these systems align with clinical best practices and ethical standards. Explainable AI refers to the ability to interpret the decision-making process of an AI model in a way that is comprehensible to non-experts, such as healthcare professionals. For instance, AI-driven clinical decision support systems (CDSS) need to not only provide a diagnosis or treatment recommendation but also explain how the system arrived at that conclusion based on patient data and its underlying algorithms. This transparency ensures that healthcare providers can assess whether the AI recommendations are medically sound and justifiable, improving the quality of patient care and reducing the potential for errors.

6.2.Informed Consent for AI Usage

Informed consent is a core principle of medical ethics that must be adapted to the context of AI in healthcare (Amann, J.,et.al,2020). Patients and healthcare providers must be made fully aware of when and how AI technologies are being used in healthcare settings. This includes understanding the role of AI in the clinical decision-making process, how AI interacts with their data, and the potential risks and benefits associated with the use of these technologies. AI systems must be transparent about their capabilities, limitations, and the data they rely on, so patients can make informed choices about their care. Healthcare providers, too, must be equipped with adequate training and knowledge about AI tools to explain their functionalities and limitations to patients. For instance, if an AI tool is being used to recommend a particular treatment or predict patient outcomes, patients should be informed about how the model works, what data it uses, and any potential risks, including biases in the model. Informed consent ensures that stakeholders, both patients and healthcare providers, are actively engaged in the AI implementation process, fostering a sense of trust and collaboration in healthcare decision-making.

6.3.Ensuring Equity in AI Implementation

As AI technologies are integrated into healthcare systems, it is critical to ensure that these improvements are applied equitably across diverse populations. While AI has the potential to revolutionize healthcare, there is a risk that it could exacerbate existing healthcare disparities if not deployed thoughtfully. Underserved and marginalized populations often have limited access to the latest medical technologies, and without careful consideration, AI-driven healthcare solutions could reinforce these inequities. For instance, AI systems trained predominantly on data from wealthier, urban populations may not perform as accurately or effectively when applied to rural or low-income groups. In such cases, AI algorithms may inadvertently exclude or misrepresent certain demographics, leading to biased outcomes. Ensuring equity in AI implementation requires that healthcare systems actively work to include diverse datasets that represent a wide range of socioeconomic, racial, and geographic groups. Additionally, stakeholders must assess the accessibility of AI-driven healthcare solutions, ensuring that all patients—regardless of their background or location—have equal access to these benefits. Healthcare policies must be put in place to ensure that AI tools are deployed in a manner that addresses health disparities rather than exacerbating them.

6.4.Responsibility and Accountability in AI Decisions

AI systems that drive operational decisions in healthcare must be accompanied by clear frameworks for responsibility and accountability. This ensures that when AI tools are used to support clinical decision-making, or when errors occur as a result of AI-based recommendations, there is clarity on who is responsible for the outcomes(Smith, H., 2021). For example, if an AI model makes an incorrect prediction about a patient's prognosis or incorrectly recommends a treatment plan, the healthcare provider must know whether the responsibility lies with the AI system, the developers of the model, or the healthcare provider who implemented the system. Establishing clear accountability frameworks is necessary to ensure that any negative outcomes resulting from AI-driven decisions are addressed and that patients' rights and safety are upheld. In addition, there must be mechanisms in place to review and challenge AI-driven decisions, ensuring that healthcare professionals can intervene when necessary(C Kishor Kumar Reddy, et.al,2024). For instance, a clinician should have the ability to override AI recommendations if they believe that the AI's decision is not in the best interest of the patient. Furthermore, healthcare organizations and policymakers must work to ensure that liability for AI-related errors is well-defined, promoting an ethical and responsible approach to AI adoption in healthcare.

The ethical considerations surrounding the use of AI in healthcare are essential for fostering trust, ensuring fairness, and safeguarding the rights of patients and healthcare providers alike. Transparency and explainability of AI models empower healthcare professionals to make informed decisions, while informed consent ensures that patients understand the risks and benefits of AI-driven interventions. Furthermore, ensuring equity in AI implementation helps prevent disparities in healthcare access and outcomes, while clear responsibility and accountability frameworks ensure that AI decisions remain ethical and justifiable. By addressing these ethical concerns, healthcare organizations can ensure that AI technologies are used responsibly and effectively, ultimately contributing to the improvement of healthcare outcomes and operational efficiencies.

7. FUTURE DIRECTIONS AND THE EVOLVING ROLE OF AI IN HEALTHCARE OPERATIONS

7.1.AI in Predictive Healthcare and Proactive Management

The future of healthcare is increasingly data-driven, with Artificial Intelligence (AI) leading the charge in predictive healthcare and proactive management of patient conditions. AI algorithms are already being employed to forecast patient outcomes, track disease progression, and predict the onset of chronic diseases. However, as AI models become more sophisticated, they will be able to provide even more accurate predictions, enabling healthcare providers to intervene earlier and more effectively. For example, predictive analytics can help identify high-risk patients who are more likely to develop conditions like diabetes, heart disease, or strokes. By recognizing these risks in advance, healthcare providers can initiate preventive measures such as lifestyle changes, medication adjustments, and closer monitoring to manage the condition before it worsens. Additionally, AI can help to optimize the treatment plans for chronic conditions, such as diabetes or hypertension, by continuously monitoring vital signs and adjusting treatment regimens based on real-time data. These AI-driven approaches will lead to more personalized care, reduce the need for emergency interventions, and ultimately improve patient outcomes while also reducing healthcare costs. Proactive management not only improves patient quality of life but also minimizes hospital readmissions and enhances overall population health management.

7.2.AI and the Future of Healthcare Staffing and Workforce Management

AI's impact on healthcare extends beyond patient care into the management of healthcare personnel. As the demand for healthcare services continues to rise, AI technologies will play an increasingly vital role in workforce management. One of the key challenges facing healthcare organizations is staff burnout and workload imbalance. Healthcare professionals often face long working hours, overwhelming patient loads, and high levels of stress, leading to burnout and reduced job satisfaction. AI systems can help address these challenges by optimizing staffing levels, predicting peak demand for services, and matching the right resources to the right tasks. AI-powered workforce management solutions can analyze historical data to predict patient volumes and staff availability, allowing healthcare organizations to adjust schedules dynamically. For example, AI tools can forecast when certain departments, such as emergency rooms or intensive care units, will be busiest and ensure that sufficient medical staff are available to meet demand. Furthermore, AI can be used to monitor healthcare workers' well-being and prevent burnout by detecting signs of stress or fatigue. This enables healthcare systems to better manage workloads, ensuring that staff are supported, improving job satisfaction, and ultimately contributing to better patient care.

7.3.The Promise of AI in Remote and Rural Healthcare Operations

AI has immense potential to address the challenges of delivering quality healthcare in remote and underserved regions. Access to healthcare services is often limited in rural areas due to a lack of medical professionals, infrastructure, and specialized care. AI can bridge this gap by providing innovative solutions such as telemedicine platforms, remote patient monitoring, and virtual healthcare assistants. Telemedicine, powered by AI, allows patients in remote areas to consult with doctors and specialists through video calls or online platforms. AI-driven diagnostic tools can assist in interpreting medical data remotely, enabling healthcare providers to make accurate diagnoses without the need for in-person consultations. Additionally, AI-powered devices like wearable sensors and mobile health apps can continuously monitor patients' vital signs, such as heart rate, blood pressure, and glucose levels. These devices can send real-time data to healthcare providers, who can monitor patients remotely, detect potential health issues early, and provide timely interventions. For rural healthcare workers, AI-based systems can act as decision-support tools, helping them to make informed decisions based on the latest clinical guidelines and best practices. By extending healthcare services to underserved regions, AI helps to bridge the healthcare access gap, improving health outcomes and reducing the disparity between urban and rural care.

7.4.Integration of AI with Emerging Technologies

The future of AI in healthcare is not isolated; it is poised to integrate seamlessly with other emerging technologies, creating powerful synergies that will revolutionize healthcare operations. Among these technologies, blockchain, the Internet of Things (IoT), and cloud computing will be particularly impactful in enhancing the role of AI in healthcare.

- **Blockchain and AI**: Blockchain technology provides a secure, transparent, and immutable record of transactions, which is highly beneficial for managing patient data. By integrating AI with blockchain, healthcare providers can ensure the privacy and security of patient records while also enabling secure data sharing across institutions. Blockchain's decentralized nature makes it ideal for supporting AI applications, ensuring that AI models use verified, real-time data for more accurate predictions and decisions. Additionally, blockchain can be used to track the provenance of medical supplies, reducing fraud and enhancing supply chain management.

- **IoT and AI**: The integration of AI with IoT is expected to be transformative for both clinical and operational aspects of healthcare. IoT devices, such as wearable health monitors, smart beds, and connected diagnostic tools, generate vast amounts of data that can be analyzed in real-time by AI algorithms. For instance, IoT devices used to monitor patient vitals can send continuous data to AI systems, which can then alert healthcare providers about abnormal readings or trends. This real-time data exchange will allow healthcare providers to act quickly, ensuring better patient care and reducing risks associated with delayed interventions.
- **Cloud Computing and AI**: Cloud computing will enable AI-driven applications to scale and operate seamlessly across multiple healthcare systems. Cloud-based AI models can process and analyze large datasets from different sources (e.g., electronic health records, imaging data, genetic information) in real-time, enabling faster decision-making and improving the accuracy of diagnoses and treatment recommendations. Moreover, the cloud offers greater accessibility and storage capacity, making AI tools more available and affordable to healthcare providers, especially in resource-constrained settings. Cloud computing also facilitates data sharing between hospitals, research institutions, and healthcare providers, promoting collaborative efforts in improving patient care and advancing medical research.

These synergies between AI and emerging technologies will not only optimize healthcare operations but also create new possibilities for patient care, data management, and medical research. The convergence of AI, blockchain, IoT, and cloud computing is set to transform the healthcare industry, making it more efficient, secure, and patient-centric. Table 5 discusses the Future Directions in AI-Driven Healthcare Operations

Table 5. Future Directions in AI-Driven Healthcare Operations

Future Direction	Description	Potential Impact
AI in Predictive Healthcare and Proactive Management	AI will evolve to forecast patient needs, disease progression, and enable early intervention for chronic conditions.	Improved patient outcomes through early detection, reduced hospital readmissions, and personalized care.
AI and Healthcare Staffing Management	AI will optimize staffing levels, predict patient demand, and help balance healthcare workloads.	Reduced burnout, improved job satisfaction, and more effective utilization of healthcare workers.
AI in Remote and Rural Healthcare Operations	AI will enhance access to healthcare in underserved regions through telemedicine, remote monitoring, and AI-powered diagnostic tools.	Increased healthcare access, particularly in remote areas, leading to better patient care and health equity.
AI Integration with Emerging Technologies	AI will integrate with blockchain, IoT, and cloud computing to enhance healthcare operations and data security.	Enhanced data security, real-time patient monitoring, and more accurate decision-making in healthcare.

The evolving role of AI in healthcare offers promising opportunities to improve patient care, optimize operations, and bridge gaps in access to healthcare services (Alowais, S.A,et.al,2023). Predictive healthcare models, AI-driven staffing solutions, and remote healthcare capabilities are set to revolutionize the way healthcare is delivered, making it more proactive, personalized, and efficient. As AI continues to integrate with emerging technologies, such as blockchain, IoT, and cloud computing, the future of healthcare will be more interconnected, data-driven, and patient-centered. These developments will shape the healthcare landscape for years to come, promising better outcomes for patients and a more sustainable, efficient healthcare system.

8. CONCLUSION

Recap of AI's Transformative Impact on Healthcare Operations

Artificial Intelligence (AI) has brought a paradigm shift to healthcare operations, creating a landscape where efficiency, precision, and patient-centered care are central to everyday practices. The infusion of AI technologies—such as machine learning (ML), natural language processing (NLP), predictive analytics, and robotic process automation (RPA)—has transformed both clinical and administrative aspects of healthcare. These technologies have optimized resource management, streamlined clinical workflows, improved patient care, and reduced operational costs.

AI-driven solutions have revolutionized the way healthcare providers manage hospital resources such as beds, equipment, and staff. They have also improved clinical decision-making by offering real-time insights and predicting patient outcomes. For instance, AI tools are now being used for predicting patient admissions, assisting in patient scheduling, and managing supply chains to reduce wastage. These improvements have not only led to better operational efficiency but also have contributed to better patient outcomes. By automating routine tasks and enabling more precise decision-making, AI has helped healthcare professionals focus more on providing personalized care rather than administrative work.

Moreover, AI's integration into healthcare has promoted a more sustainable model, where resource allocation and care delivery are optimized, thus reducing unnecessary costs. Hospitals and healthcare systems are now able to maintain optimal resource utilization, minimize errors, and improve patient care quality through AI-driven strategies. As AI continues to evolve, its impact on healthcare operations is poised to grow even further, allowing for more accurate, faster, and accessible care.

Key Takeaways on the Benefits, Challenges, and Future of AI in Healthcare Operations

While the potential of AI in transforming healthcare operations is vast, several challenges need to be addressed to fully realize its benefits.

- **Benefits**: AI has undeniably brought about significant improvements in healthcare efficiency, decision-making, and patient care. Key benefits include improved accuracy in diagnostics, better resource management, optimized patient flow, and more personalized care delivery. With AI's predictive capabilities, healthcare providers can anticipate patient needs and make proactive decisions, leading to improved patient outcomes. Furthermore, the automation of administrative tasks through AI frees up valuable time for healthcare professionals, enabling them to focus on more complex clinical work and enhancing overall productivity.
- **Challenges**: Despite the impressive benefits, AI adoption in healthcare comes with its own set of challenges. Data privacy and security concerns remain one of the most significant barriers, as healthcare organizations must comply with strict regulations like HIPAA and GDPR to protect patient information. Additionally, AI systems are not immune to biases, especially when the train-

ing data used for machine learning models are incomplete or unrepresentative. These biases can lead to discriminatory practices or unfair healthcare decisions, which can undermine trust in AI technologies. Moreover, the integration of AI into legacy healthcare systems can be complex, with interoperability issues hindering seamless deployment. There are also workforce-related challenges, including the need for healthcare professionals to be trained to use AI tools effectively and the potential for job displacement due to automation.

- **Future**: The future of AI in healthcare is filled with promise. As AI technologies continue to evolve, their ability to drive predictive, preventive, and personalized healthcare will expand. Future advancements in AI, combined with the integration of other emerging technologies such as blockchain and the Internet of Things (IoT), will enable a more interconnected and data-driven healthcare system. AI-driven solutions will continue to enhance remote and rural healthcare, ensuring that underserved populations benefit from cutting-edge technologies. Furthermore, AI will continue to play a crucial role in addressing staff shortages, optimizing workforce management, and improving employee satisfaction within healthcare systems.

The future trajectory of AI in healthcare is one where patient outcomes, operational efficiencies, and healthcare accessibility are significantly enhanced. However, to maximize these benefits, it will be essential to navigate the challenges of adoption, regulation, and workforce adaptation carefully.

Final Thoughts on Fostering Responsible AI Adoption in Healthcare

The responsible adoption of AI in healthcare requires a careful, balanced approach that upholds ethical standards, transparency, and inclusivity. Ethical considerations must be at the forefront of AI deployment to ensure that technologies do not compromise patient rights, exacerbate existing inequalities, or result in discriminatory practices. Key to this responsibility is ensuring that AI systems are explainable, and that healthcare professionals and patients can trust the decisions made by AI models. Transparent decision-making processes will build trust in AI and foster widespread acceptance across healthcare systems.

Another vital aspect of responsible AI adoption is equity. AI technologies must be deployed in ways that are inclusive and accessible to all populations, particularly underserved communities. This requires addressing biases in AI models, ensuring that the datasets used are diverse and representative of all groups. Furthermore, healthcare organizations must ensure that AI solutions do not exacerbate healthcare disparities but instead work to close gaps in access and care.

Lastly, healthcare organizations must prioritize workforce readiness and adaptability to ensure that AI adoption benefits both healthcare professionals and patients. This includes providing adequate training and support to healthcare workers, who will need to adapt to new technologies and workflows. Moreover, healthcare systems must address concerns about job displacement by developing strategies that retrain workers for roles in AI-supported healthcare environments.

Ultimately, fostering responsible AI adoption in healthcare is about ensuring that the technologies are deployed ethically, that they align with patient-centered care principles, and that they benefit society as a whole. AI's transformative potential in healthcare is vast, but its benefits can only be fully realized when it is implemented thoughtfully, responsibly, and inclusively. By doing so, AI will continue to be a powerful tool in improving healthcare outcomes, optimizing operations, and ensuring equitable access to care for all individuals.

REFERENCES

Abbasi, N., Nizamullah, F. N. U., & Zeb, S. (2023). AI in healthcare: Integrating advanced technologies with traditional practices for enhanced patient care. *BULLET: Jurnal Multidisiplin Ilmu*, *2*(3), 546–556.

Al-Anazi, S., Al-Omari, A., Alanazi, S., Marar, A., Asad, M., Alawaji, F., & Alwateid, S. (2024). Artificial intelligence in respiratory care: Current scenario and future perspective. *Annals of Thoracic Medicine*, *19*(2), 117–130.

Alowais, S. A., Alghamdi, S. S., Alsuhebany, N., Alqahtani, T., Alshaya, A. I., Almohareb, S. N., Aldairem, A., Alrashed, M., Bin Saleh, K., Badreldin, H. A., Al Yami, M. S., Al Harbi, S., & Albekairy, A. M. (2023). Revolutionizing healthcare: The role of artificial intelligence in clinical practice. *BMC Medical Education*, *23*(1), 689. DOI: 10.1186/s12909-023-04698-z PMID: 37740191

Amann, J., Blasimme, A., Vayena, E., Frey, D., & Madai, V. I. (2020). Explainability for artificial intelligence in healthcare: A multidisciplinary perspective. *BMC Medical Informatics and Decision Making*, *20*(1), 310. DOI: 10.1186/s12911-020-01332-6 PMID: 33256715

Awasthy, R., Malhotra, M., Seavers, M. L., & Newman, M. (2024). Admission prioritization of heart failure patients with multiple comorbidities. *Frontiers in Digital Health*, *6*, 1379336. DOI: 10.3389/fdgth.2024.1379336 PMID: 39015480

Comito, C., Falcone, D., & Forestiero, A. (2022). AI-Driven Clinical Decision Support: Enhancing Disease Diagnosis Exploiting Patients Similarity. *IEEE Access : Practical Innovations, Open Solutions*, *10*, 6878–6888. DOI: 10.1109/ACCESS.2022.3142100

Dhatterwal, J. S., Kaswan, K. S., & Kumar, N. (2023). Robotic Process Automation in Healthcare. In Bhattacharyya, S., Banerjee, J. S., & De, D. (Eds.), *Confluence of Artificial Intelligence and Robotic Process Automation. Smart Innovation, Systems and Technologies* (Vol. 335). Springer., DOI: 10.1007/978-981-19-8296-5_7

Dubey, A. (2024). *C Kishor Kumar Reddy, Srinath Doss and Marlia Mohd Hanafiah, "Exploring the Advancements and Future Directions of Digital Twins in Healthcare 6.0.* IGI Global.

Eswaran, U., Eswaran, V., Murali, K., & Eswaran, V. (2024). Elevating healthcare: the synergy of ai and biosensors in disease management. i-Manager's Journal on Artificial Intelligence & Machine Learning (JAIM), 2(1).

Eswaran, U., Eswaran, V., Murali, K., & Eswaran, V. (2024). Predictive healthcare analytics. In *Exploring the Advancements and Future Directions of Digital Twins in Healthcare 6.0* (p. 29). IGI Global., DOI: 10.4018/979-8-3693-5893-1.ch009

Eswaran, V., Eswaran, U., Eswaran, V., & Murali, K. (2024b). Revolutionizing healthcare: The application of image processing techniques. In *Medical Robotics and AI-Assisted Diagnostics for a High-Tech Healthcare Industry* (p. 16). IGI Global., DOI: 10.4018/979-8-3693-2105-8.ch019

Knight, D. R. T., Aakre, C. A., Anstine, C. V., Munipalli, B., Biazar, P., Mitri, G., Valery, J. R., Brigham, T., Niazi, S. K., Perlman, A. I., Halamka, J. D., & Abu Dabrh, A. M. (2023). Artificial intelligence for patient scheduling in the real-world health care setting: A metanarrative review. *Health Policy and Technology*, *12*(4), 100824. DOI: 10.1016/j.hlpt.2023.100824

Lee, D., & Yoon, S. N. (2021). Application of Artificial Intelligence-Based Technologies in the Healthcare Industry: Opportunities and Challenges. *International Journal of Environmental Research and Public Health*, *18*(1), 271. DOI: 10.3390/ijerph18010271 PMID: 33401373

Maleki Varnosfaderani, S., & Forouzanfar, M. (2024). The Role of AI in Hospitals and Clinics: Transforming Healthcare in the 21st Century. *Bioengineering (Basel, Switzerland)*, *11*(4), 337. DOI: 10.3390/bioengineering11040337 PMID: 38671759

Mitchell, M. D., Williams, K., Brennan, P. J., & Umscheid, C. A. (2010). Integrating local data into hospital-based healthcare technology assessment: Two case studies. *International Journal of Technology Assessment in Health Care*, *26*(3), 294–300. DOI: 10.1017/S0266462310000334 PMID: 20584358

Nithya, B., & Ilango, V. "Predictive analytics in health care using machine learning tools and techniques," *2017 International Conference on Intelligent Computing and Control Systems (ICICCS)*, Madurai, India, 2017, pp. 492-499, DOI: 10.1109/ICCONS.2017.8250771

Pierre, K., Haneberg, A. G., Kwak, S., Peters, K. R., Hochhegger, B., Sananmuang, T., Tunlayadechanont, P., Tighe, P. J., Mancuso, A., & Forghani, R. (2023). Applications of artificial intelligence in the radiology roundtrip: Process streamlining, workflow optimization, and beyond. *Seminars in Roentgenology*, *58*(2), 158–169. DOI: 10.1053/j.ro.2023.02.003 PMID: 37087136

Smith, H. (2021). Clinical AI: Opacity, accountability, responsibility and liability. *AI & Society*, *36*(2), 535–545. DOI: 10.1007/s00146-020-01019-6

Thorat, V., Rao, P., Joshi, N., Talreja, P., & Shetty, A. R. (2024, May 7). Role of Artificial Intelligence (AI) in Patient Education and Communication in Dentistry. *Cureus*, *16*(5), e59799. DOI: 10.7759/cureus.59799 PMID: 38846249

Chapter 9
Leveraging Artificial Intelligence for Transformative Operational Improvements in Healthcare:
Enhancing Efficiency, Patient Care, and Decision-Making

Jagadeshwari Puttanapura
https://orcid.org/0009-0008-9607-7438
Stanley College of Engineering and Technology for Women, India

Thakur Monika Singh
https://orcid.org/0009-0006-8534-9130
Stanley College of Engineering and Technology for Women, India

Shugufta Fatima
https://orcid.org/0009-0005-4396-4947
Stanley College of Engineering and Technology for Women, India

Manoj Kumar Reddy Dadireddy
Vardhman College of Engineering, India

ABSTRACT

Artificial Intelligence (AI) is transforming healthcare operations by enhancing efficiency, optimizing resource utilization, and improving patient outcomes. This chapter explores how AI-enabled technologies revolutionize workflows, streamline resource allocation, and address bottlenecks like patient wait times and supply chain inefficiencies. Key AI techniques, including machine learning, natural language processing, and robotic process automation, are discussed alongside applications in predictive analytics, administrative tasks, and decision support systems. Real-world case studies highlight benefits such as cost reduction and improved services. The chapter also examines challenges like data security, algorithmic bias, and workforce adaptation, while exploring future prospects at the intersection of AI with IoT and telemedicine, offering strategies to build more flexible, efficient healthcare systems.

DOI: 10.4018/979-8-3373-1022-0.ch009

1. INTRODUCTION

Deployment of Artificial Intelligence (AI) in health care is a real turning point in the delivery and management of medical services. The increasing demand for health care services, resource shortages, and the focus on patient-centered care create new opportunities for solving systemic problems through the adoption of new technologies in streamlining operations, optimizing the use of resources, and improving the overall efficiency of the health systems. Using advanced data analytics, machine learning algorithms, and automation depending on the future, these newly adopted innovations can help healthcare organizations overcome operational challenges while providing appropriate care standards. This chapter considers AI's influence and revolutionizing impact on health operations concerning sustainable improvements.

The creation of artificial intelligence has transformed healthcare not only in its clinical aspects but also in the non-clinical arena. Apart from being heavily promoted in personalized medicine and diagnostics, potential applications of the technology in health services operations over the next decade are equally promising. AI will provide healthcare systems with tools to predict patients' needs and automate administrative tasks so that they can manage their supply chains in new ways.

Big applications of AI in healthcare operations are:

Predictive Analytics: patient admission rates forecasting, seasonal rise in demand, and resource requirements (Ushaa, Eswaran., et al., 2024).

Automated Scheduling: Optimizing the efficiency of scheduling healthcare personnel and patients with the help of intelligent algorithms.

Inventory Management: Monitoring and replenishing medical stock as per the usage pattern (Saha, E., et al., 2019).

Revenue Cycle Management: Automating several billing processes and reducing errors in this system.

These advancements make possible cost improvements, removing operational bottlenecks, and improving the overall experience of patients in the organization.

Importance of Operational Efficiency

Effective operations are among distinct pillars holding the edifice of a healthcare system which is regarded as sustainable and high-performing. The increasing patient numbers, phenomenal costs of intervention, and limited resources test the performance of systems and their ability to achieve operational efficiency in timely and effective care. Inefficient operations can house overcrowded facilities, areas of extended wait times, resource wastage, and patient outcomes that are compromised (Ko, D-G., et al., 2019).

Artificial Intelligence has a key place in the solutions to these challenges:

Optimizing Resource Use: Having the most appropriate resources available at the right time.

Reducing Waste: Reduction of redundancies, both in terms of inventory and processes.

Increasing Staff Productivity: Automating repetitive tasks in order to free health professionals to put their efforts in the most important: the patient (Cogin, J.A., et al., 2016).

Operational efficiency is thus achieved through a decrease in costs and possible improvement in the quality of services provided to patients, which can, in turn, lead to better patient outcomes and a higher level of satisfaction for healthcare teams.

2. KEY AREAS OF OPERATIONAL IMPROVEMENTS

Healthcare systems are being stretched to the seams to deliver quality care with escalating patient numbers and resource shortages. Operational inefficiencies such as long patient wait times, workforce allocation inefficiencies, and bottlenecks in workflow can affect significantly care delivery. Artificial Intelligence (AI) offers its transformational solutions in analyzing very large data sets, detecting patterns, and automating most complex processes to streamline operations. This section delineates three areas where AI has made active strides in bringing operational improvements: scheduling and workflow optimization; resource allocation and inventory management; and patient flow and capacity planning.

2.1 Scheduling and Workflow Optimization

Scheduling efficiently in healthcare is vital for smooth operations. Poor scheduling leads to wasted resources, long patient waits, and overworked staff. AI will refashion this aspect using machine learning algorithms to analyze historical data, patient preference, and resource availability for effective dynamic optimization of appointment schedules, minimizing no-shows, and ensuring demand reflects supply (Harris, S. L., et al., 2016). For instance, predictive scheduling systems can predict peak activity based on past trends and can automatically adjust the availability of clinicians and facilities. Rescheduling patients due to cancellations is considered "smart" rescheduling by AI since it provides information about the nadir of time slots where patients can receive care. Another great benefit of the artificial intelligence technology in health care is optimizing Workflow process. It minimizes the workflow inefficiency in repetitive tasks as in patient check-ins, verification of the insurance, and data entry, leaving health care staff to focus on providing quality patient care instead of handling a lot of administrative work (Goffman, R. M., et al., 2017). The use of natural language processing (NLP) technologies will enhance this experience even further by converting spoken notes of physicians into structured data, thereby speeding documentation and lessening errors.

2.2 Resource Allocation and Inventory Management

Resource allocation is the ability to tie right personnel, equipment, and supplies at the right time and in the right place. AI is tremendous in analyzing so complicated data to make resource management more effective and responsive. The ability of machine learning models to be able to predict the demand for beds at hospitals, specific diagnostics equipment, and specialists during peak hours is what ensures optimal allocation of resources (Wu, H., et al., 2023).

The table 1 outlines the operational challenges of resource allocation and inventory management, demonstrating how AI tools such as predictive analytics and automated monitoring improve optimal resource utilization and reduce waste and timely availability of medical supplies.

Table 1. Optimizing Resource Allocation with AI

Operational Challenge	AI Tool/Technique	Outcome	Examples
Overstocking/Understocking	Predictive Analytics	Improved inventory accuracy	Inventory management systems
Resource misallocation	Machine Learning Models	Optimized resource utilization	Staff scheduling tools
Sudden demand spikes	Demand Forecasting Algorithms	Minimized supply shortages	Pandemic supply chain solutions
Expired stock issues	Automated Monitoring (IoT + AI)	Reduced waste	Smart inventory systems

AI revolutionizes the system of inventory management by facilitating real-time tracking of supplies and automating stock replenishment. An example of this would be predictive analytics, which could foretell when medicines or surgical instruments would likely run out, and then trigger the automatic reordering process. This would reduce wastage, and above all, it will be helpful during crucial shortages in emergencies, even during pandemics. AI tools schedule availability with work requirements of patients and personnel according to skill set, work load, and shift preference factors. (Nicholson, L., et al., 2004) These systems improve staff satisfaction levels with the overall quality of care while creating much better-balanced schedules.

2.3 Patient Flow and Capacity Planning

Controlling the flow of patients is very essential for reducing overcrowding and for rendering timely care. With the aid of AI-based tools, sophisticated modeling and predicting of patient flow through hospital departments can improve capacity monitoring (Munavalli, J. R., et al., 2021). For example, AI can conduct a historical trend analysis to predict the number of patients that are going to arrive on a particular day or time of day into emergency departments, thereby helping administrators allocate their resources appropriately. Thus, hospitals are also using AI to manage bed status optimization through the prediction of discharge times and identification bottlenecks in the admission process.

Figure 1 portrays an AI improving healthcare workflow optimized in patient care and resource management. Initially patient registration; AI helps in streamlining data collection and triage. The system manages patients along the care pathway, for example, diagnostics, up to consultations with specialists, and more. Real-time feedback loops keep healthcare resources such as staff and equipment in line with different patient loads for great operational efficiencies.

Figure 1. AI-Driven Patient Workflow in Healthcare Operations

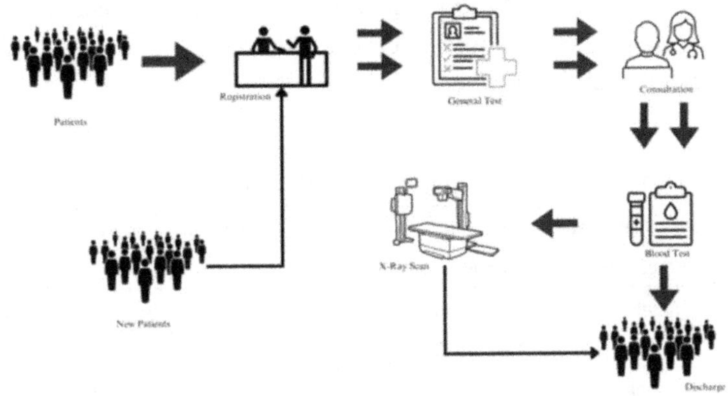

Patients flow smoothly from emergency departments into inpatient care without overloading any single department. Using artificial intelligence simulations, capacity planning enables the running of different operational strategies, like extended operating hours or increasing staff during peak times. This insight allows healthcare facilities to proactively adapt their activity to ensure that they meet patient demand and have no unnecessary costs (Mahmoudian, Y., et al., 2023).

3. AI TECHNIQUES IN HEALTHCARE OPERATIONS

AI in hospitals is the basis for transforming hospital operations to improve their production efficiencies and reduce costs. Major areas of AI techniques, such as Machine Learning (ML), Natural Language Processing (NLP), Robotic Process Automation (RPA), and Computer Vision (CV), have been of great help in solving the operational issues that health organizations face. They enhance process automation and make prediction easier, not leaving behind reducing the amount of administration thus improving patient care and organizational effect. Based on their concepts, applications, and benefits, these applications extend from resource demand forecasting to the automation of repetitive chores, bringing a paradigm shift in the management of health care.

3.1 Machine Learning for Predictive Analytics

Machine learning is known to give healthcare organizations the power of predicting operational needs. Analyzing past and present data is part of their work in forecasting patient admissions, emergency room (ER) visits, and staff allocation needs. For instance, this predictive algorithm would determine seasonal spikes in patient visits and enable hospitals to adequately fine-tune staff schedules and resources. This reduces waiting time and still gives patients a quality of care during peak times.

Another important use is in predictive maintenance of medical equipment. All ML algorithms monitor usage and performance data of the equipments, hence predicting their failures before such an occurrence (Nasrullah, Abbasi., 2024). Minimizes downtime, meaning that critical machines like the MRI scanner operate when most require them. By this, predictive insights ensure the operational continuity and avoid needless spending.

Below table 2 indicates machine learning models and their applications in health care, such as forecasting patient admission, monitoring chronic diseases, and predicting disease outbreaks, as well as the operational benefits accrued from them.

Table 2. Machine Learning Models for Predictive Analytics in Healthcare

Machine Learning Model	Healthcare Application	Key Benefits	Example Use Cases
Linear Regression	Forecasting patient admissions	Reduced overcrowding	Seasonal flu admission prediction
Decision Trees	Identifying high-risk patients	Proactive care delivery	Chronic disease management
Clustering (e.g., K-Means)	Grouping similar patient profiles	Personalized treatment plans	Cancer patient categorization
Neural Networks	Disease outbreak prediction	Early warning for outbreaks	COVID-19 case surge predictions

AI indeed supports the financial forecasting aspects of healthcare in an indirect way. Predictive models are used for analyzing patient billing trends along with the trends in insurance claims and even the operational expenses of a healthcare entity in order to give an accurate budget prediction. This analysis helps the healthcare administrators to come up with informed decisions regarding resource allocation and maintain financial stability within the organization.

3.2 Natural Language Processing in Administrative Tasks

The use of Natural Language Processing changes administrative processes in health care. One of the prime uses of NLP is in automating medical transcription and documentation whereby speech or handwritten notes are converted through an NLP algorithm into an electronic health record (EHR). By reducing the workload of health care professionals, the latter has more time to spend with patients (Thakur, G. K., et al., 2024).

Likewise, it improves inter-patient communication. Chatbots and virtual assistants powered by NLP serve as instant assistants to schedule an appointment, answer frequently asked questions, or remind follow-ups. It lessens the load on the administrative staff, while also increasing patient satisfaction and engagement.

NLP also allows analyzing unstructured data in EHR. By extracting material from physician notes, discharge summaries, and clinical reports, NLP tools help to extract trends, risks, and opportunities for operational improvement. Such capability smoothens decision making and is overall enhancement in healthcare delivery (Janowski, A., 2023).

3.3 Robotic Process Automation (RPA) in Billing and Documentation

RPA-Robotic Process Automation alleviates repetitive administrative tasks, significantly improving efficiency in operations at healthcare's end. For instance, within billing, the automation processes tasks like claims processing, coding, and tracking of reimbursement by RPA bots. With such systems eliminating human errors and rushing up cycles of revenue by defining accuracy and speed, they become handy instruments for institutions (Dhatterwal, J. S., et al., 2023).

This Venn diagram in figure 2 is an illustration of how Machine Learning, Natural Language Processing and Robotic Process Automation come together in healthcare operations, with their distinct and shared contributions to enhancing the efficiency of operations and increasing the decision-making capacities.

Figure 2. Integration of AI Techniques in Healthcare Operations

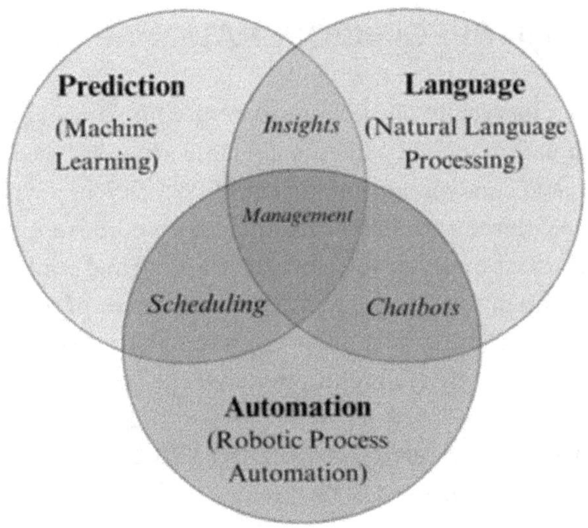

RPA is used for the organization of the patient records in documentation for automation of data, upload, and compliance checks. For instance, RPA tools can fill forms, check for consistency of data, and ensure compliance with regulators like HIPAA. (Udo, Backhaus., et al., 2023) It's manual workload maintenance for administrative staff-hence, the protection of data integrity.

Robotic Process Automation also enables integration of disparate systems within healthcare organizations. RPA can act as a link between the legacy systems and new EHR platforms, ensuring proper migration of information as well as synchronization of information on both ends. Furthermore, they enhance the interoperability of these operational workflows, thus ensuring the processes are integrated and more efficient.

3.4 Computer Vision in Operational Efficiency

Computer Vision (CV) places itself in some parts of automating visual tasks in the healthcare operation. Radiological CV algorithms get to analyze medical images, such as X-rays, CT, and MRI, and enhance the efficiency of abnormality detections. The resultant less workload enables quicker diagnoses that translate to speedier patient care (Mohanarangan, Veerappermal, Devarajan., et al., 2024).

Now video footage along with a real-time computer vision can improve the stock level managements as a part of inventory management in hospitals. Health facilities employ cameras and computer vision algorithms to ensure that real-time monitoring is done for drug inventory, surgical instruments, and consumables. This further helps the organization in reducing manual counting errors, avoiding stockouts, and ensuring that the essential supplies are always available.

Real-time monitoring and quality assurance through CV come into play in surgical settings. (Zizheng, Hua., et al., 2023) The adoption of AI-powered cameras makes visible any stages involved in procedures from which compliance with sterilization protocols and further reduction of infection risks can be achieved. Such technology can lead to an increase in the safety of the operating environment and improved patient outcomes.

4. APPLICATIONS OF AI IN SPECIFIC OPERATIONAL CHALLENGES

AI in healthcare operations has really carved out to deal with some of the most complex problems in healthcare. Especially optimizing the activities in a healthcare work environment, making improved patient experience outcomes, and finally maximizing resource efficiency will be the hassles that one has to tackle with in this regard. With the actionable insights and predictive capabilities of an AI-powered system, the bottleneck barriers can be successfully broken through and contribute to the overall enhancement of performance. The section of this communication covers three of the main application areas of AI to hospitals: effective patient throughput time reduction, emergency department efficiency improvement, and lastly, supply chain and logistics efficiency improvement.

4.1 AI in Patient Flow Management: Reducing Wait Times and Enhancing Emergency Care

Effective patient flow management is one of the pillars in healthcare delivery upon which patient satisfaction and clinical outcomes hinge. Associated problems such as prolonged waiting times and congested emergency department (ED) facilities impose costs on the health system and degrade care quality. The revolutionizing medium that brings together these interrelated matters is artificial intelligence (AI), which optimizes scheduling, improves triage management, and distributes resources effectively.

4.2 AI Solutions in Patient Flow

AI-enabled system for setting appointments has an engine of predictive analytics. This engine helps balance patient flow demand against the capacity use in healthcare facilities. These systems create appointment schedules adjusted and optimized dynamically using historical data, show patterns on patients failing to attend, and the seasonal context through minimizing the bottlenecks. AI, for example, prioritizes urgent cases or reschedules routine check-ups during peak hours to avoid overworking staff by maintaining physicians' flow (Cecula, P., et al., 2021).

Automated check-in systems and virtual assistants greatly enhance the patient experience by collecting initial information from patients and guiding them through the registration process. These systems reduce the administrative burden of staff while minimizing the initial waiting time. Real-time analytics platforms, too, are important in this regard, as they point out waste in workflows, thereby enabling administrators to make specific adjustments, such as improved diagnostic pathways or better utilization of staff.

4.3 Emergency-Specific Applications

The miscellaneous challenges presented by the emergency department could be unpredictability in the influx of patients plus the speed at which a decision has to be made. AI-enhanced triage tools use real-time data regarding a patient's symptoms and vitals to determine which cases are most serious and, therefore, should be seen first. This results in immediate care for those patients in critical condition while maintaining an orderly flow for less severe patients.

Another significant application of such models would involve forecasting the influx of patients to the emergency department, using outside data such as local events or weather patterns. Such models would allow the managers of the emergency department to make changes in staffing levels and allocate resources to various services in anticipation of surges to minimize delays and increase the preparedness of such services during busy periods. Furthermore, AI-powered dashboards also present an emergency department in real time, focusing on congestion points and possible actions to be taken, such as redirecting non-emergency cases to other clinics (Aityan, S. K., et al., 2024).

4.4 Case Studies and Outcomes

Hospitals employing AI technology for patient flow management as well as emergency care actually witnessed a lot of improvement. As, for example, hospitals using scheduling systems driven by AI have substantially reduced average wait times, while predictive triage tools have actually improved the prioritization of treatment leading to better outcomes for serious cases. Again, AI-enabled forecasting and resource allocation have led to less overcrowding and the shorter length of stay among patients in emergency departments.

Combining AI capabilities for reducing patient waiting time and improving efficiency in emergency departments will help the health system create a seamless and responsive environment for care delivery. Such developments will uphold patient satisfaction and empower providers to deliver quality care under varying operational conditions.

4.5 Enhancing Supply Chain and Logistics

All healthcare professionals today know there is so much complexity inside the healthcare supply chain that it could only demand an exact coordination of inventory, procurement, and distribution. With AI in health optimization, it can work wonders with predictive analysis and automation. Forecasting demand accurately happens through machine learning analysis of usage patterns so that there is availability when needed of medical supplies, pharmaceuticals, and equipment without excessive overstocking.

AI-powered inventory management systems keep a record of stock levels as well as expiration dates, which helps minimize any further waste and costs (Chirag, Kalaria., et al., 2023). Just like the ability of anticipating shortages, the systems are programmed to trigger reorder automatically as well, so that operations will remain uninterrupted. Hospitals used to save money through practice with this innovation as well as greatly improve supply chain dependability.

AI improves logistics by providing the best routes for medical supplies and equipment. AI algorithms can consider traffic and weather conditions and how urgently it's needed to determine the best delivery route to a health facility. In case of emergencies like natural calamities, AI can prioritize the distribution of critical supplies, thus minimizing casualties. AI can improve the resilient and responsive healthcare systems for dealing with all types of insurgencies and making resource flows seamless and without inefficiencies.

5. AI-DRIVEN DECISION SUPPORT SYSTEMS

AI-enabled decision support systems (DSS) are forging their pathways into the hospitals-the revolutionary implement in their health care act. They do enhance the decisioning process, making decisions by insightful, plausible actions and various data sources. Sophisticated algorithms are used through machine learning and predictive analytics to give evidence to physicians, clerks, or even the chief executive officers of hospitals in making timely decisions. After proper integration of the infrastructure into the existing healthcare systems, the widest possible optimization will occur in every process and experience, from patient care to operations. AI in strategic planning, clinical decision-making, and resource management is altering health care for future generations into one that is driven to improve health outcomes, decrease costs, and be responsive to shifting demands.

5.1 Role of AI in Strategic Planning

AI has transformed strategic planning in healthcare, that is provided with the best tools possible to analyze extensive data volumes quickly and accurately. Most planning methods rely on what has happened in the past and manual forecast processes where inefficiencies and errors can occur. Much of the present AI analytical tools provide information managers with real-time data and predictive models for actionable insight for more effective resource allocation and future planning. For example, machine learning algorithms can analyze patient data, operational trends, and financial aspects of demand forecasting, workforce scheduling management, and infrastructure planning. This enables health organizations to make data-driven decisions by capturing the reality at greater levels of precision (Salhout, S. M., 2024).

Table 3 compares methods that are based on the age-old decision-making processes with those that have been AI-enabled in certain strategic areas, most notably, resource allocation, infrastructure expansion, and financial planning, and illustrates the measurable differences AI makes in efficient and accurate performance.

Table 3. AI-Driven Strategic Planning in Healthcare

Strategic Decision Area	Traditional Approach	AI-Enhanced Approach	Impact of AI
Resource Allocation	Based on historical usage	Predictive analytics	Accurate resource planning
Infrastructure Expansion	Manual surveys and statistics	AI-driven geospatial analysis	Optimized location and scale
Policy Design	Rule-based systems	Data-driven decision-making	Improved efficiency and fairness
Financial Planning	Excel-based financial models	AI-based cost optimization	Increased ROI and cost savings

Moreover, AI enablement in scenario modeling allows healthcare leaders to capriciously present a host of "if-then" scenarios based on assumptions and different possible outcomes. (Fayaz, M., et al., 2024) AI tools will allow scenario synthesis with various strategic options, particularly in complicated, fast-changing environments such as those where patient volumes fluctuate abruptly or in the event of sudden changes in regulatory policies, and they will pinpoint the most efficient action choice. Therefore, health care executives can work toward proactively addressing all these resources and ensuring organizational goals meet the most efficient way possible.

Figure 3 is depicting how AI is vital in facilitating strategic planning in health systems. It actually improves operational efficiencies and proactive patient care, addiction sustainability through predictive insights. This is about growth in market share and profitability through process optimization and improved resource management. Indeed, these advancements increase the resilience of health organizations in facing challenges and holistically elevating their strategic approaches toward the attainment of objectives.

Figure 3. Role of AI in Strategic Planning: Key Benefits for Healthcare Operations

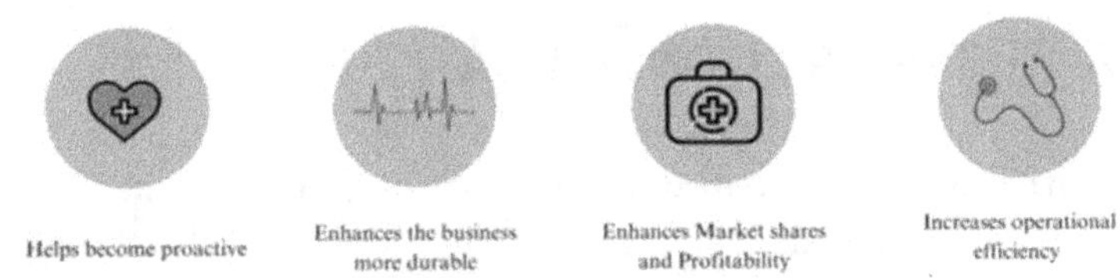

The AI's contributions to strategic planning are also related to long-term planning, such as growth and expansion. For example, by analyzing demographic changes, trends in healthcare demand, and socio-economic factors, AI will then be able to forecast future healthcare needs and assist in the planning of new facilities, new or expanded specialties, or expansion into new geographic areas. Such insights allow organizations to invest in the appropriate technologies and services at the opportune times, thereby affording them a competitive advantage. Aligning operational objectives more effectively with longer-term healthcare objectives through AI-supported strategic planning is clearly a major advance in managing healthcare institutions.

5.2 Case Studies on AI Implementation

Across the globe, numerous health organizations have started implementing an AI approach for developing decision-supporting systems. The report notes how such initiatives yield impressive results in operational efficiency improvement and clinical outcomes, citing, among others, the Mayo Clinic. (Wen, A., et al., 2019) At Mayo Clinic, AI-powered predictive models predict the number of patients that will visit to enable optimizing the staffing levels for any given day in real-time. Eventually, train-their-own, integrated with the existing hospital management system, have cut down waiting times and enhanced patient movement across the departments. The AI system considers historical and current data and alters assignment of human and material resources per the projected patient demand. Hence, effectively delivering care, lower operational costs, and higher patient satisfaction.

An AI at the Cleveland Clinic has become another good case in the application of AI to clinical decision-making. By deploying AI-based diagnostic decision aids, Cleveland Clinic has brought about early disease diagnosis, especially in cancer and heart cases. (Adenekan, T. K., 2024) The AI reads patient records and laboratory and imaging results, then delivers evidence-based treatment recommendations to clinicians. The speed of decision-making in the provision of timely, personalized services to patients improved outcome scenarios. Thereby, AI-efficient clinical services at Cleveland Clinic are a serious mind game for strategic planning in the operational process against patient care objectives.

The most recent example of this kind of situation is that of AI functioning in public health management in different countries in Asia. Singapore, one of the countries in this category, has partly adopted AI in predictive analytics for handling disease outbreaks. (Sarker, S., et al., 2021) During the COVID-19 pandemic, AI models were used to study the outbreak and optimize resource allocation, such as ventilators, ICU beds, and PPE. These data were taken from health authorities, hospitals, and even social media to predict infection trends, allowing the government and healthcare to prepare in advance for spikes in cases. This is how AI can not only determine support in day-to-day healthcare operations but also play a significant role in crisis management and in the long-term public health strategy.

6. CHALLENGES AND ETHICAL CONSIDERATIONS

Data privacy and security concerns stand to be the most important issues to be tackled with AI in health care operations. Sensitive patient data in huge amounts are entrusted to the health care organization, and a surety that these would be secured from hackers and viruses is of greatest significance (Swathi, Ganesan., et al., 2024). In this increased use of AI, progressive processing and analysis of sensitive information often go through machine learning algorithms, which risks further these in cases wherein health institutions lack competent security protocols. Breach in data access, illegal accessing or misuse of patient information-consequences can lead to harm to the patient and severe legal and/or reputational damage. Thus, strict measures must be enforced in ensuring protection of data. Encryption can be done end to end; another could be two-factor authentication to keep patient private data steering clear of breach or misuse by any outsider while still upholding regulatory compliance like HIPAA (Health Insurance Portability and Accountability Act).

In addition, the sheer volume of the healthcare data processed through AI systems complicates it further when it comes to security. The training of AI models generally requires huge amounts of data, and such data are typically scattered across manifold locations or cloud systems. Due to this reason, the high incidence of data dispersity in storage and processing creates an even more lenient environment for vulnerabilities. Therefore, the healthcare organization must focus not only on protecting data at rest but also those in transit. As now, AI is integrated into electronic health record (EHR) systems; this makes every data breach and mishandling dangerous to patient confidentiality and safety. The use of AI applications in automation of tasks, such as billing and appointment scheduling, exposes sensitive private and financial information and needs to be handled securely.

To remedy such matters, healthcare providers need to take proactive approaches toward cybersecurity. (Burrell, D. N., et al., 2023) AI systems can be part of the solutions, identifying possible vulnerabilities from detection of unusual activity to real-time-threat response. Healthcare organizations are also able to improve their cyber monitoring and defending capabilities by incorporating AI-powered security tools with their infrastructures. However, improvement requires investments in required technologies and skilled personnel and their constant vigilance. Regular auditing, continuous monitoring, and compliance with national and international data protection standards are among crucial steps to maintain an ultimately secure AI-driven healthcare environment.

6.1 Addressing Bias in AI Models

Adverse effect of artificial intelligence bias is yet another big area of challenge in the healthcare sector. AI is a set of computer program or algorithm being trained on the data from history, and if that historical data is biased either by race, gender or even socio-economic status, then it is likely for this model to propagate or even aggravate that particular bias (Abràmoff, M. D., et al., 2023). It can be seen that such 'biased' Artificial Intelligence systems, as in the case of healthcare, will usually generate differences in the level of care received by patients. For instance, if the determined risk level by such biased algorithms is lower for some minority groups, or if it underestimates the needs of underrepresented populations, it will lead to less than optimal treatment and unequal access to care. Such unethical biases would raise serious ethical and practical issues as they pose further clinical decisions in their wake.

AI seems to be a double-edged sword because of its historical data, especially in health care. Many health datasets have long-embedded systemic inequalities so that AIs can learn to copy the patterns unless supervised closely. Training datasets lack diversity, which increases the issue. Limited or biased datasets could lead to underperforming models, failing to generalise to the broad patient population. This is very important in medical diagnostics, where AI decisions can have a high impact on health outcomes achieved for patients. Hence, to ensure that AI systems are fair and inclusive, the healthcare institution should conduct data auditing, find possible bias, and retrain processes accordingly.

This requires a multiple prong approach to mitigate biases on AI models. First, healthcare providers need to ensure that the datasets they feed their algorithms are sufficiently diverse and a true representation of the populations that they serve. In other words, such datasets should include information from a very wide variety of demographic groups, such as different races, genders, and socioeconomic backgrounds. Second, there is a requirement for constant monitoring and auditing of AI models to detect any emerging bias and correct it each time it arises during deployment (Ueda, D., et al., 2024). Transparency in AI algorithms and decision-making processes also aids the proper identification of sources of bias as well as providing remedies to mitigate them. Finally, the developing models should prioritize equity and fairness in patient care through a fruitful collaboration from healthcare practitioners, data scientists, and ethicists.

6.2 Workforce Adaptation and Training

In countries across the globe, AI imbues a change in professionalism towards the workforce; especially integration, training, and use of AI tools by healthcare stakeholders such as physicians, nurses, and administrative personnel. It requires a shift in a new mindset configuring a healthcare worker or a consultant on the perceived risk of using the AI in achieving their jobs or tasks. AI can automate many clinical and administrative tasks, yet places the onus of critical decision making, interpreting results, as well as couples human services delivery on compassionate care. As AI eventually takes care of much more routine items, professionals have a duty to adapt through training in those areas of the profession that require high levels of empathy, judgment, and creation. Changes like this might result in a reallocation or even modification of job functions and skills, thus making specialized continuous development of the workforce necessary (Lopes, M. A., et al., 2015).

Further, the introduction of AI creates concerns regarding job substitutions. The implementation of AI may provide support but a fear when it comes to redundancies of certain jobs. Often, automation works specifically with jobs that are directed toward administration. Because certain workers may never learn to use or work with AI, this may be translating to losing employment opportunities. Thus, it requires investments on healthcare institutions for transforming human resources. Training-and-qualification programs should be framed and followed by an MBA candidate to enable workers to learn how to interact with AI, interpret AI's outputs, and deal with having their roles changed. With this endeavor, the health organizations can make sure that their workforce can continuously adapt to the changing environments and leverage AI to on one course regarding improving patient care.

Table 4 considers the obstacles in adapting healthcare organizations' workforce to the use of AI and presents AI-based solutions, such as training workshops and personalized learning, to better align the workforce and speed up the use of AI tools.

Table 4. Workforce Adaptation to AI in Healthcare

Challenge	Proposed Solution	AI Support	Outcome
Lack of AI knowledge	Training workshops	AI-assisted learning platforms	Improved skill levels
Resistance to change	Leadership initiatives	AI insights on employee engagement	Better workforce alignment
High learning curve for new tools	Intuitive AI-powered interfaces	Simplified user experience	Faster adoption rates
Unequal access to training	Remote training programs	AI-driven personalized learning paths	Equitable skill distribution

Beyond that, it is the continuous overcoming of resistance to change by healthcare professionals that is the successful use of AI in healthcare. Many a worker would normally shy away in doubt of AI as even seen as a threat to their professional expertise or encroach upon their independence. Hence it becomes pertinent for the healthcare organizations to sell what AI can do in benefit of human workers as not seen as a possible replacement, but an enhancement in the different ways to deliver quality care. Clear communication, hands-on training, and active involvement of healthcare staff in the implementation process can help ease this transition. Besides this, the AI systems must also be designed to complement human expertise, thus, ensuring that the healthcare professionals will be mainly responsible for the most critical aspects of patient care while using AI systems in improving speeds and decision-making (Heba, Mohtady, Ali., et al., 2022).

7. FUTURE DIRECTIONS AND INNOVATIONS

The future of AI in healthcare will involve revolutionary transformations triggered by new emerging technologies, which tend to disrupt current norms in managing the healthcare model and how medical care is delivered. Disruptive innovations, such as AI-powered IoT solutions, the impact of AI on population health management, and AI-enabled telemedicine, will soon allow healthcare systems to become more efficient, personalized, and accessible. All these advances will not only help to improve patient outcomes but may well reduce the cost, optimize resource allocation, and create streamlined healthcare processes. With the developing AI technology with time, it is expected to engrave itself further into healthcare as the next driver of operational improvements and major shifts in global healthcare delivery.

7.1 Integration of AI with IoT and Wearable Devices

The convergence of Artificial Intelligence (AI) with Internet of Things (IoT) devices as well as wearables can add a new dimension to healthcare by making it possible to provide real-time personalized care. Wearables, such as smartwatches and fitness trackers, actually allow the continuous collection of data on relevant health markers, including heart rate, saturation of oxygen in the blood, exercise levels, and sleep patterns. With AI, such devices could analyze online data in addition to forecasting health problems and providing early warnings to patients as well as health workers. This gives rise to smart proactive health care, thus minimizing emergencies and hospitalizations (Joshi, H., et al., 2024).

The appointment between AI and IoT will promote the benefit of developing smart healthcare systems, which provide personalized suggestions. For example, AI can offer customized insights for managing chronic conditions such as diabetes, hypertension, and asthma through the analysis of data from IoT-connected devices like wearables and environmental sensors. Furthermore, AI-based IoT devices can monitor patient adherence to medication, remind patients of missed doses, and adjust treatment plans based on continuous data input-all working together to improve patient outcomes and enhance the overall effectiveness of healthcare delivery.

Figure 4 outlines a process of three steps for personalized healthcare, namely: collecting data from genetics, medicine, and personal wearable devices; analyzing it with the aid of AI to produce insights; and analyzing the individual information to give an appropriate recommendation on what medication one should undertake, lifestyle changes, or surgery.

Figure 4. AI-Powered Personalized Healthcare Framework

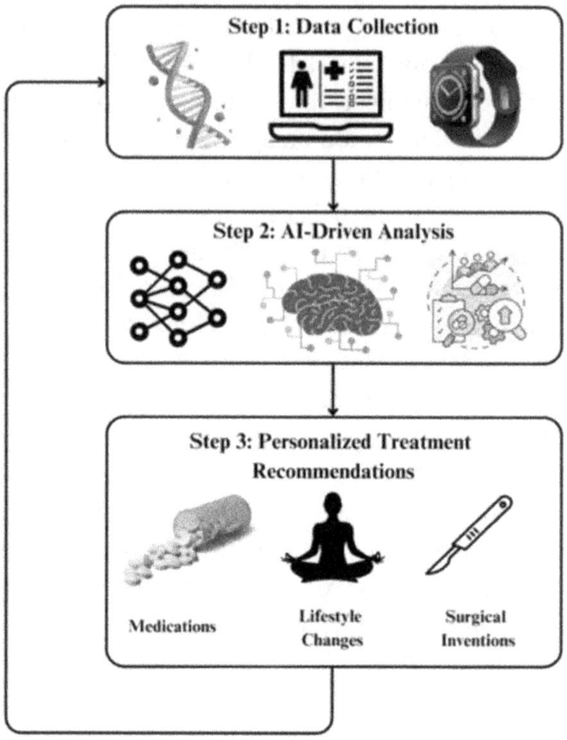

Integration of AI and IoT has given rise to promising applications in intelligent homecare systems. Now caregivers can monitor patients remotely in their homes through the development of smart devices that track vital signs, movements, and overall health metrics and provide immediate care or changes in the patients' health regimens. Thus, innovative homecare solutions can help reduce the burden on hospitals, making long-term conditions more manageable and giving way to the aged in better and less stressful environments.

7.2 Role of AI in Population Health Management

In simple terms, population health management works to improve health outcomes for people and the cost and resource controls around their care. AI plays a pivotal role via analyzing several terabytes of health data for identifying trends, predicting behavior, and optimizing intervention strategies. Further, machine learning models and big data analytics can predict outbreaks of diseases, high-risk individuals, and more effective intervention targeting. Health systems can shift from a reactive model to proactive, preventive disease management, thus considerably mitigating overall burdens on healthcare.

Identify patients who could experience such chronic diseases like heart disease, diabetes, and cancer. Bringing all health data available through different channels like electronic health records (EHRs), genetic information, and lifestyle attributes, an AI-enabled model can also produce actionable health insights from its study of these data for use by health providers in early interventions. This early detection would make possible better treatment and decrease long-term health costs as well as disease severity in the population.

By understanding and analyzing massive amounts of data, AI will optimize resource allocation in PHM. (Singh, T. M., et al., 2024) For example, it will assist healthcare systems decision-making based on the prediction of future population groupings requiring further care in the area of staffing, resource distribution, and program implementation. At a broader level, AI can help inform policies in public health through future projection of healthcare requirements and supporting evidence to shape efficient strategies toward improving population health outcomes, resulting in more equitable and effective health systems.

7.3 Potential of AI-Driven Telemedicine

Over the recent years, telemedicine has grown leaps and bounds, responding particularly to the verdict of the COVID-19 pandemic. (Reddy, C. K. K., et al., 2024) The idea is to leverage and integrate AI into telemedicine and transform the whole delivery of services to remote consultations, making them more productive and accurate. AI-powered tools such as virtual health assistants and diagnostic algorithms enhance telemedicine platforms, which provide immediate, evidence-based support for healthcare professionals. Tasks performed by AI include triaging patients, interpreting symptoms, and offering potential diagnoses, enabling real-time decision-making by clinicians during consultations.

Table 5 highlights some of the features on which AI-powered telemedicine platforms are built, such as virtual consultations, remote monitoring, and real-time language translation, as well as how they facilitate access to chronic care and efficient utilization of healthcare resources.

Table 5. Transforming Telemedicine with AI

Telemedicine Feature	AI Application	Operational Impact	Examples
Virtual Consultations	AI-powered diagnostic tools	Faster and accurate consultations	Symptom-checker apps
Remote Patient Monitoring	AI-driven alerts	Improved chronic care	Diabetes monitoring systems
Language Translation	NLP for real-time translations	Increased accessibility	Multilingual telehealth platforms
Patient Triage Systems	AI for priority determination	Efficient resource utilization	Emergency triage apps

AI brings a major change in patient engagement and monitoring in telemedicine. An AI virtual health assistant could walk the patient through the medical process, answer questions about symptoms or medications, and provide emotional support as needed. In addition, patients' data collected by wearable devices like smartwatches or m-health applications can also be monitored by AI algorithms. They measure progress, identify abnormalities, or alert health care providers of disturbing changes, which enable continuous care even outside of the clinic.

AI-powered telemedicine has fantastic prospects for eliminating disparities with respect to access to healthcare services in remote areas and other underserved areas. Telemedicine powered by AI allows patients to have appointments with specialists from the comfort of their homes, reducing travel time, costs, and waiting time to get the care they need. With such inclusiveness, high-quality care is available to almost everyone and improves overall equity in healthcare.

7.4 AI-Driven Personalized Medicine

Personalized medicine essentially customizes medical treatment by individual patient characteristics, like their genetic makeup, lifestyle, and environment. Each person is diverse from one another. AI is very significant across the world toward the improvement of personalized medicine because healthcare providers can design more targeted treatments. AI algorithms can analyze large amounts of patient data, genetic sequences, electronic health records (EHRs), and clinical histories to identify patterns and predict how individuals will react to interesting therapies. Such precision can enhance the effectiveness of therapies with reduced adverse effects offering patients care designed to be unique to their needs (Yogeshappa, V. G., 2024).

Machine learning models are extremely proficient in predicting genetic markers associated with disease, allowing healthcare providers to determine disease risk, optimize preventive care, and, perhaps most critically, tailor treatment to the individual's genetic profile. For instance, oncologists can design personalized cancer treatments by using AI to analyze tumor genetics of the patient and determine the best drug regimens that are most likely to be effective, enhancing the chances for a successful outcome. In addition to oncology, AI-powered personalized medicine has potential applications in other branches, such as cardiology and neurology, or in rare diseases, where treatments tend to be limited or less effective without a customized approach.

The role of AI in personalized medicine stretches treatment planning beyond the drug discovery and clinical trials. AI can cross over to analyzing large datasets to recognize prospective drug candidates while completely predicting how they would behave in the human body; thus there is a considerable reduction in the time a drug would take to develop. AI-based optimization can lead to better design for clinical trials, making it possible to identify candidates based on genetic profiles, and also predict how such individuals will respond to new treatments. All this ensures quicker clearance time for drugs into the market and gives the patient's perfect medicine tailored toward his unique informative characteristics.

CONCLUSION

AI can really improve operational processes in the health systems so that healthcare become more efficient and effective. The analysis of machine learning can optimize the scheduling of patients, resource allocation, flow management, and overall patient management, which in turn will help reduce waiting time and increase demand. Besides, the health system will be aided by predictive analytics to forecast demand and manage the volume of patients, thereby maintaining operational smoothing and minimizing inefficiencies. Moreover, even the AIs that are meant for decision support for clinical staff and administrators can lead to even better clinical decision making in a given patient population based on higher quality and speed of information that is processed. These changes indicate savings in overhead costs, resource improvement, and enhanced patient satisfaction. AI can also be used to automate and shuttle tasks such as billing, documentation, and the processing of claims, freeing up employees to concentrate on providing better patient care. Last but not least, it adds the linking role in optimizing supply chains in the health care service industry, thereby ensuring that the needed resources are available with the least amount of waste.

Adoption of phased and strategic approaches to scaling, integrating, and sustaining AI-improvements can make or break healthcare organizations. Investment in a technological infrastructure that ties into existing systems like the electronic health record (EHR) becomes significantly more crucial. Custom solutions targeted at specific operational needs must be developed with the guidance of AI experts, as well as policies regarding governance of data for security and compliance. Staff must be counseled on, trained in, and prepared for acceptance of AI technologies and change management strategies that reduce natural resistance. Continuous performance monitoring of AI implementation by leadership and real-time data-informed steering will go a long way toward successful and strategic implementation of AI in healthcare organizations. Through meticulous planning and elicit engagement, freedom is given to AI to delve into improving healthcare operations, rendering them more efficient, effective, and patient-centered.

REFERENCES

Abràmoff, M. D., Tarver, M. E., Loyo-Berrios, N., Trujillo, S., Char, D., Obermeyer, Z., Eydelman, M. B., & Maisel, W. H. (2023). Considerations for addressing bias in artificial intelligence for health equity. npj. *Digital Medicine*, *6*(1), 170. DOI: 10.1038/s41746-023-00913-9 PMID: 37700029

Adenekan, T. K. (2024). *AI-Driven Diagnostic Models for Cardiovascular Health: Exploring Security and Business Analytics in Aortic Stenosis Detection*. ResearchGate.

Burrell, D. N., Burton, S. L., Nobles, C., Springs, D., Huff, A. J., Brown-Jackson, K. L., Richardson, K., Wright, J. B., Muller, S. R., & Jones, A. J. (2023). The Managerial Ethical and Operational Challenges of Hospital Cybersecurity. In Burrell, D. (Ed.), *Transformational Interventions for Business, Technology, and Healthcare* (pp. 444–458). IGI Global Scientific Publishing., DOI: 10.4018/979-8-3693-1634-4.ch026

Cogin, J. A., Ng, J. L., & Lee, I. (2016). Controlling healthcare professionals: How human resource management influences job attitudes and operational efficiency. *Human Resources for Health*, *14*(1), 55. DOI: 10.1186/s12960-016-0149-0 PMID: 27649794

Dhatterwal, J. S., Kaswan, K. S., & Kumar, N. (2023). Robotic process automation in healthcare. In S. Bhattacharyya, J. S. Banerjee, & D. De (Eds.), Confluence of artificial intelligence and robotic process automation (pp. 157–175). Smart Innovation, Systems and Technologies (Vol. 335). Springer, Singapore. https://doi.org/DOI: 10.1007/978-981-19-8296-5_7

Eswaran, U., Eswaran, V., Murali, K., & Eswaran, V. (2024). Predictive Healthcare Analytics. In Exploring the Advancements and Future Directions of Digital Twins in Healthcare 6.0 (pp. 171-199). IGI Global.

Fayaz, M., Amin, M., & Iqbal, M. (2024). Artificial intelligence in decision-making: A descriptive analysis of its impact on strategic planning. *Journal of Business and Management Research*, *3*(2), 222–235. http://jbmr.com.pk/index.php/Journal/article/view/228

Goffman, R. M., Harris, S. L., May, J. H., Milicevic, A. S., Monte, R. J., Myaskovsky, L., Rodriguez, K. L., Tjader, Y. C., & Vargas, D. L. (2017). Modeling patient no-show history and predicting future outpatient appointment behavior in the Veterans Health Administration. *Military Medicine*, *182*(5-6), e1708–e1714. DOI: 10.7205/MILMED-D-16-00345 PMID: 29087915

Harris, S. L., May, J. H., & Vargas, L. G. (2016). Predictive analytics model for healthcare planning and scheduling. *European Journal of Operational Research*, *253*(1), 121–131. DOI: 10.1016/j.ejor.2016.02.017

Heba, M. (2022). Healthcare Workers' Resilience Toolkit for Disaster Management and Climate Change Adaptation. *International Journal of Environmental Research and Public Health*, *19*(19), 12440–12440. DOI: 10.3390/ijerph191912440 PMID: 36231739

Janowski, A. (2023). Natural Language Processing Techniques for Clinical Text Analysis in Healthcare. *Journal of Advanced Analytics in Healthcare Management*, *7*(1), 51–76. https://research.tensorgate.org/index.php/JAAHM/article/view/37

Joshi, H., Kumar Reddy, C. K., Ouaissa, M., Mohd Hanafiah, M., & Doss, S. (2024). Intelligent systems and IoT applications in clinical health. In IGI Global. https://doi.org/DOI: 10.4018/979-8-3693-8990-4

Kalaria, C., Singh, S., & Prajapati, B. G. (2023). Intelligent Healthcare Supply Chain. Human-Machine Interface: Making Healthcare Digital, 449-481.

Ko, D.-G., Mai, F., Shan, Z., & Zhang, D. (2019). Operational efficiency and patient-centered health care: A view from online physician reviews. *Journal of Operations Management*, *65*(4), 353–379. DOI: 10.1002/joom.1028

Lopes, M. A., Almeida, Á. S., & Almada-Lobo, B. (2015). Handling healthcare workforce planning with care: Where do we stand? *Human Resources for Health*, *13*(1), 38. DOI: 10.1186/s12960-015-0028-0 PMID: 26003337

Mahmoudian, Y., Nemati, A., & Safaei, A. S. (2023). A forecasting approach for hospital bed capacity planning using machine learning and deep learning with application to public hospitals. *Healthcare Analytics*, *4*, 100245. DOI: 10.1016/j.health.2023.100245

Mohanarangan, V. Devarajan., Rajya, Lakshmi, Gudivaka., Basava, Ramanjaneyulu, Gudivaka., Raj, Kumar, Gudivaka., T., Ganesan., Priyan, Malarvizhi, Kumar. (2024). Computer Vision-Based Radial Basis Function Networks in Healthcare Applications. DOI: 10.2139/ssrn.4809360

Munavalli, J. R., Boersma, H. J., Rao, S. V., & van Merode, G. G. (2021). Real-time capacity management and patient flow optimization in hospitals using AI methods. In Masmoudi, M., Jarboui, B., & Siarry, P. (Eds.), *Artificial intelligence and data mining in healthcare*. Springer., DOI: 10.1007/978-3-030-45240-7_3

Nasrullah, A. (2024). Utilizing Machine Learning for Predictive Analytics. *Advances in Healthcare Technology.*, *1*(1), 57–67. DOI: 10.60087/japmi.vol01.issue01.p67

Nicholson, L., Vakharia, A. J., & Erenguc, S. S. (2004). Outsourcing inventory management decisions in healthcare: Models and application. *European Journal of Operational Research*, *154*(1), 271–290. DOI: 10.1016/S0377-2217(02)00700-2

Reddy, C. K. K., Pujala, N., & Doss, S. (2024). From Industry 4.0 to 5.0: Navigating the human-tech symbiosis in the era of COVID-19. In Ethical artificial intelligence in power electronics. CRC Press Taylor and Francis. https://doi.org/DOI: 10.1201/9781032648323

Saha, E., & Ray, P. K. (2019). Modelling and analysis of inventory management systems in healthcare: A review and reflections. *Computers & Industrial Engineering*, *137*, 106051. DOI: 10.1016/j.cie.2019.106051

Sarker, S., Jamal, L., Ahmed, S. F., & Irtisam, N. (2021). Robotics and artificial intelligence in healthcare during the COVID-19 pandemic: A systematic review. *Robotics and Autonomous Systems*, *146*, 103902. DOI: 10.1016/j.robot.2021.103902 PMID: 34629751

Singh, T. M., Reddy, C. K. K., & Lippert, K. (2024). Advancing human-centric solutions: The future trajectory of soft computing in modern society. In Kumar, N., Pal, S., Agarwal, P., Rosak-Szyrocka, J., & Jain, V. (Eds.), *Human-machine collaboration and emotional intelligence in Industry 5.0* (pp. 1–18). IGI Global., DOI: 10.4018/979-8-3693-6806-0.ch001

Swathi, G. (2024, August 29). Navigating the Integration of Machine Learning in Healthcare: Challenges, Strategies, and Ethical Considerations. *Journal of Computational and Cognitive Engineering*. Advance online publication. DOI: 10.47852/bonviewJCCE42023600

Thakur, G. K., Thakur, A., Khan, N., & Anush, H. (2024). The role of natural language processing in medical data analysis and healthcare automation. *2024 International Conference on Knowledge Engineering and Communication Systems (ICKECS)*, Chikkaballapur, India, 1–5. https://doi.org/DOI: 10.1109/ICKECS61492.2024.10616749

Udo, B. (2023). Robotic Process Automation (RPA) in Healthcare. *International Research Journal on Advanced Science Hub*, *5*(05S), 229–235. DOI: 10.47392/irjash.2023.S030

Wen, A., Fu, S., Moon, S., El Wazir, M., Rosenbaum, A., Kaggal, V. C., Liu, S., Sohn, S., Liu, H., & Fan, J. (2019). Desiderata for delivering NLP to accelerate healthcare AI advancement and a Mayo Clinic NLP-as-a-service implementation. npj. *Digital Medicine*, *2*(1), 130. DOI: 10.1038/s41746-019-0208-8 PMID: 31872069

Wu, H., Lu, X., & Wang, H. (2023). The application of artificial intelligence in health care resource allocation before and during the COVID-19 pandemic: Scoping review. *JMIR AI*, *2*, e38397. DOI: 10.2196/38397

Yogeshappa, V. G. (2024). AI-driven precision medicine: Revolutionizing personalized treatment plans. [IJCET]. *International Journal of Computer Engineering and Technology*, *15*(5), 455–474. DOI: 10.5281/zenodo.13843057

Zizheng, H. (2024, February). Computer vision-aided mmWave communications for indoor medical healthcare. *Computers in Biology and Medicine*, *169*, 107869. Advance online publication. DOI: 10.1016/j.compbiomed.2023.107869

Chapter 10
Artificial Intelligence in Transforming Healthcare Operations and Enhancing Clinical Efficiency

M. Manickam
https://orcid.org/0009-0006-7621-9588
SRM Institute of Science and Technology, India

A. Divya
Sathyabama Institute of Science and Technology, India

D. Sungeetha
Saveetha University, India

G. Michael
Saveetha University, India

S. Ramesh
SRM Institute of Science and Technology, India

Raj Kumar Masih
Jazan University, Saudi Arabia

ABSTRACT

Some have even gone so far as to call AI the most revolutionary technology of the 2000s. AI is the study and practice of developing smart devices and systems, especially Artificial Intelligence (AI). The diversity of AI's uses demonstrates the pervasiveness of this technology. In discussions about AI in healthcare, the vast databases that hospitals and physicians have access to might include knowledge that could save lives. Medical professionals may benefit from AI algorithms if they were to use them to develop better methods and treatment plans for their patients. Traditional medicine's three pillars—diagnosis, prognosis, and therapy—are all enhanced by AI. In this chapter, we will go over the basics of AI in healthcare, including how it works, different systems for collecting and storing data, preprocessing medical data, algorithms for healthcare, methodology for medical while medicinal diagnosis, feature selection and extraction, disease diagnosis, medical image processing, and AI-powered patient care and treatment.

DOI: 10.4018/979-8-3373-1022-0.ch010

1. INTRODUCTION

To be more specific, the research found that AI could reliably identify ailments 87% of the time, but human healthcare providers could only manage an 86% success rate. Deep learning approaches achieved an accuracy of 93%, which is higher than the 91% achieved by people (Taliento, 2023). Deep learning has the potential to significantly improve its diagnostic accuracy in the next years as AI technology progresses (Al-Dmour et al., 2025). In a recent collaboration, pharmaceutical giant Bayer and digital startups developed software to aid in the diagnosis of rare and odd illnesses and the development of novel treatments for these conditions. They have also been working with medical facilities and academics to determine what other factors AI should use when determining a patient's health state. Symptom data, illness causes, test findings, medical pictures, doctor reports, and a plethora of other sources provide the data that the AI processes (Swain et al., 2022). Computers can analyze data obtained from the diagnosis of various chronic diseases like Alzheimer's, cardiovascular disease, diabetes, and many types of cancer (e.g., breast cancer, colon cancer, etc.), and artificial intelligence aims to make computers more efficient at solving difficult healthcare problems. It makes it possible to identify a range of chronic illnesses, which in turn reduces healthcare costs and slows the course of these conditions. To minimize human error and monitor illness progression, several computational systems and devices are used. These include ASL-MRI, biomarkers, Arterial Spin Labeling (ASL) Imaging, Brain-Computer Interfaces (BCIs), and a plethora of other approaches. To assist clinicians in decreasing inter- and intra-observer variability, computer-aided decision-support systems, diagnostics, expert systems, and software integration are available (Nianga, 2024) (Patil & Shankar, 2023).

In particular, AI methods aim to streamline the diagnostic process. It is possible to handle many kinds of medical data using ANN and Fuzzy methods (Khan et al., 2024b). When it comes to designing clinical support systems, the ANN technique is efficient and can uncover hidden relationships and patterns in medical data. The use of AI allows for rapid and accurate interpretation of the data. There are four main types of chronic illnesses that are not caused by a virus or other infectious agent: cardiovascular disease, cancer, chronic obstructive pulmonary disease, and diabetes. It would be very helpful in lowering disease compilations if any non-communicable illnesses could be identified efficiently. It helps in formulating treatment plans. Numerous identification and treatment techniques have shown that AI is beneficial to healthcare. Computers may be programmed to solve healthcare issues, and data collected from the diagnosis of various chronic illnesses can be examined with the help of AI (Suboyin et al., 2024).

Figure 1. Testing and Training Models

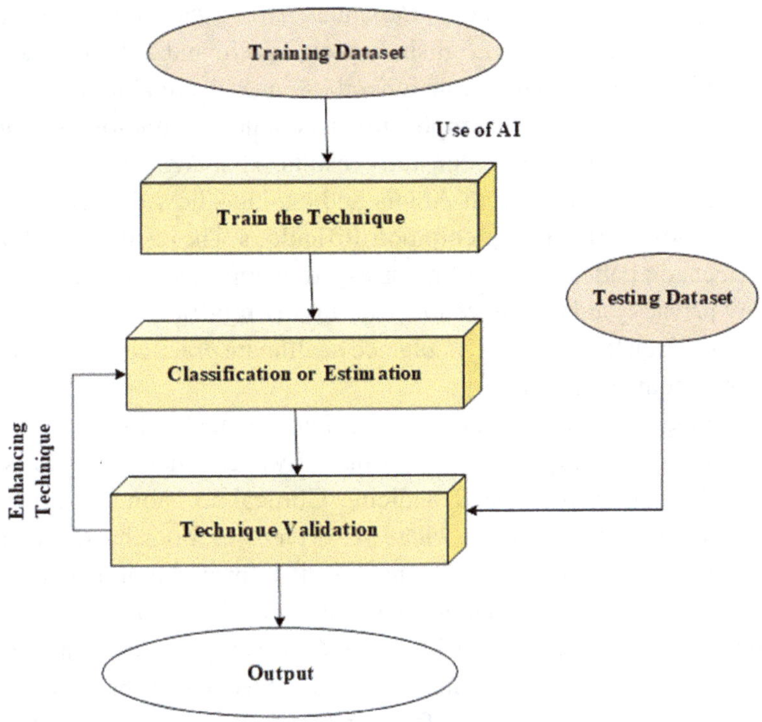

By defining a number of methods, AI makes it possible for systems to carry out tasks more successfully and efficiently. As more and more data is collected digitally, AI approaches are becoming more important in healthcare and wellness enterprises. Machine learning (ML), as well as AI, may provide useful results by combining many tasks simultaneously and improving upon prior results, especially as the dataset becomes larger by the day. These strategies may be used for the collection, storage, and analysis of many types of healthcare data, ranging from inpatient histories to diagnostic procedures. Afterward, it offers smart ways to discover potential healthcare solutions. Cardiology, strokes, diabetes, cancer, and other diseases may all benefit from the early detection and treatment made possible by AI techniques (Rawas et al., 2024).

While AI finds its most common use in medical diagnosis, it is also employed for prediction and treatment, the three mainstays of conventional medicine. You can see the medical diagnostic-therapeutic cycle in Figure 1. Assessment and evaluation of the patient, gathering of relevant data from the patient, analysis of that data in light of the physician's clinical expertise, and finally, the development of a diagnosis and treatment plan comprise the standard medical diagnostic cycle. Let's compare the medical diagnostic cycle to an intelligent agent system. We can see that the practitioner is the agent, patient data is the input, and the diagnosis is the output. There is a wide variety of ways in which AI may mimic this diagnostic procedure and aid doctors in making diagnoses (Ara & Mifa, 2024).

2. STATE OF THE ART

Generative AI model, CoSpeak (Agrawal & Poovaiah, 2021) was created and deployed, enabling Spanish, voice-to-voice communication in English, French, Hindi, and Telugu, among other languages. In order to provide adaptive and tailored interactions, these agents are able to interpret and empathize with human emotions. To comprehend the complex impacts of new technologies on healthcare delivery, (Zhang & Kamel Boulos, 2023)compiles recent study results. That analysis focuses on healthcare innovations that have been implemented in Saudi Arabia and explains how they have improved healthcare quality, streamlined processes, and addressed common difficulties. The results show that new technologies have many positive effects on patient care along with system administration. Still, they also bring new problems with security privacy, and they have to spend more on infrastructure. The analysis highlights the need for continuing research to successfully enhance healthcare practices and negotiate the challenges of technology adoption (Yadav et al., 2025).

Based on ever-improving deep learning and machine learning technologies, (Iliashenko et al., 2019) study considers the major possibilities given by AI, particularly in enhancing diagnosis accuracy, optimizing planning therapy, and enabling customized medicine. Clinical decision support, predictive analytics, and large-scale medical imaging are all areas where AI-driven solutions have shown encouraging performance, giving doctors greater opportunities to make well-informed judgments. When integrating AI into healthcare facilities, there are substantial hurdles that must be tackled. Problems with data privacy, algorithmic bias, and the lack of visibility into AI decisions are only the tip of the iceberg. Additionally, accountability is important because usage ethics are at the forefront of the debate around the deployment of artificial intelligence in healthcare, and few legal frameworks address that issue. Therefore, the assessment has recognized that thorough policy formulation, ethical norms, and regulations are urgently required to enable the secure and effective implementation of AI. Emerging developments in AI that are poised to improve patient care include telemedicine, remote patient monitoring, and robotic surgery with AI enhancements. The prospect of AI in healthcare is bright. Although there has been a lot of focus on the healthcare applications of AI, it is essential to tackle the ethical, legal, and operational issues that come with AI systems before we can fully use their capabilities.

The article (Olawade et al., 2024) introduces a paradigm for AI-powered service delivery that can optimize operations on its own, boost customer happiness, and drive company development. In order to automate issue management, anticipate operational interruptions, and improve client experiences, the article makes use of AI algorithms. Enhancements in service efficiency and operational cost reduction of 30%, along with customer satisfaction ratings of 30% have been seen in real-world applications across the retail, healthcare, as well as technology industries. In order to revolutionize the delivery of complicated, scalable, and dependable services, that paper suggests AI-driven service innovations.

The paper delves into the revolutionary effects of cloud computing and artificial intelligence on the retail, healthcare, and mobile banking industries (Valaboju, 2024). We investigate how these technologies are transforming innovation, consumer experiences, and operational efficiency by conducting an in-depth study of industry-specific applications. We study how scalable cloud infrastructure and continuous integration/continuous delivery automation may improve healthcare system dependability and patient care (Qamar et al., 2023). Supply chain optimization and consumer insights powered by AI are the primary areas of attention in the retail industry's study. We take a look at blockchain's use in real-time analytics and fraud detection as it pertains to mobile financial services (Ango et al., 2024) (Masih et al., 2023). Across all three sectors, the results show considerable increases in operational effectiveness, decision-making speed, and customer happiness. However, we also see possibilities and threats that are sector-specific. Industry experts and policymakers may gain useful insights from that essay as they navigate the integration of AI with cloud technology in their respective disciplines. It also adds to the increasing body of research on digital transformation (Shuaib et al., 2023).

That article takes a look at the many facets of AI in healthcare, including topics such as real-time data analysis, patient interaction platforms, operational efficiency gains, therapeutic advantages, and future advances. The paper highlights notable progress in healthcare accessibility, customization of patient care, and diagnostic accuracy achieved using AI-powered technologies. That article shows how several healthcare organizations have used AI to improve patient outcomes, administrative procedures, and clinical decision-making. Additionally, it discusses the important role AI plays in lowering healthcare inequities by allowing underprivileged populations to access high-quality medical treatments via telemedicine (Singh et al., 2022)

Examining short-term operational gains and long-term cost savings, the essay assesses the financial ramifications of AI deployment in healthcare systems. The article's study sheds light on the complementary nature of artificial intelligence and telemedicine, providing a foundation for comprehending how these two technologies could influence healthcare delivery in the years to come.

Examines the creation and launch of Doctolib, an AI-powered healthcare platform meant to resolve these concerns, in (Deepa et al., 2024). To improve the effectiveness of appointment management, Doctolib uses complex algorithms and real-time scheduling with predictive analytics. Important features include a chatbot powered by artificial intelligence that provides round-the-clock patient assistance, a safe way to integrate telemedicine for distant consultations, and tools to optimize demand for improved resource allocation. Extensive testing of the platform revealed significant improvements to operational operations and patient satisfaction rates. Doctolib can revolutionize digital healthcare with its unique and scalable solutions, as shown by these results.

That article examines the portrayal of AI and ADM in news and industrial media as well as its present uses in Australian healthcare settings (Watson & Wozniak-O'Connor, 2025). It classifies the most popular uses of AI and ADM, which include tracking and monitoring, handling and analyzing data, cloud computing, and robots. By looking at the ways AI and ADM are portrayed in connection to healthcare procedures, it examines the optimism that is shown in these ways. The last section of the essay considers the consequences of promissory discourses on the comprehension and incorporation of technology into healthcare practices and locations.

A comprehensive analysis of the ways in which AI is improving healthcare systems' operational efficiency and the results for patients is presented in (Polevikov, 2023). Numerous areas of healthcare delivery are incorporating AI via the use of complex algorithms, including diagnoses, individualized treatment plans, and administrative duties. Improving diagnosis accuracy is a key area of attention. In terms of identifying and diagnosing medical conditions, AI-backed diagnostic technologies like picture recognition software and prediction models have surpassed conventional approaches. For example, AI algorithms have shown to be very adept at evaluating medical imagery, leading to more precise diagnosis and early identification of illnesses such as cancer, cardiovascular issues, and neurological disorders. These improvements not only make it possible to intervene quickly, but they also greatly decrease the number of cases when a false diagnosis is made, which improves patient prognosis and dramatically lowers healthcare expenses.

The purpose of the research was to examine the impact of AI techniques and HRM practices that encourage creativity on the successful functioning of organizations (Ghaffar et al., 2024). Its stated goal was to investigate how progressive HR practices and AI deployment work together to boost productivity and other performance indicators for businesses. Staff members of private hospitals in Lahore, Pakistan, were surveyed using a cross-sectional method for that research. In order to determine the connections among AI execution of strategies, creativity-oriented HRM practices, and organizational effective performance, 144 valid replies were examined applying Partial Least Squares Structural Equation Modeling. Composite reliability, Cronbach's alpha, and average variance extracted metrics were used to assess the constructs' reliability and validity (Singh et al., 2025).

3. AI METHODOLOGY FOR MEDICAL AND MEDICINAL DIAGNOSIS

Many industries have begun to use AI techniques, particularly ML and DL since they are both very efficient and accurate, and they can replace manual labor. Since AI uses a scaled noise level to quantify the mapping among known and unknown (Karthik, Aalam, et al., 2024), it outperforms more conventional methods like characteristics extraction. A more effective method for solving complicated issues may be achieved by combining old and current learning algorithms.

The use of AI in healthcare has grown in prominence in the last few years. There seems to be a great deal of promise for the use of AI in healthcare. These days, computers can learn from experience and respond to specific inputs by predicting outcomes, identifying objects, and even suggesting next steps. With the help of AI, medical professionals may be able to treat patients more effectively and with more accuracy. There are several potential benefits for healthcare industry advancements in using AI for medical diagnostics. Artificial intelligence software may diagnose a patient's condition before any outward signs of illness show up (Karthik, Hamatta, et al., 2024).

3.1 Digital Imaging

Laboratory testing using AI is much more efficient when smart equipment with digital imaging capabilities is used (Poloju & Rajaram, 2024). The use of artificial intelligence in medical diagnostics has the potential to reduce diagnosis times compared to more traditional methods of microscopic analysis.

3.2 Cloud-based Platform for Interaction

Through AI-based medical diagnosis, pathologists may electronically transmit pictures and data to experts all over the world, greatly enhancing research, diagnosis, and collaborative diagnosis; this eliminates the need to transfer samples from one place to another physically. Physical inspections are prone to human mistakes; however, automated AI technologies, such as AI for medical research, significantly lessen this challenge (Aqeel et al., 2023) .

Automated Diagnosis

Thanks to AI, the automated design of digital pathology allows pathologists to significantly boost their productivity by eliminating manual procedures and laborious elements of generating pathology reports. Machine learning allows for faster and more accurate diagnosis.

3.3 AI Lab Testing

AI in the lab means smart algorithms that can identify patterns, both broad and detailed, and use that information to make reasonable and reliable diagnoses of patient illnesses. Automated testing techniques in AI-based medical diagnostics provide for a faster reaction time than traditional microscopic tests (Syamala et al., 2024).

3.4 Image Analysis

There will likely be a dramatic shift when AI-powered medical diagnoses replace glass with pixels that can be transmitted for specialist study anywhere in the world, making digital pathologists obsolete. AI in medical testing uses image analysis methods to automate detection based on software-generated research and recorded data (Reddy et al., 2024).

3.5 Predictive Analytics

AI systems use predictive analytics technology to aid doctors in early illness vulnerability detection. That encourages people to focus on prevention rather than therapy after the fact. Intelligent machine learning identifies patients with a history of a specific illness susceptibility, allowing doctors to monitor their long-term health better. AI is a game-changer for pathologists when it comes to medical diagnosis. It can spot unusual things in all sorts of bodily fluids, including blood, urine, and other tissues . Using AI, medical diagnostic tools might automatically identify abnormalities in bodily fluids and tissues (Khan et al., 2024a).

3.6 Selection and Extraction of Features Using AI

Several research works have focused on the issue of variable selection, with datasets including hundreds or even thousands of variables for purposes such as classification, clustering, and function approximation. There are two separate ways to characterize the subset of input variables that might be considered:

- **Feature Selection:** By picking out a subset of the real input variables, feature selection aids in dimensionality reduction.
- **Feature Extraction:** The process of feature extraction changes the real variables into more valuable features. When dealing with data that has a lot of characteristics, it's better to reduce them so that the data can be studied better.

The curse of dimensionality issue arises when the number of variables exceeds the number of samples available; this causes the learning technique's accuracy to decrease as the number of features increases. It may happen in extreme instances. The primary rationale for attempting data reduction is the need to shorten the computational effort of the given learning technique, improve its accuracy, and increase the understanding and knowledge of the problem at hand by identifying the factors that directly impact it.

3.7 Disease Diagnosis with AI

Correctly diagnosing illnesses calls for years of medical education. Even then, the diagnostic process is lengthy and intricate. There is a severe shortage of qualified individuals in various fields. As a result, physicians are already under a lot of stress, and patients sometimes have to wait longer for life-saving diagnoses (Reddy C et al., 2024). Automatic illness diagnosis has lately made great strides with the use of AI, especially DL methods, which has made diagnosis more accessible and economical. Computer programs will eventually be able to recognize patterns in the same way that humans can. One key distinction is the large number of specialized examples required for algorithmic learning (Alqahtani et al., 2023). Furthermore, these examples must be digitalized in a seamless manner since computers are unable to read the fine print in textbooks. When a physician can access digital versions of the medical records they utilize for patient care, AI becomes even more valuable. Here are a few examples:

- Cancer of the lung and strokes may be discovered with computed tomography imaging.
- Assessing the risk of sudden cardiac death or other cardiac diseases using electrocardiogram (ECG) and magnetic resonance imaging (MRI) of the heart.
- Skin condition classification using skin photos.
- Signs of diabetic retinopathy may be seen in ocular pictures.

Diagnostic methods are evolving to match the efficacy of professionals in these cases, thanks to the availability of high-quality data available. The difference is that the methods could be easily copied all around the world and could provide the outcomes in a matter of seconds. Eventually, everyone will be able to affordably access the same high-quality radiological diagnostic professionals from across the globe.

4. AI PARADIGM FOR HEALTHCARE

4.1 Data Collection

Data collection is all about gathering and analyzing specific variable information. This information helps find the right solution and analyze the outcomes. Primary and secondary sources of information are the two main ways in which data may be collected.

Figure 2. Medical diagnostic–therapeutic cycle

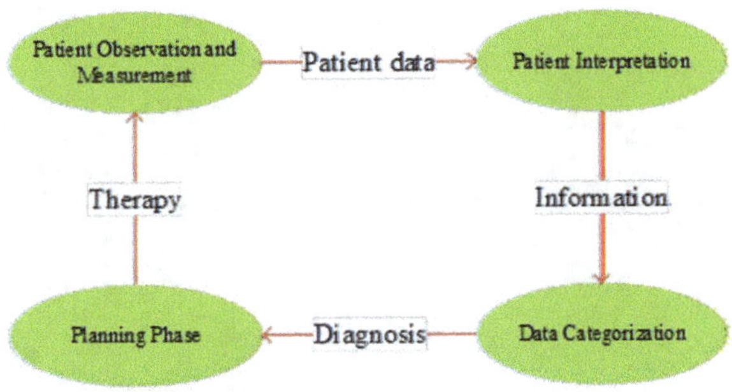

- Primary data collection: It is also known as primary data. Observation, surveys, interviews, and focus groups are some examples.
- Secondary Data: Information that has already been gathered and examined by another party. Sources such as research articles, the Internet, and libraries are examples. There is a dearth of useful information in the healthcare industry's massively produced data.

Data may be collected for healthcare research and administration in a variety of ways. The varied nature of healthcare data makes it feasible to gather information from a variety of different sources, both primary and secondary. With their well-established gathering and reporting of data information systems, well-trained staff, and familiarity with quality enhancement tools, hospitals are always prepared to gather demographic information from their patients (Alam et al., 2023; Khubrani & Alam, 2021). Multiple organizations, including CHCs, physicians, health plans, and hospitals, use a wide variety of public and commercial data-gathering methods, such as health reviews, organizational registration, accounting records, and medical information. Data collection, both from patients and on their behalf, is an integral aspect of healthcare, particularly when analysis of that data is critical to providing the most effective and optimal therapy. Due to the proliferation of online disease registries, healthcare providers now have access to a wealth of data that allows them to process more patients' information in less time with more trustworthy findings, ultimately leading to faster treatment. All providers, no matter how big or little, need a plan for gathering data and then processing it.

Figure 3. AI-based Healthcare Model

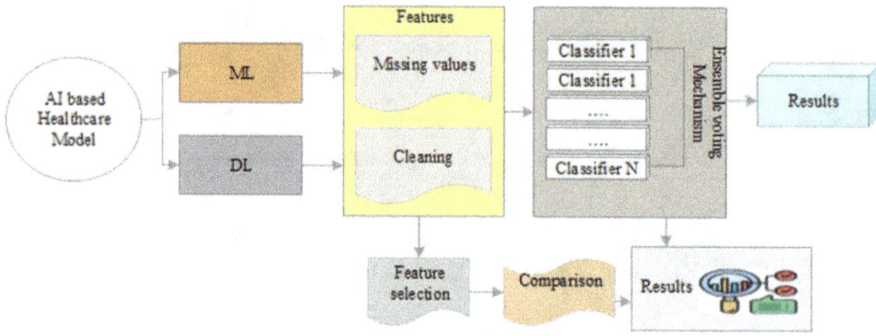

4.2 Medical Data Pre-processing

Data pre-processing and data collection are the two most important components of data mining because they allow for the selection of high-quality, final data that is suitable for further processing. Healthcare institutions collect a wide variety of data, some organized and others unstructured, including information about patients, doctors, hospitals, and medical records. All sorts of visual and auditory information are a part of medical records. These massive and varied datasets need efficient pre-processing technologies for integration and translation into a single format. As medical data continues to grow at an exponential rate, data mining has gained significant traction in the healthcare sector. When it comes to assessing and discovering useful medical data, data mining is perhaps the best approach. The healthcare industry relies heavily on data pre-processing. Missing values, inconsistent data, noisy data, etc., are the results of the lack of strict regulation of the data-gathering procedure. The analytical method may provide unpredictable results when dealing with such data kinds. For this reason, the processing format of the data is essential for accurate output. Consequently, prior to doing any analysis, it is essential to ensure that the data is accurately represented and of high quality. Cleansing, normalizing, transforming, selecting, and extracting features are all part of data pre-processing. Data pre-processing yields the final training set. There is a high degree of noise, unpredictability, and missing numbers in raw data. Among the most critical steps in data mining—which is all about getting the original information ready for analysis—is data pre-processing, which is ideal for enhancing data quality. Mistakes abound when it comes to medical data, which is often lacking, inconsistent, or incomplete. Sometimes, there is not enough information in the raw medical records to make the right judgments.

Regardless, the outcomes produced by the pre-processing techniques are precise. Healthcare companies nowadays generate a diverse array of data forms, including unstructured, structured, and semi-structured data. Information on patients' health has been compiled from a variety of sources, including online databases, medical facilities, doctors' notes, and patient records. Using ETL tools or typical pre-processing procedures, large and varied data may be combined from several sources. It includes Excel, SQL databases, and more. Then, a number of pre-processing tools and procedures are already in existence to convert them into a single standard format. The success of healthcare decisions and treatments depends on healthcare knowledge data. Standard data preparation procedures, such as cleaning, integrating, transforming, and reducing data, are also followed in medical data pre-processing. The real-time nature of medical data makes its handling a formidable obstacle. Data There are four main types of pre-processing methods:

- Data cleaning— managing databases containing information on cardiac disorders and other ailments, including those with missing values, inconsistent data, and noisy data.
- Combining information from many sources, such as patient records, test results, and doctors' notes, is known as data integration.
- Data transformation is the process of converting many data formats into one common one.
- Reducing Data - Converting Large Data Sets into a Small Number of Condensed Reports.

4.2.1 Data Cleaning

It goes without saying that a comprehensive or noise-free dataset is essential for many data mining approaches. Data collected in the actual world is far from perfect. Data pre-processing techniques for noise removal or partial data filling (i.e., impute) are actually widely used. There are a lot of blanks in medical records that patients must fill out because of emergencies, and the data that is gathered isn't always clean and clear.

4.2.2 Missing Values Imputation

Completing the medical records with missing information is a complex process. Improper handling of missing values may swiftly result in inaccurate data extraction and perhaps erroneous conclusions. It has been shown that knowledge extraction becomes inefficient due to missing values. Especially in healthcare, the wrong value substitution leads to the wrong decisions and treatments.

4.2.3 Noise Treatment

Research into data pre-processing techniques for noise treatment in data mining often employs two key approaches. The noisy numbers are first corrected through data-cleaning procedures. Even minimal noise correction is thought to work, but it's a difficult procedure and is usually only applied to very small amounts of noise. Second, you may use noise filters to identify and remove noisy examples from the training data; this approach doesn't need any changes to the data mining techniques.

4.2.4 Data Integration

Problems arise when trying to integrate EMR, HER, and PHR data sets, including patient information. Medical records detailing specific patients and biological records detailing our genome are both affected by the problem of database heterogeneity. When it comes to data models, data schemas, query languages, and recognized terminologies, databases are among the most diverse examples of this kind of software. The goal of many database management systems is to bring together disparate databases by providing standard conceptual schemas that address representational heterogeneities and querying capabilities that bring together dispersed data. Research in this area has made extensive use of databases as well as information mining methods, such as term mapping, query translation, query optimization, semantic data modeling, and ontology building.

4.2.5 Data Transformation

Data is transformed from one format into another using this procedure. Information about health is collected from a variety of sources in a variety of forms, including database files, Excel spreadsheets, and XML documents. Data mapping is the first step in transforming data. In order to translate data from one application to another before loading it into another, data mapping must first establish the relation among the data parts of both applications. Prior to converting the data itself, data mapping creates vital information. A number of transformation techniques are presented for the purpose of converting formats. Those people are:

- Smoothing: Eliminates data noise.
- Data cube building and summarization are examples of aggregation.
- Generalization: the idea of moving up the corporate ladder.
- « Normalization » means to scale the data so that it falls within a certain range.
- Building features or attributes.

When it comes to medical data, not all transformation strategies currently available are up to the task. Treatment decision-making and analysis rely on data.

4.3 Dimensionality Reduction

The curse of dimensionality issue affects data mining methods when datasets are enormous in terms of the number of samples or predictor variables. Since this would cause the computational cost of various data mining methods to rise, it is a major concern. Based on the partition produced in Feature Selection, along with techniques based on space transformation, this phase might highlight the most essential dimensionality reduction strategies. Every example is crucial to several other analyses, making medical data reduction a bit of a challenge. Hospital administration, fraud detection, patient care, diagnostics, etc., are all made possible by data analysis.

4.4 Feature Selection

This strategy is all about identifying and removing superfluous data. The goal is to extract a subset of attributes that accurately characterize the underlying problem while retaining its essence. The advanced study has shown further advantages; hence, this subgroup is extensively employed in learner training. By removing superfluous or irrelevant information, Feature Selection improves the generalizability of learning algorithms by reducing the likelihood of accidental similarities. Time, money, detection, sample, and personnel might all be saved during data collecting using Feature Selection (ARIF et al., 2024).

4.4.1 Space Transformation

Reducing the number of magnitudes is one way to cope with the curse of dimensionality; feature selection is only one of several. Instead of picking the most desirable traits, spatial transformation methods combine them to build a whole new set of attributes. A number of conditions must be satisfied in order to produce such a compilation. Initial techniques rely on linear methodologies such as Principal Component Analysis (PCA) and Factor Analysis.

4.4.2 Instance Reduction

One popular approach to dealing with very big data sets is to use instance reduction methods. They reduce the dimensionality of the data set without lowering the quality of the information that might be retrieved. It is an optional task related to feature selection. It reduces the data set by either removing or adding new examples.

4.4.3 Instance Selection

Choosing the right examples is seen as crucial right now. The biggest obstacle is sorting through a massive amount of instances to locate relevant ones to use as data mining inputs. To achieve the goal of a data mining application—namely, to remove noisy and useless examples from the actual training data—the selection of instances process comprises a series of procedures that should be prepared to choose a subset of data that may replace the original dataset. In contrast, instance-creation techniques might not only select data but also generate new data to replace the old data. Using this approach may either cover portions of the issue domain without real-data examples or compress a large number of examples into a small number of cases. Since the false examples produced often reflect a region or subset of the real instances, techniques for generating instances are also called methods for generating prototypes.

4.5 Classification and Prediction

AI is now attempting to revolutionize a number of sectors, the healthcare industry being one of them. The medical field has recently seen a meteoric rise in the utilization of ML and DL. Machine Learning is a subfield of artificial intelligence, and deep learning is a subfield of Machine Learning. It employs an algorithmic interpretation of the data via the use of layered architecture. Machine learning is an approach to computer programming that relies on algorithms to automatically generate outputs from inputs by applying statistical processes. There is still a need for regulation and guidance of machine learning methods despite their steadily improving performance. However, using neural networks, a deep learning algorithm can independently assess the veracity of a prediction. To train a machine learning algorithm to recognize patterns in data, a person with technical and subject expertise must first convert the data into a form the computer can comprehend. In contrast, deep learning may build its own representations from unprocessed data in order to find patterns with minimal data pretreatment approaches. So far, the healthcare sector has been wary of deep learning techniques and has instead advocated for more conventional machine learning approaches, which are easier to explain. However, deep learning's popularity has been on the increase recently, especially for image-based jobs. Presently, the healthcare system is receiving an overwhelming amount of data, the majority of which is unintelligible due to incorrect labeling and subjective feature selection. Thoroughly analyzing and evaluating such data is crucial. Due to its design, a deep-learning network is able to identify this kind of data. When other techniques for machine learning are to be employed, developers would have to manage data processing and filtering, but this method handles it all. Deep learning algorithms learn features indirectly as data passes through its layers; this allows for the identification of valuable data points, which in turn increases a model's accuracy as it analyzes more data and learns from its previous findings (Bajpai et al., 2024). Deep learning models and machine learning models both learn in their unique ways:

- In supervised learning, doctors train an algorithm by assigning labels to clinical symptoms and then selecting a set of diagnoses to use.
- In the early stages of drug discovery, for example, an algorithm is required to establish its assumptions, which is known as "unsupervised learning." It involves detecting patterns in data without expectations.

In the medical field, the most popular AI algorithms include.

Discovering and building systems that can learn from data and generate predictions is the domain of Machine Learning (ML), a branch of AI. Some also claim that ML makes computers smart enough to learn on their own without human intervention.

4.5.1 Machine Learning

ML finds use in domains where it is difficult or impossible to develop and code high-performance explicit methods. Email filtering and intrusion detection are two examples of ML's many uses. ML is also involved with computational statistics, a branch of statistics that primarily deals with computer-based prediction. Machine learning encompasses the four popular approaches outlined below:

- **Supervised:** When the target result is known, supervised learning algorithms may be trained using labeled data to produce the intended output.
- **Unsupervised:** Without previous labels, an algorithm must deduce the meaning of the input in unsupervised learning. The same tasks that supervised learning are good for also apply to semi-supervised methods. It contains training data with labels and without labels.
- **Reinforcement Learning:** The optimal policy mechanism is the basis of the reinforcement learning algorithm's operation. The agent, their surroundings, and their behaviors are the three main parts of this algorithm. The goal is for the participant to maximize the predicted reward within a certain time frame by selecting activities. By adhering to sound policy, the agent will accomplish the task somewhat more quickly.

4.5.2 Deep Learning

Hierarchical learning, deep structured learning, and deep machine learning are all terms used to describe deep learning, a subfield of machine learning. Without any input from a human, deep learning can automatically extract features. This method is based on an artificial neural network, which mimics the way the human brain works.

- Artificial Neural Network (ANN): It addresses challenges that, when determined through human or statistical criteria, would be insurmountable. Artificial neural networks (ANNs) are computer systems that attempt to mimic the way the human brain processes and analyzes data. Recurrent Neural Networks (RNNs), Multilayer Perceptrons (MLPs), and Convolutional Neural Networks (CNNs) are the three subsets of ANN.

- Multilayer Perceptrons (MLPs): They warp the input space so that data classes may be separated linearly. These kinds of neural networks are called feed-forward neural networks, and they need a tiny dataset with three layers: an inner layer, a hidden layer, and an outer layer.
- Convolutional Neural Networks (CNNs) or ConvNet: Are created in the form of several arrays. For example, consider a basic picture with three 2D arrays. Image and video processing, NLP, and recommender systems are just a few of the several areas that might benefit from CNNs.

Figure 4. CNN Model

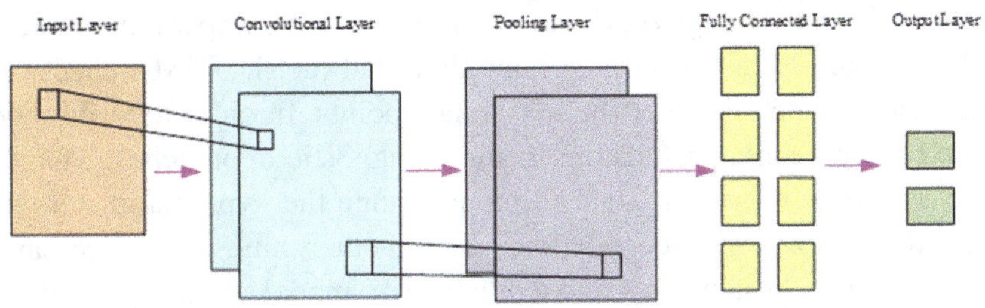

- Recurrent Neural Networks (RNNs): For tasks that need language or voice inputs in a sequential fashion, recurrent neural networks operate well. It finds usage in programs that deal with language modeling, machine translation, and voice recognition.

4.5.3 Explainable AI

How readily humans can grasp the model's conclusions and the method of making the technology/system accessible is what the word "explainability" alludes to. Additionally, that's when they know for sure whether the results are correct or if they need to reconsider. Constructing learning algorithms that humans can understand is one approach to XAI. The boundary between explainable and interpretable machine learning algorithms is blurry. While an explainable algorithm makes it easy to understand how each node works, an interpretable algorithm clarifies the reasoning behind each result. Additionally, an algorithm will be more explainable if it can be understood. When it comes to self-driving automobiles, for example, it's possible to precisely forecast the reason behind creating the output (Fig. 7) if we can monitor each car's behavior (i.e., if each car's behavior can be clearly described in many circumstances). On the other hand, an interpretable model is the same as an explainable one, and more accurate simulations are complex to interpret.

There is a cost to adopting interpretable ML models like Regression & Decision Trees (DT), but doing so may reduce the requirement for black box models. One example is linear regression, which uses a mixture of input characteristics with different weights to produce the output feature. However, when characteristics are strongly associated, it's doubtful that using regression alone can provide beneficial results. In contrast, DT uses a threshold value to categorize characteristics and attempts to establish hierarchical connections between them. While DT does not need a direct or inverse relationship between the variables, regression must. However, the feature's weight is determined by its placement in the tree's elevation, and any modification to the feature's properties significantly alters the prediction outcome. DT is essentially a re-creation of if-then rules, and many studies that have used them have shown that they can decipher sparse variable relationships, which are notoriously tough for regression models to grasp. In order to comprehend the connection between the non-linear data, another class of interpretable models called Generalized Additive Models (GAMs) utilizes a flexible function called a spline. This spline-based smoothing function uses linear regression model coefficients to generate both straight and wavy curves for data analysis and interpretation. The combination of splines forms the GAM.

In contrast to PDP, the ICE plots provide results from local prediction analyses. In contrast to ICE, which displays every instance of change against the result, PDP presents the average impact of the characteristics on the output. LIME illustrates the impact of individual predictions on the total output of black box models. LIME uses changes to the input data points to compare the model's behavior with that of the original and changed data points. As an additional metric, LIME checks how closely the updated data points' results match those of the initial data points. In order to build models that can be understood, more and more people are turning to model-agnostic approaches. These techniques can automatically create ensemble as well as stacked models, tune the hyperparameters, comprehend the features' relevance, and visualize partial correlations, among other things. It is necessary to examine the models in addition to the facts. As it evolves into a reliable ML model, an interpretable one generates an explainable one. The questions answered, the algorithms used, and the methods for data evaluation all benefit greatly from a robot response that can explain itself. A self-explanatory software is a hallmark of an understandable artificial intelligence.

5. CONCLUSION

Disease detection, chronic condition management, health service delivery, and drug development are just a few of the many applications of AI in healthcare and research. Potentially limiting AI's capacity to solve critical health problems is the lack of high-quality health data currently accessible, as well as AI's lack of empathy and other human traits. A lot of the social and ethical concerns brought up by AI use cases coincide with those brought up by information as well as healthcare tech in general. Future AI governance will face the formidable task of encouraging and pushing innovation in the field while simultaneously guiding its development and application in a transparent and compatible manner with the public interest.

6. THE FUTURE OF AI

Artificial intelligence systems will certainly evolve and learn to do more and more jobs on their own in the not-too-distant future. Some have speculated that this would necessitate the development of “ethical” AI capable of making moral judgments. A lot of philosophical thought has gone into this, with many people wondering if and how machines can ever learn or be programmed to act ethically, who ought to choose on these values if machines should be required to carry out human duties, or if new ethical principles are necessary.

REFERENCES

Agrawal, R., & Poovaiah, R. (2021). CoSpeak: Peer Feedback on Voice Stories to Inform Learning Spoken English. *Companion Publication of the 2021 Conference on Computer Supported Cooperative Work and Social Computing*, 1–4. DOI: 10.1145/3462204.3481750

Al-Dmour, R., Al-Dmour, H., Basheer Amin, E., & Al-Dmour, A. (2025). Impact of AI and big data analytics on healthcare outcomes: An empirical study in Jordanian healthcare institutions. *Digital Health*, *11*, 20552076241311052. DOI: 10.1177/20552076241311051 PMID: 39777060

Alam, S., Bhatia, S., Shuaib, M., Khubrani, M. M., Alfayez, F., Malibari, A. A., & Ahmad, S. (2023). An overview of blockchain and IoT integration for secure and reliable health records monitoring. *Sustainability (Basel)*, *15*(7), 5660. DOI: 10.3390/su15075660

Alqahtani, N., Alam, S., Aqeel, I., Shuaib, M., Mohsen Khormi, I., Khan, S. B., & Malibari, A. A. (2023). Deep belief networks (DBN) with IoT-based Alzheimer's disease detection and classification. *Applied Sciences (Basel, Switzerland)*, *13*(13), 7833. DOI: 10.3390/app13137833

Ango, R., Masih, R. K. R. K., Kishor Kumar Reddy, C., Shuaib, M., Monika Singh, T., Alam, S., Reddy, C. K. K., Shuaib, M., Singh, M., Alam, S., Kishor Kumar Reddy, C., Shuaib, M., Monika Singh, T., & Alam, S. (2024). Fraud Detection in Banking using the Kaggle Credit Card Dataset and XGBoost Model. *2024 International Conference on IoT Based Control Networks and Intelligent Systems (ICICNIS)*, 968–973. DOI: 10.1109/ICICNIS64247.2024.10823227

Aqeel, I., Khormi, I. M., Khan, S. B., Shuaib, M., Almusharraf, A., Alam, S., & Alkhaldi, N. A. (2023). Load Balancing Using Artificial Intelligence for Cloud-Enabled Internet of Everything in Healthcare Domain. In *Sensors* (Vol. 23, Issue 11). DOI: 10.3390/s23115349

Ara, A., & Mifa, A. F. (2024). Integrating artificial intelligence and big data in mobile health: A systematic review of innovations and challenges in healthcare systems. *Global Mainstream Journal of Business, Economics. Development & Project Management*, *3*(01), 1–16.

Arif, M., Adak, M., Ahmad, A. A., Nayak, C., Aqeel, I., Alam, S., & Siddiqua, A. (2024). Energy optimization approach based machine learning on linear reflector systems. *Journal of Theoretical and Applied Information Technology*, *102*(6).

Bajpai, A., Srivastava, V., Shuaib, M., Jaiswal, A., Bharany, S., Alam, S., & Ahmad, S. (2024). An Efficient Hybrid Model to Summarize the Text Using Transfer Learning. In *Lecture Notes in Electrical Engineering* (Vol. 1146). LNEE., DOI: 10.1007/978-981-97-0037-0_5

Deepa, P., Badrinath, P., Mohanaprasanth, N., Pranesh, S., & Sriram, E. (2024). AI-Powered Doctolib: Revolutionizing Healthcare Appointment Management. *Asian Journal of Basic Science & Research*, *6*(4), 90–102. DOI: 10.38177/AJBSR.2024.6407

Ghaffar, A., Arshad, A., Siddqiue, M. U., & Nasir, A. (2024). AI Strategy in Healthcare CHRM: Analyzing the Influence Organization Effective Performance Evidence from the Private Hospitals of Lahore Pakistan. *Journal of Health and Rehabilitation Research*, *4*(1), 639–645. DOI: 10.61919/jhrr.v4i1.339

Iliashenko, O., Bikkulova, Z., & Dubgorn, A. (2019). Opportunities and challenges of artificial intelligence in healthcare. *E3S Web of Conferences, 110*, 2028.

Karthik, A., Aalam, S. S., Sivakumar, M., Sundari, M. V. R., Rose, J. D., Elangovan, M., & Rajaram, A. (2024). Improving brain tumor treatment with better imaging and real-time therapy using quantum dots. *Biomedical Signal Processing and Control*, *95*, 106286. DOI: 10.1016/j.bspc.2024.106286

Karthik, A., Hamatta, H. S. A., Patthi, S., Krubakaran, C., Pradhan, A. K., Rachapudi, V., Shuaib, M., & Rajaram, A. (2024). Ensemble-based multimodal medical imaging fusion for tumor segmentation. *Biomedical Signal Processing and Control*, *96*, 106550. DOI: 10.1016/j.bspc.2024.106550

Khan, A., Zubair, S., Shuaib, M., Sheneamer, A., Alam, S., & Assiri, B. (2024a). Development of a robust parallel and multi-composite machine learning model for improved diagnosis of Alzheimer's disease: Correlation with dementia-associated drug usage and AT (N) protein biomarkers. *Frontiers in Neuroscience*, *18*, 1391465. DOI: 10.3389/fnins.2024.1391465 PMID: 39308946

Khan, A., Zubair, S., Shuaib, M., Sheneamer, A. A. M., Alam, S., & Assiri, B. (2024b). Development of a robust parallel and multi-composite machine learning model for improved diagnosis of Alzheimer's disease: Correlation with dementia-associated drug usage and AT (N) protein biomarkers. *Frontiers in Neuroscience*, *18*, 1391465. DOI: 10.3389/fnins.2024.1391465 PMID: 39308946

Khubrani, M. M., & Alam, S. (2021). A detailed review of blockchain-based applications for protection against pandemic like COVID-19. *Telkomnika*, *19*(4), 1185–1196. DOI: 10.12928/telkomnika.v19i4.18465

Masih, R. K., Alam, S., Tabassum, S., Shuaib, M., & Ahmad, S. (2023). An Analysis of the Significant Role Played by Mobile Cloud Forensics and its Key Obstacles. In *2023 International Conference in Advances in Power, Signal, and Information Technology, APSIT 2023*. DOI: 10.1109/APSIT58554.2023.10201715

Nianga, Z. W. (2024). Leveraging AI for Strategic Management in Healthcare: Enhancing Operational and Financial Performance. *Journal of Intelligence and Knowledge Engineering (ISSN: 2959-0620), 2*(3), 1.

Olawade, D. B., David-Olawade, A. C., Wada, O. Z., Asaolu, A. J., Adereni, T., & Ling, J. (2024). Artificial intelligence in healthcare delivery: Prospects and pitfalls. *Journal of Medicine, Surgery, and Public Health*, *3*, 100108. https://doi.org/https://doi.org/10.1016/j.glmedi.2024.100108. DOI: 10.1016/j.glmedi.2024.100108

Patil, S., & Shankar, H. (2023). Transforming healthcare: Harnessing the power of AI in the modern era. *International Journal of Multidisciplinary Sciences and Arts*, *2*(2), 60–70. DOI: 10.47709/ijmdsa.v2i1.2513

Polevikov, S. (2023). Advancing AI in healthcare: A comprehensive review of best practices. *Clinica Chimica Acta*, *548*, 117519. https://doi.org/https://doi.org/10.1016/j.cca.2023.117519. DOI: 10.1016/j.cca.2023.117519 PMID: 37595864

Poloju, N., & Rajaram, A. (2024). Transformation with yolo tiny network architecture for multimodal fusion in lung disease classification. *Cybernetics and Systems*, •••, 1–22. DOI: 10.1080/01969722.2024.2343992

Qamar, S., Amaan, M., Rahman, M. I., Aqeel, I., Shuaib, M., Khormi, I., & Alam, S. (2023). Cloud data transmission based on security and improved routing through hybrid machine learning techniques. *Soft Computing*. Advance online publication. DOI: 10.1007/s00500-023-08417-0

Rawas, S., Tafran, C., AlSaeed, D., & Al-Ghreimil, N. (2024). Transforming Healthcare: AI-NLP Fusion Framework for Precision Decision-Making and Personalized Care Optimization in the Era of IoMT. *Computers, Materials & Continua*, *81*(3), 4575–4601. DOI: 10.32604/cmc.2024.055307

Reddy, C. K. K., Rangarajan, A., Rangarajan, D., Shuaib, M., Jeribi, F., & Alam, S. (2024). A transfer learning approach: Early prediction of Alzheimer's disease on US healthy aging dataset. *Mathematics*, *12*(14), 2204. DOI: 10.3390/math12142204

Reddy, C. K. K., Reddy, P. A., Janapati, H., Assiri, B., Shuaib, M., Alam, S., & Sheneamer, A. (2024). A fine-tuned vision transformer based enhanced multi-class brain tumor classification using MRI scan imagery. *Frontiers in Oncology*, *14*, 1400341. DOI: 10.3389/fonc.2024.1400341 PMID: 39091923

Shuaib, M., Alam, S., & Reegu, F. A. F. A. (2023). Blockchain-based self-sovereign identity for COVID-19 medical passports and immunity certificates. *AIP Conference Proceedings*, *2587*(1), 070003. Advance online publication. DOI: 10.1063/5.0150394

Singh, A., Joshi, K., Alam, S., Bharany, S., Shuaib, M., & Ahmad, S. (2022). Internet of Things-based Integrated Remote Electronic Health Surveillance and Alert System: A Review. *2022 IEEE International Conference on Current Development in Engineering and Technology (CCET)*, 1–6. DOI: 10.1109/CCET56606.2022.10080629

Singh, A., Nagabhooshanam, N., Kumar, R., Verma, R., Mohanasundaram, S., Manjith, R., & Rajaram, A. (2025). Deep learning based coronary artery disease detection and segmentation using ultrasound imaging with adaptive gated SCNN models. *Biomedical Signal Processing and Control*, *105*, 107637. DOI: 10.1016/j.bspc.2025.107637

Suboyin, A., Sreedeth, D., Rahman, M. M., Diaz, S., Kannan, J., Sreedeth, H. S., Rehman, A., Valiyapalathingal, M., Noor, Y., & Somra, B. (2024). Transforming Strategy with AI-Augmented Personas for Sustainability, Data Management, Regulatory Frameworks, Healthcare and Compliance. *Abu Dhabi International Petroleum Exhibition and Conference*, D011S016R005.

Swain, S., Oyekola, P. O., & Muduli, K. (2022). Intelligent technologies for excellency in sustainable operational performance in the healthcare sector. [IJSESD]. *International Journal of Social Ecology and Sustainable Development*, *13*(5), 1–16. DOI: 10.4018/IJSESD.313963

Syamala, M., Chandrasekaran, R., Balamurali, R., Rani, R., Hashmi, A., Kiran, A., & Rajaram, A. (2024). Evaluating generative adversarial networks for virtual contrast-enhanced kidney segmentation using Res-UNet in non-contrast CT images. *Multimedia Tools and Applications*, •••, 1–24. DOI: 10.1007/s11042-024-19626-6

Taliento, M. (2023). AI in Healthcare Management and Accounting: Novelties and Trends from a Literature Review and Illustrative Cases. *Proceedings of the 42nd International Business Information Management Association Conference*, 1685–1696. DOI: 10.5171/2023.4252023

Valaboju, P. K. (2024). *Transformative Impact of AI and Cloud Technologies: A Comparative Analysis across Healthcare*. Retail, and Mobile Financial Services.

Watson, A., & Wozniak-O'Connor, V. (2025). The promise of artificial intelligence in health: Portrayals of emerging healthcare technologies. *Sociology of Health & Illness*, *47*(1), e13840. DOI: 10.1111/1467-9566.13840 PMID: 39311476

Yadav, G., Ubaidullah Bokhari, M., Alzahrani, S. I. I., Alam, S., Shuaib, M., Bokhari, M. U., Alzahrani, S. I. I., Alam, S., Shuaib, M., Ubaidullah Bokhari, M., Alzahrani, S. I. I., Alam, S., & Shuaib, M. (2025). Emotion-Aware Ensemble Learning (EAEL): Revolutionizing Mental Health Diagnosis of Corporate Professionals via Intelligent Integration of Multi-Modal Data Sources and Ensemble Techniques. *IEEE Access : Practical Innovations, Open Solutions*, *13*, 11494–11516. DOI: 10.1109/ACCESS.2025.3529032

Zhang, P., & Kamel Boulos, M. N. (2023). Generative AI in Medicine and Healthcare: Promises, Opportunities and Challenges. In *Future Internet* (Vol. 15, Issue 9). DOI: 10.3390/fi15090286

Chapter 11
Ensuring Security and Privacy in Internet of Things-Enabled Healthcare Ecosystems

B. Arunsundar
https://orcid.org/0009-0001-2641-635X
SRM Institute of Science and Technology, India

Nirmalkumar S. Benni
RNS Institute of Technology, India

Praveenkumar S. Challagidad
Nagarjuna College of Engineering and Technology, India

S. Ranjith
Jeppiaar Engineering College, India

D. Prabakar
SRM Institute of Science and Technology, India

C. Ranjeeth Kumar
Ashoka Women's Engineering College, India

ABSTRACT

Modern technology has made data protection paramount, especially in the face of threats posed by the dark web along with hackers. There is a threat to the online healthcare data collection and analysis systems. It is the responsibility of the data handler to guarantee the secrecy of all patient information entrusted to healthcare organizations. Every step of the data lifecycle—from collecting to using, storing, and transmitting—to sensitive personal health information. Cybercriminals may be able to access data kept on cloud-based platforms due to the proliferation of Internet-connected gadgets and the increasing prevalence of new technology. It all comes down to the data's security and how effectively it's kept secret. This chapter examines the difficulties, dangers, worries, and problems associated with healthcare data, as well as potential solutions to these issues. In this article, we examine numerous case studies in this healthcare domain and attempt to comprehend how the different IT businesses deal with these concerns while preserving the data's integrity.

DOI: 10.4018/979-8-3373-1022-0.ch011

1. INTRODUCTION

Everywhere you look, the healthcare system is making a big splash. Thanks to the exponential rise of information and communication technologies, the healthcare industry has come a long way from the days of purely empirical practices to the modern era of evidence-based medicine. Even the healthcare industry on a worldwide scale is not immune to the influence of technology. In the past, doctors were the primary point of contact for patient information in the healthcare system, which relied on paper records. Healthcare has evolved from a paper-based system to one that is data-centric as a result of technological advancements and the replacement of manual record-keeping with digital systems (Singh et al., 2022). Electronic Health Records (EHR), Personal Health Records (PHR), Electronic Medical Records (EMR), and Electronic Health Data (EHD) are only a few of the many digital record formats that have been developed (F. A. Reegu et al., 2021). All relevant healthcare providers, patients' loved ones, legal guardians, or patients themselves have access to these types of documents, which aid in the preservation of comprehensive patient medical histories. In addition to reducing the need for physical storage space and the number of employees needed to maintain them, digitizing records helps keep data open and accessible to both clients and healthcare providers (Heart et al., 2017). Among the many pieces of information stored in these digital records are patients' demographics, medications, medical histories, test results (both positive and negative), bank account information, and any financial transactions that may have been incurred to pay for the patients' hospital bills. When compared to manual storage, the benefits of digitizing healthcare records are tremendous. Improved clinical decision-making, less manual reporting of clinical errors, and increased patient safety are all benefits of digital record maintenance. Roughly 90% of healthcare institutions have implemented e-healthcare services as a result of the rising tide of technological innovation (Nadakuditi et al., 2024).

Figure 1. Secure Data Transmission in IoT

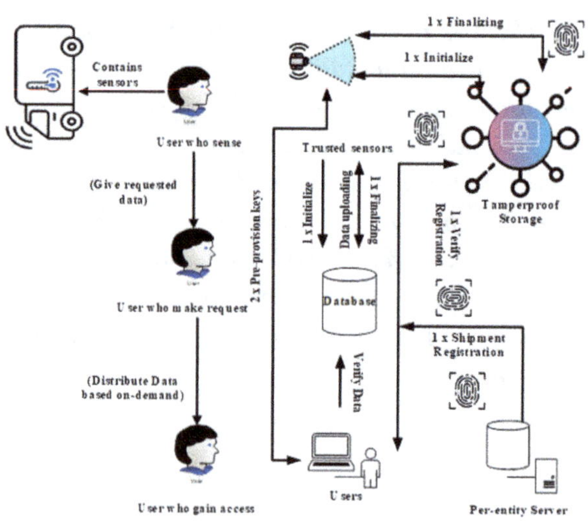

Online medical care is now seeing explosive growth in popularity. Improved healthcare system management has resulted from using EHD and EPR. When it comes to servicing healthcare systems throughout the world, EPR, RPM, and a plethora of other integrated system ideas and methodologies have been the most effective. In regards to e-healthcare, the vast majority of healthcare providers have developed their own individualized online platforms. Using this web portal, patients and physicians may have online conversations. At the same time, EPRs can be shared and accessed conveniently via websites using the login credentials of the patients or their caregivers. One example of a healthcare website built through the University of California, San Diego, is the Patient-Centered Access to Secure Organizations Online (PCASSO). You will be able to view all of your patient's medical records, including electrocardiograms (ECGs), lab results, demographic information, and payment histories, on these websites. Doctors are able to enhance treatment methods and contribute to improved healthcare facilities when patient clinical trial data are correctly stored. As part of e-healthcare offerings, several computational techniques are being used to collect data in order to comprehend the patient's sickness. These approaches, which include Cloud Computing, AI ideas, and data mining, are having a significant influence on remotely tracking patients as well as healthcare groups (Qamar et al., 2023). Therefore, being able to contact medical specialists and maintain a healthy lifestyle easily has been made simpler as a result of healthcare system modernization. But now, there's a huge problem: protecting the confidentiality of patients' medical records. Every healthcare provider has a significant obligation to ensure the privacy and security of their patient's medical records. After providing a high-level overview of the information flow across the healthcare system, this chapter will go on to address the most pressing concerns related to the privacy and security of patient data. In order to gain a better understanding of how the healthcare industry has met the present demands for protecting the privacy of patient's medical records, this chapter also covers healthcare information security problems, various methods to strengthen data security, and case studies on the subject (Kumar et al., 2024). Every healthcare organization and institution must maintain patients' health data and ensure the privacy and security of their health information. One of the moral obligations of medical practitioners is to provide patients, their families, or caregivers with information about their health in a way that is both transparent and discreet. The current healthcare system relies on digital records as the primary means of transmitting patient information. They come in several forms, including EPRs, PHRs, EMRs, and EHDs.

Users have the option to restrict access to their data to a select group of friends and family. Patients with mental illness or HIV cannot have their health records (PHRs) shared with anybody other than the government's health survey department or the individual with whom the patient gives permission. The reason is that this is personal information about patients and might inadvertently lead to prejudice in our culture. Therefore, protecting the confidentiality of patients' medical records is of the utmost importance in these situations (Selvam et al., 2025). The healthcare system's information flow follows a standard graphical flow, considering the numerous security and privacy regulations in place. A graphical representation of the flow of patient information throughout the healthcare system is shown in Figure 1. Here, only a specific approved resource body has access to the patient's information. A tremendous shift has occurred in the healthcare sector within the last few decades [6]. A well-organized set of patient medical records is required under the Healthcare Insurance Portability and Accountability Act of 1996 (HIPAA) (F. Reegu et al., n.d.). Only specific groups, as defined by HIPAA along with other national health security and confidentiality acts, such as health bank groups, the Extended Health Enterprise (which includes subgroups like pharmacists), and insurance companies (which assist in maintaining patients' health insurance records), are authorized to access patients' medical records. Government, as well as health department authorities, considers regional health information organizations as part of public policy to regulate health disasters and diseases, offer national health information security, improve decision-making in the health sector, and keep a complete overview of disease and health reports for particular areas. These organizations also keep complete medical records from health enterprise groups. The confidentiality and integrity of patient's medical records have also been the focus of several legislative initiatives and policy statements aimed at this end.

Figure 2. Security Checking in IoT

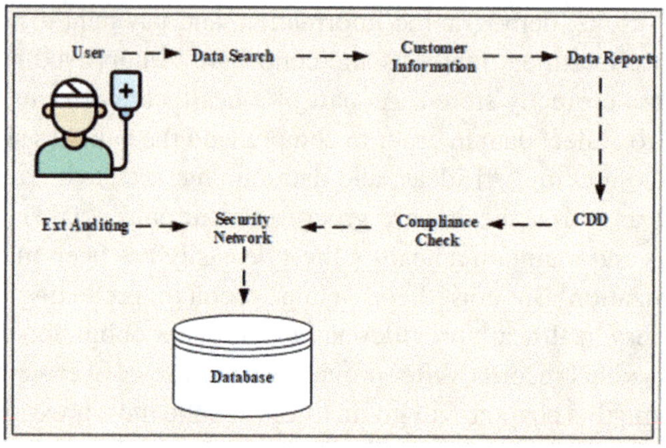

1.1. Motivation

Many industries, including healthcare, farming, transportation, smart homes, supply chains, etc., are using blockchain technology to protect user data (Alam, 2023; M. Khubrani & Alam, 2023; M. M. Khubrani & Alam, 2021). Nobody else should be allowed to view the patient's private medical records because of how important and delicate they are. Healthcare information is the most particular information sent over the internet, making data security and privacy a difficult problem (Alam et al., 2023; Shuaib et al., 2023). With the advent of cutting-edge technologies like blockchain, the IoT, edge computing, and AI, an intelligent healthcare system that has been plagued by issues like security breaches, unreliability, high costs, centralized systems, and excessive latency has made tremendous strides forward. Along with improving security, dependability, and transparency, the suggested healthcare system also makes use of a decentralized design, which helps to overcome the issues mentioned above. Secure information sharing between healthcare institutions, protection of patient privacy, data integrity, and resilience against single-point-of-failure vulnerabilities are all outcomes of this study that will give birth to blockchain-based solutions. Healthcare sector stakeholders also gained from the study, which helped them better manage healthcare systems. It causes a shift from the current healthcare system, which is focused on hospitals, to a digital one, which is patient-centric. Additionally, this activity contributes to the advancement of scientific knowledge by providing opportunities for other researchers to expand their research.

2. CURRENT SECURITY AND PRIVACY SCHEMES IN IOT

In order to provide a safe and private solution for healthcare applications that the IoT enables, suggests a unique hybrid strategy (Waheed et al., 2023) that combines blockchain technology with federated learning. Blockchain technology verifies the authenticity of local model modifications. It establishes responsibility and control over who has access to what, while their method makes use of a public-key cryptosystem to secure these updates semantically. By using federated learning, sensitive patient data may be safely aggregated without compromising security (Reddy et al., 2024). They show that their suggested approach successfully preserves data security and confidentiality while keeping computation efficient by implementing it and evaluating it utilizing EMNIST datasets. Based on the findings, it seems like their hybrid method may significantly improve the creation of safe and privacy-preserving healthcare apps that are enabled by the Internet of Things (Kaza et al., 2024). That points to an excellent route for future study in that area.

Figure 3. Security Method for Healthcare

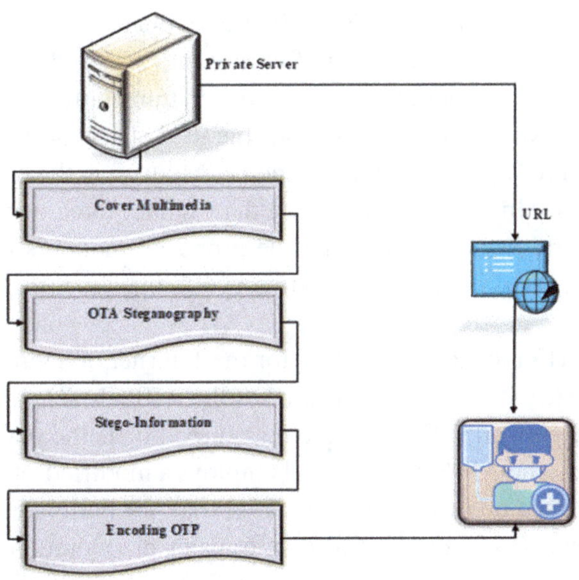

Incorporating a SE technique and forward privacy and verifiability, the paper suggests an IoT cloud-enabled health information system (Wang et al., 2021). They make the resultant data seem to the attacker as random, meaningless data by using a trapdoor permutation function. The system achieves forward secrecy or privacy because the adversary can't determine the connection between a newly added record and a previous search token. Their proposed method utilizes a pseudo-random algorithm to validate multi-keyword searches. In the top-k search case with incomplete results, their method resolves the problem of checking the accuracy of search results. Their technique accomplishes forward privacy preservation, as shown in a formal security analysis, which may aid in guaranteeing the privacy of healthcare data. In addition, their solution is effective and efficient according to a performance review, and it provides a system for data security to protect patient privacy in healthcare systems that are enabled by the Internet of Things.

Create a healthcare data analytics and privacy protection solution for the IoT using deep learning (Bi et al., 2021). They get raw data from users and store it in a privacy-isolation zone to protect their personal information. On the back end, they build a refined security module using a convolutional neural network and conduct analyses on health data without revealing any user private information. They further test the prototype system's efficacy and resilience by deploying and evaluating it.

The research study (Siddiqui, 2023)aims to investigate the possibility of creating a Smart Quarantine Environment by combining blockchain technology, wireless sensors, and the IoT. The SQE's stated goal is to make quarantine protocol maintenance more efficient while also enhancing privacy and security. In order to shed light on the practicality and advantages of introducing such a system, that study will examine pertinent case studies and review the current research. The use of wireless sensors and Internet of Things devices makes it possible to gather data and monitor it in real-time. Integrating blockchain technology, which guarantees the integrity of data, transparency, and user control, supports that strategy. That integration of technology improves the system's overall performance by resolving issues with privacy and security.

To solve that issue, researchers in (Du & Xie, 2024)combined the Secure Hash Algorithm, Rivest Cipher 4, and the Elliptic Curve Digital Signature Scheme into a hybrid security scheme. That scheme would guarantee the privacy and authenticity of medical data transmitted by healthcare systems that the IoT enables. To execute exclusive OR procedures inside the RC4 encryption technique, that hybrid model makes use of the Elliptic Curve Digital Signature Scheme. Modifying the encryption key that improves the RC4 encryption procedure. In addition, incoming data is encrypted using SHA-256 to ensure data security. A study of real-world data confirms that the proposed model is better. The encryption time for that framework is 846 ms, and the decryption time is 627 ms, resulting in a data transmission rate of 11.67 MB/s.

An innovative AIBS-IoTHS blockchain method for the Internet of Things healthcare systems is introduced in (Escorcia-Gutierrez et al., 2024). The goal of the AIBS-IoTH paradigm is to ensure safe and efficient data transfer in IoT networks. Gathering medical records is the main use case for IoT devices. To improve energy efficiency, the AIBS-IoTH model employs a modified sunflower optimization-based clustering approach that is based on metaheuristics. After that, for both inter- and intra-cluster communication, the blockchain-enabled secure medical data transfer procedure is executed. Finally, in order to ascertain the presence of illnesses, the Classification Enhancing Generative Adversarial Networks algorithm diagnoses the protected medical data. That study is innovative because of the way MSFOC and CEGAN procedures are designed. The suggested AIBS-IoTH model outperformed the competing approaches in a comprehensive experimental study of the benchmark dataset.

Figure 4. Secure Data Transmission in IoT

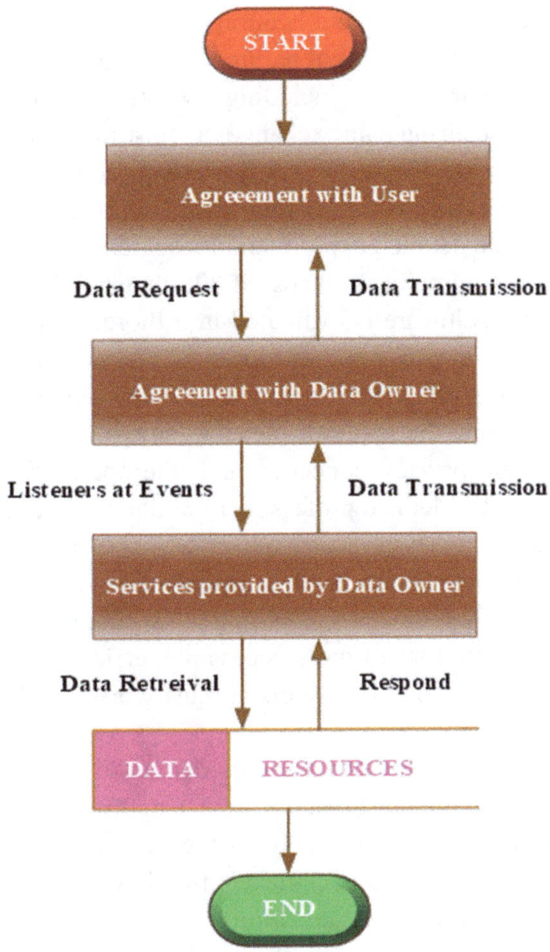

By combining blockchain with the IoT, the (Rattanawiboomsom et al., 2023) project aims to decentralize healthcare data storage while also improving data security and privacy. Despite the fact that centralized processing and storage pose concerns such as data manipulation along with privacy issues, the deployment of IoT devices enables the real-time gathering and analysis of patient sensory data. That research looks at the feasibility of building a blockchain-based decentralized IoT e-healthcare system that accounts for these concerns. Furthermore, the article highlights how smart contract technologies have been expanded via the usage of blockchain. IoT smart contracts provide accountability, auditability, and data integrity via secure user identification. Improved data interoperability, patient-centered care, streamlined administrative processes, and more transparent transactions are some of the revolutionary uses of blockchain technology that the research explores. In light of blockchain's critical impact on patient safety and welfare, the paper also emphasizes the importance of technology in controlling pharmaceutical supply chains. Supply chain disruptions or breaches may have far-reaching consequences, making effective management a must-have in the healthcare industry.

For IoT device authentication, identification, and verification, fog computing incorporates a hybrid mathematical framework: Elliptic Curve Cryptography with Proxy Re-encryption using an Enhanced Salp Swarm Algorithm, as described in a research publication (Corthis et al., 2024). The PR algorithm uses ESSA to find the best key size and PR algorithm parameters. To be more precise, the ESSA improves both its global and local search capabilities by including a Whale Optimization Algorithm into the traditional Salp Swarm Algorithm. Securing data exchange in real-time services is the primary goal of the mathematical model that has been developed. In comparison to conventional cryptographic methods, the suggested model almost halved the processing time (from 60 ms to 18 ms) and increased reliability (from 25% to 3%), according to the detailed experimental research. In the area of security analysis, the suggested model also achieves a communication cost of 4260 bits while using 680 bytes of memory.

The influence of the IoT on healthcare is evaluated in a thorough review of research (Habibur et al., 2024) that synthesizes data from peer-reviewed journals, industry reports, and case studies. Topics covered include the function of automated medical devices, remote tracking of patient systems, and wearable sensors. They examine the main obstacles to smooth integration and provide solutions, including security of information, privacy concerns, and interoperability. Findings: The Internet of Things can revolutionize healthcare. Medical professionals and patients alike benefit from the real-time data provided by devices like insulin pumps, pacemakers, as well as smart baby monitors. The IoT revolutionizes many fields, including pediatric care, surgical aid, and the treatment of chronic diseases. Data leaks and gadget incompatibility, however, continue to be major problems. In conclusion, the IoT represents a sea change in healthcare toward more accessible, efficient, and patient-centered services. Policymakers, medical professionals, and IT developers must work together to solve security, privacy, and system compatibility issues.

Authors in (Alam et al., 2022) explained the quantum danger to healthcare IoT security, explaining how broken encryption might lead to privacy breaches, device malfunctions, and tampered medical data, among other possible consequences. In order to address their use in healthcare IoT devices, including telemedicine systems, monitoring tools, and pacemakers that have limited resources, it presents post-quantum cryptography with quantum-resistant algorithms such as quantum key distribution. That chapter delves deeper into the difficulties of implementing these solutions, examines international initiatives to reduce quantum concerns, and provides recommendations for appropriate PQC primitives for different healthcare applications (Shuaib et al., 2022).

3 CHALLENGES IDENTIFIED IN HEALTHCARE INFORMATION SECURITY AND PRIVACY

Ensuring Healthcare Safety Every healthcare institution has a significant problem managing the flow of information while upholding its policy on privacy and security. Every day, millions of health records are sent all over the globe by every health organization as the digital health system develops. Unfortunately, there has been a steady growth in both the abuse and corruption of these records. Integral to any comprehensive healthcare system is the adoption of an e-healthcare system, which places a premium on data protection. Additionally, the e-healthcare system expands the use of Internet-connected electronic and telecommunications technologies in healthcare. The primary goal of the e-healthcare framework is to increase the quality of services while also increasing the effectiveness and efficiency of managing healthcare. It has had a significant impact on treating patients who are located in distant areas. As a result, all data is now stored digitally, making data security a top priority. When comparing the conventional healthcare system with the e-healthcare system, it becomes clear that the latter has a significant advantage when it comes to treating patients and keeping accurate health records via the use of electronic devices, which ultimately leads to improved decision-making. However, concerns about privacy and security of patient data sometimes outweigh the advantages of electronic health records. There are a number of security concerns with the e-healthcare system, including software viruses and worms, data loss, hackers using patients' medical records for their gain, and privacy concerns. The parts that follow will go over a few of the problems with healthcare information security.

3.1 Threats to Information Privacy and Security

There are many ongoing investigations of healthcare institutions' data privacy and security practices. There are two main categories of potential dangers to data privacy and security: organizational risks and systemic threats. Emergencies Facing the Company Internal agents of the company or external agents exploiting information system vulnerabilities might misuse permitted access to patient data, posing an organizational danger. These dangers can manifest in various ways, such as when an authorized employee of a healthcare organization misuses the data for personal gain or when outsiders, like hackers, take advantage of security holes in healthcare information systems to access the data for their own financial or non-financial gain. Threats to organizations may be better understood by breaking them down into their defining characteristics, which include theme, resource, accessibility, and technological capabilities. Any danger to an organization is based on the economic and non-economic advantages to the adversary. For example, criminals may exploit patients' personal information for their financial gain, or they may have some other motive unrelated to money, such as being in a personal connection with patients. As a function of the technological skills of the attacker/hacker, the organizational danger level is high. There are a number of reasons why the risk level of organizational risks is high, including:

- Unintentional exposure of patient data (for instance, when a healthcare provider accidentally sends a patient's medical information to the incorrect address).
- An inside agent of the company commits a data breach (for instance, a healthcare institution insider passing patient information to an outside party for their gain or vengeance).
- An external actor physically invades a healthcare institution in order to steal sensitive information (for instance, an outsider using physical force to coerce an insider into giving them access to sensitive medical records).
- Criminals break into healthcare organizations' computer systems (for example, a former employee attempted to exact vengeance on the firm by hacking its computer systems).
- An insatiable need for knowledge (thinks of an insider in a healthcare company who uses their position to obtain patient information illegally)

3.2 Systemic Threats

Misuse of patient information by any entity in the healthcare industry's information flow chain poses a systemic risk. When it comes to protecting sensitive patient information, every healthcare provider and business follows standard privacy and security procedures. Systemic risks may arise whenever this healthcare firm rejects these regulations.

3.3 Privacy Concerns among Patient's Health Records

Maintaining the privacy of patients' medical records is of the utmost importance. Disclosure of some of the patient's private medical information could lead to prejudice in the community. For instance, in the case of a patient with a mental illness or a human immunodeficiency virus (HIV) infection. In the event that their medical records are made public. Some patients may die as a result of the trauma they experienced as a result of society's bias against them. Therefore, it is difficult to keep patients' health records private.

4. LIGHTWEIGHT CRYPTOGRAPHY

For as long as security experts have been involved, cryptography has been the only debatable option for conveying data via both encrypted and unencrypted channels. Bells Systems was the birthplace of the idea of communication under secrecy systems, which outlines the process of translating a collection of plaintext data into a set of potential ciphers. Symmetric encryption is a popular approach for secure data transfer (ALAM, 2013). The block cipher is NIST-approved for its ability to enable many modes of operation that ensure secrecy. Many individuals involved in private communication must share a secret key for the aforementioned method to work. Allowing the encryption method to be publicly available while secretly storing the key is the primary goal of an asymmetric encryption technique. Data is encrypted and sent from one location to another using a secret key (Fig. 4), and then, at the other end, an identical shared private key is used to reverse-engineer the data.

- ***AES:*** At the application layer, devices with limited resources often employ the standardized algorithm known as Advanced Encryption Standard (AES). Three standardized versions of the Rijndael encryption make up the Advanced Encryption Standard (AES), a symmetric block cipher. Different versions of AES use different block sizes: 128 bits, 192, and 256 bits. Whether the key size is 128 bits or less determines the inner state. A 128-bit internal state built as a 4-4 structure of bytes of cryptography standards is what encryption entails, along with the related chores. It incorporates ShiftRows, MixedColumns, and SubBytes, with Add-RoundKey into every byte. Whole rounds of AES can be broken via biclique while man-in-the-middle attacks, and the maximum key size that AES allows is 128/192/256 bits .
- ***CHAM-64/128:*** A novel and lightweight block cipher named CHAM has been suggested by the authors, with a focus on devices with limited resources. With CHAM-128/128-bit and CHAM-128/256-bit, the input blocks are of a fixed size of 64 bits, while the key sizes are 128 bits along with 256 bits, respectively. CHAM uses a generalized Feistel system using A-addition, R-rotation, and X-XOR operations to generate the ciphertext. Whole ciphertext generation in CHAM-64, CHAM-128/128, and CHAM-128/256 takes 80, 96, and 96 rounds, respectively, due to the design.
- ***CLEFIA:*** CLEFIA is a 128-bit classic block cipher; its base size changes from 128 to 192 to 256 bits, correspondingly. Digital rights management (DRM) solutions are the focus of Sony Corporation's CLEFIA encryption method, a unique symmetrical lightweight block cipher algorithm.
- ***FeW:*** FeW is a novel block cipher that is both lightweight and engineered for use in software-based systems. It takes 32 iterations on 64-bit plaintext to produce 64-bit ciphertext. To improve

protection against elementary cryptographic attacks, FEW uses a hybrid of Feistel and extended Feistel structures. Additionally, FEW shows that it can withstand zero correlation and linear assaults, which means that the design is well-protected.

- ***HIGHT:*** Devices with limited resources may benefit from the HIGHT algorithm. Key brightening is applied to the ARX-based GFS coordinate HIGHT. Most notably, bitwise rotations and XOR are used. The F0 and F1 subfunctions XOR have three separate information pivots. Eight bytes of whitening keys are generated in the array using the master key and one hundred twenty-eight subkeys.
- ***KASUMI:*** KASUMI meets the mobile network security requirements—including GSM, EDGE, UMTS, and GPRS. KASUMI is compatible with the 3GPP integrity method and 3GPP confidentiality. It accepts a 64-bit block as input and uses a 128-bit key size. The Feistel function generates ciphertext after eight iterations. After splitting the input into two 32-bit strings, each half is sent through a round operation to generate the 32-bit ciphertext.
- ***MIDORI:*** Midori is perfect for use in medical implants since it was designed to work with low-power sources. You get Midori64 and Midori128 with this bundle. A 128-bit key is generated using 16 iterations on 64-bit blocks and 20 iterations on 128-bit blocks, respectively.
- ***KHUDRA:*** For FPGAs, the innovative lightweight block cipher Khudra was developed. The minimum key size is 10 bytes, while the maximum block size is 8 bytes. By using the Feistel function, which generates ciphertext by performing substitution-permutation and diffusion on input blocks, the Feistel network is able to function. In order to create ciphertext, the outside structure of khudra employs 18 rounds, whereas the inside mechanism needs six rounds.
- ***KATAN and KTANTAN:*** The hardware-arranged stream cipher is simple and well-structured. A small, immutable 80-bit key may be implanted into a KATAN or KTANTAN device just once. In order to create the intricate ciphertext, both KATAN and KTANTAN used distinct key scheduling methodologies. Bits are sent from registers to two nonlinear Boolean capabilities in every cycle. Registers get the bare minimum of crucial bits (after shifting) from the boolean capability. There are 254 iterations of the figure to ensure proper mixing.
- ***LBLOCK:*** Renowned for its outstanding implementation, LBlock is a cryptographic computation that targets both software and hardware benchmarks. Its primary use case is in Feistel development, which first uses two 4-byte twigs and then swaps them. By effectively rotating it by one byte, the F task's XORed yield is altered. The algorithm's computing function includes a permutation shuffling of 4-bit words, an 8×4 S-box layer, and an XOR operation using subkeys.
- ***ITUbee:*** With a total execution duration of 29,37 cycles and a code footprint of 586 bytes, ITUbee is a very efficient software encryption. Many believe this encryption method to be the smallest. Each key and block is the same size, 80 bits. To alleviate software overload, round-dependent variables are used rather than key scheduling.
- ***LED:*** The LED Block Cipher uses AES as the foundation for its SPN. The key is XORed in between each 48-slice increment during encryption [30]. The XOR operation on an AES panache round creates a single round. While an 8-byte key is XORed using an internal state, a 16-byte key is split into two 8-byte subkeys. Power consumption increased as a result of ad hoc assaults (12 rounds of LED-08-bytes, 32 slices of LED-16-bytes).
- ***PRESENT:*** The current iteration of the method relies only on the straightforward, efficient, and bit-orientation-focused SPN structure. Unassuming wiring formed the basis of the PRESENT

hardware implementation. Nevertheless, implementing software may be a real pain. A tiny S-box with good cryptographic characteristics and a small hardware footprint was hand-picked for this.

- ***QTL:*** With key sizes ranging from 8 to 12 bytes, QTL has just emerged as a novel 8-byte cipher surplus. A generalized Feistel pattern summarizes another variation, QTL. With QTL-128-bit, the ciphertext is generated after 20 rounds, whereas with QTL-64-bit, it takes 16 rounds. There are two additional rounds inside the internal framework for each specialized round. The rapid dissemination of SPNs, or QTL, strengthens the Feistel network's security measures. QTL employs just 22 GE and utilizes 4×4 S-boxes to offer suitable security. Furthermore, it employs a constant function that differs from the round function.
- ***RECTANGLE:*** Bit-slice is a solid foundation for RECTANGLE block cipher for both implementation types. It had two revisions throughout its design. For a full 25 rounds, RECTANGLE-8-bytes with a 10-byte key and RECTANGLE-12-bytes with a 12-byte key are operational. RECTANGLE uses S-Box and operates on key sequencing in a matrix. There is a 19-round vulnerability in RECTANGLE.
- ***SIMON & SPECK:*** Authors from the National Security Agency (NSA) introduce SIMON and SPECK, a family of block ciphers designed to provide security to devices with little power. Algorithm design is simple, secure, and versatile. In order to create the ciphertext, the SIMON algorithm can handle blocks with sizes ranging from 32 bits to 128 bits and keys from 64 bits to 256 bits.
- ***TEA (Tiny Encryption Algorithm):*** Using a 128-bit key, the TEA encryption method uses 64-bit blocks to encrypt the data. It takes 64 rounds that add together to make a complex ciphertext. Roger Needham and David Wheeler developed TEA in 1994 at the Cambridge Computer Laboratory with a focus on simplicity. An enhanced version known as XTEA is based on TEA, which is enhanced via a related-key attack on the complete cipher. There are, nonetheless, 2355 gate equivalents needed for TEA equipment performance, regardless of how simple the basic round capacities are.
- ***TWINE:*** Among the many lightweight algorithms built on GFS having sixteen 4-bit twigs, TWINE stands out as particularly adaptable and robust. Along with the key sequence and s-box, the Feistel function runs for 32 rounds. With a 10-byte key size, TWINE uses 1779 GE, and with a 12-byte key size, it uses 2285 GE. Diffusion to each sub-block now takes fewer rounds, thanks to this newer step. TWINE-80-bit and TWINE-128-bit versions are both vulnerable to zero-correlation attacks; the former for 23 rounds and the latter for 25 rounds, respectively.
- ***XTEA:*** Just like ARX, XTEA is a lightweight block cipher that uses the minimum amount of publicly accessible source code to create its software. Particularly embedded in the Linux kernel was XTEA. An earlier effort, TEA, had similar goals but had several flaws; XTEA is an improved version of it. Through the use of XOR operations, left shift activities, convenient shift processes, and modular procedures for addition (modulo 232), the round function processes input plaintext. It produces encrypted ciphertext at the conclusion of rounds.

Figure 5. AES with ECC Algorithm for Data Encryption (a). Typical model

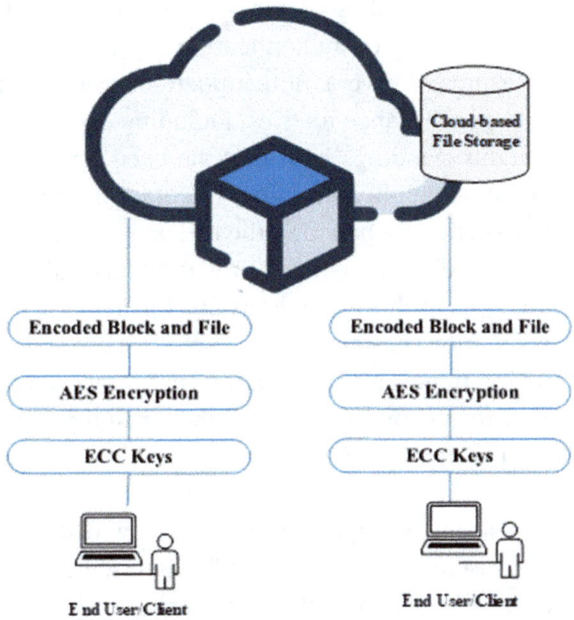

Figure 6. AES with ECC Algorithm for Data Encryption (b). Detailed Picture

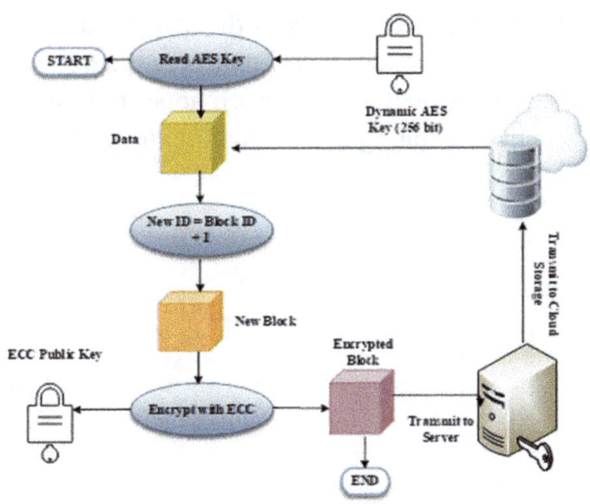

5. SUMMARY

Highlighting the crucial significance of these devices in minimizing IoT security flaws, this article offers a thorough assessment of strategies for authenticating IoT networks. The research analyses the formal and informal security measures of several authentication systems that have been established in the last ten years. It also evaluates performance metrics, including energy usage, communication costs, and computing activities, thoroughly. Findings highlight the need for a unified set of technologies to construct an innovative authentication architecture. This integration seeks to solve significant security concerns and increase privacy protection by boosting the efficacy of the IoT identification mechanism. The current state of IoT security, as well as associated threats and assaults, are thoroughly examined in this paper, which also offers solutions to these problems. To further explain the schemes' comparative analysis and make complicated situations easier to grasp, we made use of tables, figures, and additional visual aids. These graphics provide important information that might aid academics and practitioners in identifying research gaps and subjects by highlighting the advantages and disadvantages of various methods. The following is the last section of this paper:

- This study discovers that not a single suggested scheme can withstand every possible assault type; instead, each scheme can withstand specific attacks but is susceptible to others.
- To authenticate nodes, most early systems relied on secret key exchanges. And yet, there are new technologies out there (such as blockchain, ML, etc.) that can authenticate nodes at much-reduced communication and processing costs.
- The IoT security issue is crucial to its success; if resolved, its widespread use and acceptance would boost smart applications, lifestyles, modes of engagement, and conveniences in many areas of life. This study makes a substantial addition to the field of Internet of Things security. It lays out a plan for future studies that aim to enhance authentication algorithms in devices with limited resources that are part of the IoT. In addition to improving the trustworthiness and confidentiality of data exchanged between IoT devices, this research hopes to hasten the creation of more secure and effective IoT networks by integrating and evaluating the pros and cons of different solutions.

REFERENCES

Alam, S. (2023, February). Security concerns in smart agriculture and blockchain-based solution. In 2022 OPJU international technology conference on emerging technologies for sustainable development (OTCON) (pp. 1-6). IEEE.

Alam, S., Bhatia, S., Shuaib, M., Khubrani, M. M., Alfayez, F., Malibari, A. A. A., & Ahmad, S. (2023). An Overview of Blockchain and IoT Integration for Secure and Reliable Health Records Monitoring. *Sustainability (Basel)*, *15*(7), 5660. DOI: 10.3390/su15075660

Alam, S., Shuaib, M., Ahmad, S., Jayakody, D. N. K., Muthanna, A. S., Bharany, S., & Elgendy, I. A. (2022). Blockchain-Based Solutions Supporting Reliable Healthcare for Fog Computing and Internet of Medical Things (IoMT) Integration. In *Sustainability (Switzerland)* (Vol. 14, Issue 22). DOI: 10.3390/su142215312

Bi, H., Liu, J., & Kato, N. (2021). Deep learning-based privacy preservation and data analytics for IoT enabled healthcare. *IEEE Transactions on Industrial Informatics*, *18*(7), 4798–4807. DOI: 10.1109/TII.2021.3117285

Corthis, P. B., Ramesh, G. P., García-Torres, M., & Ruíz, R. (2024). Effective Identification and Authentication of Healthcare IoT Using Fog Computing with Hybrid Cryptographic Algorithm. *Symmetry*, *16*(6), 726. DOI: 10.3390/sym16060726

Du, L., & Xie, T. (2024). Towards Secure Internet of Things-Enabled Healthcare: Integrating Elliptic Curve Digital Signatures and Rivest Cipher Encryption. *International Journal of Advanced Computer Science and Applications*, *15*(8). Advance online publication. DOI: 10.14569/IJACSA.2024.0150858

Escorcia-Gutierrez, J., Mansour, R. F., Leal, E., Villanueva, J., Jimenez-Cabas, J., Soto, C., & Soto-Díaz, R. (2024). Privacy preserving blockchain with energy aware clustering scheme for IoT healthcare systems. *Mobile Networks and Applications*, *29*(1), 1–12. DOI: 10.1007/s11036-023-02115-9

Habibur, M., Hasan, M. H., Sadik, M. S., Estehad, M., Rahatul, M., Kumar, P., & Rahman, A. (2024). Impact of Internet of Things (IoT) on healthcare in transforming patient care and overcoming operational challenges. *Journal of Angiotherapy*, *8*(11), 1–8. DOI: 10.25163/angiotherapy.81110041

Heart, T., Ben-Assuli, O., & Shabtai, I. (2017). A review of PHR, EMR and EHR integration: A more personalized healthcare and public health policy. *Health Policy and Technology*, *6*(1), 20–25. DOI: 10.1016/j.hlpt.2016.08.002

Kaza, V. S. V. S., Alamer, A. M. A. A., Alam, S., Shuaib, M., Basudan, S., Sheneamer, A. A. M., Kishor Kumar Reddy, C., Kaza, V. S. V. S., Madana Mohana, R., Alamer, A. M. A. A., Alam, S., Shuaib, M., Basudan, S., & Sheneamer, A. A. M. (2024). Detecting and forecasting cryptojacking attack trends in Internet of Things and wireless sensor networks devices. *PeerJ. Computer Science*, *10*, e2491. DOI: 10.7717/peerj-cs.2491 PMID: 39650421

Khubrani, M., & Alam, S. (2023). Blockchain-Based Microgrid for Safe and Reliable Power Generation and Distribution: A Case Study of Saudi Arabia. *Energies*, *16*(16), 5963. DOI: 10.3390/en16165963

Khubrani, M. M., & Alam, S. (2021). A detailed review of blockchain-based applications for protection against pandemic like COVID-19. *Telkomnika, 19*(4), 1185. DOI: 10.12928/telkomnika.v19i4.18465

Kumar, V., Ali, A. A., Mittal, P., Aqeel, I., Shuaib, M., Alam, S., & Aalsalem, M. Y. (2024). E2SVM: Electricity-Efficient SLA-aware Virtual Machine Consolidation approach in cloud data centers. *PLoS ONE, 19*(6 June). DOI: 10.1371/journal.pone.0303313

Nadakuditi, S., Kumar, B., & Kumar, T. (2024). AI and Machine Learning in Healthcare-Applications, Challenges and Ethics. *International Journal of Health Sciences*, *7*(4), 36–43. DOI: 10.47941/ijhs.1949

Qamar, S., Amaan, M., Rahman, M. I. M. I., Aqeel, I., Shuaib, M., Khormi, I. M., & Alam, S. (2023). Cloud data transmission based on security and improved routing through hybrid machine learning techniques. *Soft Computing*. Advance online publication. DOI: 10.1007/s00500-023-08417-0

Rattanawiboomsom, V., Korejo, M. S., Ali, J., & Thatsaringkharnsakun, U. (2023). Blockchain-Enabled Internet of Things (IoT) Applications in Healthcare: A Systematic Review of Current Trends and Future Opportunities. *International Journal of Online & Biomedical Engineering*, *19*(10), 99–117. DOI: 10.3991/ijoe.v19i10.41399

Reddy, K. K., Badam, R., Alam, S., & Shuaib, M. (2024). IoT-driven accessibility: A refreshable OCR-Braille solution for visually impaired and deaf-blind users through WSN. *Journal of Economy and Technology*, *2*, 128–137. DOI: 10.1016/j.ject.2024.04.007

Reegu, F., Daud, S. M., & Alam, S. (n.d.). BLOCKCHAIN AND INTEROPERABLE STANDARDS FOR EHR-A COMPREHENSIVE REVIEW. *Turkish Journal of Physiotherapy and Rehabilitation, 32*(2).

Reegu, F. A., Daud, S. M., Alam, S., & Shuaib, M. (2021). *Blockchain-based Electronic Health Record System for efficient Covid-19 Pandemic Management*. DOI: 10.20944/preprints202104.0771.v1

Selvam, P., Karthikeyan, P., Manochitra, S., Sujith, A., Ganesan, T., Ayyasamy, R., Shuaib, M., Alam, S., & Rajendran, A. (2025). Federated learning-based hybrid convolutional recurrent neural network for multi-class intrusion detection in IoT networks. *Discover Internet of Things*, *5*(1), 39. DOI: 10.1007/s43926-025-00130-8

Shuaib, M., Alam, S., & Reegu, F. A. F. A. (2023). Blockchain-based self-sovereign identity for COVID-19 medical passports and immunity certificates. *AIP Conference Proceedings*, *2587*(1), 070003. Advance online publication. DOI: 10.1063/5.0150394

Shuaib, M., Hassan, N. H., Usman, S., Alam, S., Sam, S. M., & Samy, G. A.-L. N. (2022). Effect of Quantum computing on Blockchain-based Electronic Health Record Systems. *2022 4th International Conference on Smart Sensors and Application (ICSSA)*, 179–184. DOI: 10.1109/ICSSA54161.2022.9870964

Siddiqui, S. T. (2023). Integrating IoT and blockchain-enabled device-to-device communication to improve privacy in intelligent quarantine environments. *2023 7th International Conference on Computation System and Information Technology for Sustainable Solutions (CSITSS)*, 1–7.

Singh, A., Joshi, K., Alam, S., Bharany, S., Shuaib, M., & Ahmad, S. (2022). Internet of Things-based Integrated Remote Electronic Health Surveillance and Alert System: A Review. *2022 IEEE International Conference on Current Development in Engineering and Technology (CCET)*, 1–6. DOI: 10.1109/CCET56606.2022.10080629

Waheed, N., Rehman, A. U., Nehra, A., Farooq, M., Tariq, N., Jan, M. A., Khan, F., Alalmaie, A. Z., & Nanda, P. (2023). Fedblockhealth: A synergistic approach to privacy and security in iot-enabled healthcare through federated learning and blockchain. *GLOBECOM 2023-2023 IEEE Global Communications Conference*, 3855–3860.

Wang, K., Chen, C.-M., Tie, Z., Shojafar, M., Kumar, S., & Kumari, S. (2021). Forward privacy preservation in IoT-enabled healthcare systems. *IEEE Transactions on Industrial Informatics*, *18*(3), 1991–1999. DOI: 10.1109/TII.2021.3064691

Chapter 12
Leveraging Blockchain Technology for Secure and Transparent Medical Data Exchange

Praveenkumar S. Challagidad
https://orcid.org/0009-0001-8914-8890
Nagarjuna College of Engineering and Technology, India

T. R. Chenthil
https://orcid.org/0000-0001-9692-5195
Jeppiaar Engineering College, India

M. Manickam
SRM Institute of Science and Technology, India

D. Sungeetha
Saveetha University, India

B. Arunsundar
SRM Institute of Science and Technology, India

Raj Kumar Masih
Jazan University, Saudi Arabia

ABSTRACT

The financial platforms have been the primary focus of blockchain research. We must also investigate the potential of blockchain in other fields. When data privacy and authenticity are paramount, blockchain technology is the way to go. The potential applications of blockchain technology in healthcare have been the focus of our investigation. Similar measures are required for healthcare data due to its high criticality. Thus, healthcare data security would reach new heights with the use of blockchain technology and the healthcare cloud idea. A healthcare cloud, built using cloud computing technologies, is our new method for protecting the sensitive patient information. Blockchain technology verifies the data stored in this cloud. Data kept in a single healthcare cloud is both protected and uncompromised by this method.

DOI: 10.4018/979-8-3373-1022-0.ch012

1. INTRODUCTION

The world over, technological progress has been the driving factor. The healthcare industry has recently benefited from technological advancements. It has enhanced healthcare in numerous ways, including the system as a whole, illness prevention, medication efficacy, longevity, and many more. A single platform is necessary for productivity and interoperability in healthcare technology since several bodies regulate it. It is seen, for instance, when a patient visits a healthcare provider that uses a different paradigm than an accountable care organization. The result is a breakdown in data processing necessary for offering value-based care and an end to interoperability. Healthcare services must be efficient in order for value-based care to be implemented. In light of this, we have implemented the concept of a healthcare cloud (Alsharif & Nabil, 2020) that has gathered information from every healthcare provider organization. Next, we will suggest using blockchain technology to ensure the safety of your data. The information would be immutable since every transaction would be recorded on a blockchain (Bhan et al., 2023). There was a comprehensive inventory of all the studies and solutions that were considered for using blockchain for IoT or verification. Despite that, blockchain use in healthcare has been considered. Our study suggests using blockchain technology in healthcare data. Critical health data has to be protected in this way to ensure its validity and integrity. The goal of blockchain technology is to facilitate interoperability, which in turn decentralizes data ownership and makes it accessible to anybody who needs it. One may find private blockchain, public blockchain, and consortium blockchain. Private blockchain are available exclusively to those who have been allowed access by the administrator of the blockchain, whereas public blockchain are open to everyone and everyone, and consortium-based blockchain have limited access with hybrid access. Fig 1 shows a flow of blockchain models. The creation of a block, which includes encrypted information as well as its hash, is followed by the processing and approval of the transaction. This block is then added to the chain.

Figure 1. Blockchain Model

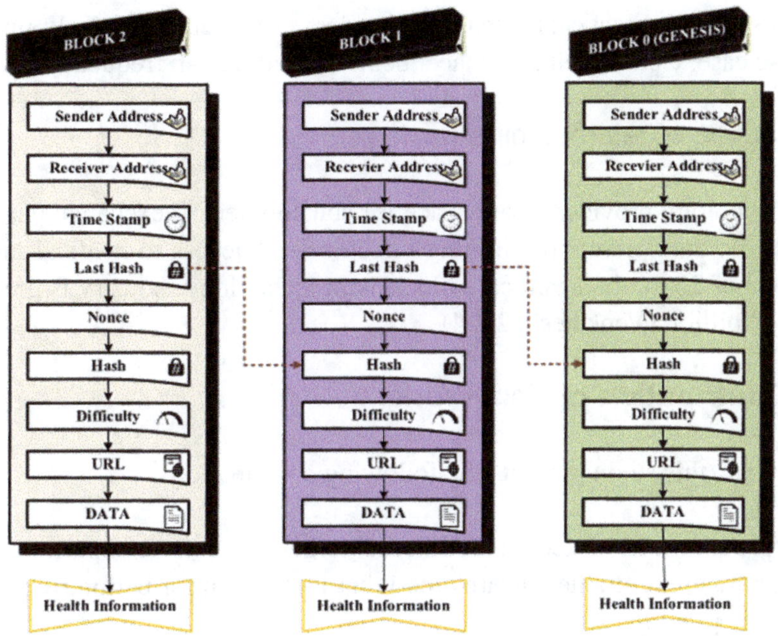

1.1 Blockchain technology for healthcare

The healthcare industry is ripe with opportunities for blockchain technology. Supply chain management with patient data security is only two of its many potential applications . When it comes to blockchain technology, healthcare data security and privacy management is where it's at (Hoang et al., 2022).

1.1.1 Data privacy and security

- Recently, patient data privacy has become a significant topic of discussion in the healthcare sector. The simple reason is that healthcare data is now open to both internal and external threats due to the prevalence of technologies such as the Internet of Things (IoT), the cloud, and smart devices in healthcare systems. data indicates that more than 100 million medical records have been compromised (Xia et al., 2021).
- Blockchain technology offers additional protection for sensitive patient information. This system creates a transparent, distributed, and incorruptible record of patient information. Healthcare data privacy is ensured by using complicated and secure codes to mask an individual's identity, even while the data is exposed. As a result, consumers, healthcare providers, and physicians may all safely access and share the decentralized data. Additionally, the period that data is susceptible is minimized with rapid data transfers. Additionally, blockchain technology allows for the secure administration and storage of healthcare information and operations and properly identifies potentially harmful errors in medical records.

1.1.2 Safe Clinical Trials

- Clinical studies that use blockchain technology to increase openness and eliminate data tampering are another use case. Counterfeit pharmaceuticals are reduced in frequency.

1.1.3 Secure practice of telemedicine

- Blockchain technology provides a safe space for stakeholders to exchange patient data and helps keep telemedicine data private by limiting unauthorized access to medical information. This is why, by the end of 2036, the healthcare blockchain technology industry is predicted to be worth more than $215 billion (Venkatesh, 2024).

1.2 Research Contribution of This Work

In light of the above, this study presents the following contributions:

- A web-based program was hosted on the Internet to get data for our experiments and research;
- this application was part of a healthcare cloud that included information from all healthcare suppliers and service providers.
- Healthcare data security uses blockchain technology, a private blockchain network setup on the AWS cloud, and an algorithm to hide data before data mining.
- A method to get the initial data is by reversing the production process.

1.3 Organization

Here is the outline of the paper. Section 2 explains the system model and how to formulate the issue. Section 3 provides illustrations of the proposed system. Section 4 delves into the topic of performance assessment. Section 5 finishes the essay by discussing potential future research.

2. STATE OF THE ART: BLOCKCHAIN MODELS

According to (Ozturk et al., 2024), medical treatments may be accessed remotely using the application of cloud computing and IoT devices. Healthcare 4.0 is based on the tenet that health records should be routinely and regularly collected, integrated, transmitted, shared, and stored. Preventing hackers from gaining unapproved access to patients' sensitive and confidential data is no easy feat. Even for authorized parts of E-healthcare systems, the security of medical information about patients acquired, stored, and distributed in the cloud must be a top priority to avoid unauthorized access or compromise. Many different cryptographic methods have been developed to ensure the safe transmission, reception, and subsequent evaluation of private medical records in CSP contexts. It has been difficult for conventional approaches to provide rapid computing, user-side verification, solid security, independence from an unbiased third party, and harmonious integration of these features into electronic health record security solutions. There has been a significant uptick in the interest in security solutions that use blockchain technology. These technologies make data storage and exchange processes more secure, and they do so with few processing resources. The researchers' only emphasis was on blockchain technology, namely Bitcoin. Right now, many are concentrating on ways to use blockchain technology to manage patient data safely. Irrespective of cloud computing, that research offers a thorough examination of existing blockchain-based methods for protecting medical records. That study employs and evaluates a number of blockchain-based technologies. That paper proposes an architecture called Medical-edge-blockchain, or MEdge-Chain, which utilizes blockchain technology with edge computing to manage large amounts of medical data (Abdellatif et al., 2021). The proposed framework outlines a healthcare system that aims to merge several health organizations into one national healthcare system by enabling the quick and secure transmission and storage of medical data. Efficient remote surveillance and the identification of critical medical events are made possible by that system using a blockchain architecture to enhance the flow of medical data across several parties. Their team develops a blockchain-based optimization strategy to enhance healthcare delivery's efficiency and security further. With that methodology, they want to reduce the time and effort needed to process medical data transfers between different hospitals as much as possible. They first describe the benefits of the proposed intelligent health system, and then they show how well their system adjusts to a number of critical events.

The authors of (Rosa et al., 2023) present a small implanted device that does not need batteries and can measure biopotential (30 dB gain, 16 Hz bandwidth), arterial pulse oximetry, and temperature (0.12 °C precision), all of which are important for assessing the function of neurons, hormones, and the cardiovascular system. The proposed device uses just 0.9 mW of power when operating at full power at depths of up to 1 cm below the skin and is powered by the near-field communication interface of an external mobile phone. Encrypting physiological signals in real-time using data stream hopping along with a lightweight symmetric-key distribution strategy protects sensitive information as it is sent between patients and trustworthy third parties. To round out the system, there is a medical blockchain consortium that incorporates important participants in the healthcare sector for data storage, processing, and recovery.

The primary goal of the research is to empower consumers with more control over their personal data and to assist healthcare companies in enhancing their data security mechanisms (Shuaib et al., 2023a) . The use of big data and blockchain technology improves the accessibility, interoperability, and security of medical records. According to the report, healthcare practitioners are well aware of the need to protect patient information by using blockchain technology and big data to improve accessibility, interoperability, and security. Consequently, patient data is handled more efficiently and affordably, and concerns regarding data manipulation are reduced. Medical records administration becomes more efficient and affordable when concerns about data manipulation are reduced. In (Aqeel et al., 2023), researchers present a novel protocol for mobile cloud-based EMR sharing that integrates blockchain technology into the decentralized Interplanetary File System (DIFS). The notion seems to offer a workable solution to protect sensitive patient data from potential dangers and ensure the security of data transfers on mobile clouds, based on the results of the experiment. Results from that efficiency and security evaluation show significant improvements compared to earlier information exchange models in areas such as data privacy safeguards, low latency in the system maximum security stages, and lightweight access control technique.

In order to construct a system capable of managing sensitive data and facilitating collaborative research, that study aims to learn how decentralized networks might be used (Colace et al., 2022). The primary focus of a recently established framework is healthcare organizations, such as hospitals and research institutes, as they were the first to face the demanding conditions brought about by the COVID-19 epidemic (M. M. Khubrani & Alam, 2021a). Some have raised the possibility that decentralized systems may improve interactions across different types of organizations, which might lead to more fair real-time information exchange and less personal data leaking. The paper (Vidhya et al., 2024) proposes a novel approach to facilitate the secure exchange of medical information by combining blockchain technology with advanced encryption algorithms with privacy safeguards. Setup, data processing, and authentication are the three legs of the suggested system. The hybrid Feistal-Shannon homomorphic encryption technique is recommended for encrypting medical data in order to ensure its confidentiality, integrity, and availability. By incorporating ring signatures into the system, participants' identities may be more protected and their anonymity enhanced during data exchanges. In addition, the created smart contract establishes a time seal, verifies the user's identity, and validates the ring signature. The system is now more secure and private, and it can withstand both external and internal assaults, thanks to that update. A comprehensive security research is conducted to assess the proposed technique in contrast to existing ones. According to the findings, private health data stored on the blockchain is successfully protected by the proposed solution. Studies propose dynamic, lightweight encryption methods that are enabled by blockchain (Aruna & Sahayadhas, 2024). For the purpose of safeguarding blockchain network data and fending off different attacks, the logistic Advanced Encryption Scheme is provided. That scheme uses chaotic logistic maps. By deploying the model on the Ethereum blockchain and evaluating the computation, transaction time, and other parameters, they were able to compare its performance to that of other current blockchain-inspired encryption approaches.

The execution of the NIST experiment further showed the recommended technique. Both the security and transaction time metrics are surpassed by the proposed method, which clocks in at 0.964 seconds. And lastly, the proposed approach may generate highly dynamic keys, which are ideal for defending blockchain against unforeseen attacks. To ensure data secrecy during transactions and construct secure HIE systems, researchers have been focusing on cutting-edge technology [19] (Merhej et al., 2024). In order to enhance the privacy and security of HIE systems, researchers are focusing on two key technologies: blockchain and artificial intelligence. These technologies can identify potentially dangerous transactions. Even if HCF can link up via the blockchain decentrally, AI models provide an extra layer of security to the transfer of patient information. They begin with a brief overview of HIE systems and the problems they face before moving on to categorize the state-of-the-art methods that show how AI and blockchain may improve these systems. That study provides an overview of HIE structures having a dual purpose.

A secure design backed by blockchain and solid-pod technology is proposed in [(Alam et al., 2023). Because of that, the ability of an intelligent healthcare system to transmit electronic medical records in the event of an emergency is significantly impaired. Prioritizing privacy and security, users may set transparent, immutable, along with finely-grained data access restrictions using solidity-based smart contracts (Singh et al., 2025). They evaluate the performance of their proposed system by looking at the results of processing and storing using solid pods.

3. SYSTEM MODEL AND PROBLEM FORMULATION

In this paper, we present the idea of using blockchain technology in healthcare cloud infrastructure. The basic premise of this approach is to establish a standard mechanism to ensure the safety of medical records. For regulatory and compliance purposes, we have also proposed hiding patients' medical records. The proposal makes use of the following definitions prior to problem formulation.

Problem Statement: In addition to more conventional, in-person approaches, the epidemic has shifted healthcare providers' attention to Internet resources. It has led to the transfer of massive volumes of patient information via various means, including the cloud, third-party systems, and on-site storage. The confidentiality and integrity of patient's medical records have become hot topics in light of this massive digital data interchange. The term "healthcare data privacy" describes measures taken to safeguard sensitive patient information from unauthorized access and use. There is a framework in place to protect patient's personal information and medical records from unauthorized access in the healthcare sector. Disjointed medical records, inaccurate data, inefficient supply chains, problems with interoperability, and security breaches involving patient data are just a few of the shortcomings of traditional healthcare systems. The intended outcomes of medical research cannot be achieved due to several reasons, including but not limited to fraud, data fabrication, and trial misconduct. For these reasons, healthcare organizations have been dealing with issues related to the security and privacy of patient information. Now we have blockchain technology in the medical field.

3.1 Private Blockchain

Access constraints with limited network access are the foundation of private blockchains (Alam, 2023a, 2023b). No one other than the parties involved in a transaction would be able to see its details on a private blockchain[30]. As indicated in Eq. 1, let's assume that a set of n transactions t creates b blocks, bringing the length of the blockchain to l:

$$\int_{i=0}^{n-1} t_i = \sum_{x=0}^{l} (b_0 + b_1 + b_2 + \ldots + b_l)$$

3.2 Masking

Because of the important nature and sensitivity of healthcare data, it is not advisable to let data flow on a shared ledger architecture without security. For this reason, it must be sent to a blockchain without losing its criticality and sensitivity. This derives from the mathematical deductions made in Equations 2 and 3:

$$\text{Data}_{\text{transaction}} \leftarrow \sum_{\text{initial}}^{\text{live}} \text{Committed}_{\text{Transaction}} \cdot \text{Data}_{\text{masked}} \leftarrow \int_{\text{dummydata}}^{\text{maskedata}} \text{Data}_{\text{transaction}}$$

Below is an example of data masking Algorithm 1, which makes the original data unrecognizable to miners. After data mining is complete, the data may be unmasked to obtain the original data. Compliance and security need this action.

3.3 Encryption

We advise encrypting data in order to prevent data mining security breaches. Therefore, data that is encrypted would be accessible to miners. This encrypted data would be mined in order to prevent any disclosure. The time elapsed is stated in Eq. 5, and Eq. 4 shows that the transaction data is encrypted using AES before it is transmitted. It maintains privacy while being honest.

$$\text{Data}_{\text{masked}} \leftarrow \int_{\text{cleartext}}^{AES} \text{Data}_{\text{transaction}}$$

$$\sum_{t=0}^{\infty} \text{Time}_{\text{total}} = \int_{e=0}^{\infty} \text{Data}_{\text{transaction}} + \text{Data}_{\text{masked}}$$

3.4 Hashing

One of the most crucial parts of blockchain technology is hashing. Hashing the value ensures the data's integrity. As far as blockchain hashing algorithms go, SHA256 is where it's at. It is a one-way conversion process that accepts input and creates output. An input of any length may be "hashed" into a string of text of a predetermined length through the use of a mathematical formula. Messages may be hashed by using a special function known as a hash function; the output of this operation is the hash value. To be useful, a cryptographic hash function has to have specific properties. Hashes generated by the output must be unique. It should be impossible to derive the same hash value from different inputs when using an input to compute the hash value; hence, a single message should always yield the same hash value. In the distributed ledger, this hash is recorded. Data integrity is ensured by feeding this hashed value into the distributed ledger. The goal of this method is to make sure that the selection of variables' numbers is entirely random so that it can't be undone by using rainbow tables or brute force. Equation 6 expresses the blockchain hash function.

$$\sum_{\text{data}=1}^{\text{data}=\text{hash}} f(x) \leftarrow \text{Data}_{\text{masked}} + \sum_{t=0}^{\infty} \text{Time}_{\text{total}}$$

3.5 Cost of Operation

It is important to consider the cost approximation aspect while implementing our suggested architecture's complete infrastructure on the cloud. Because in addition to the EHR input component, the healthcare cloud is designed to use a great deal of software and hardware resources. That is why we have also considered the approach's operational costs. Cloud computing incurs infrastructure fees, masking costs, and encryption costs, all of which add up to the overall cost. Equation 7 may be used to determine this, as shown below:

$$\sum_{c=o}^{\text{Cost}} \text{Total}(c) = \text{Cos}_{\text{Masking}} + \text{Cost}_{\text{Encryption}} + \text{Cost}_{\text{Infra}}$$

3.6 Decentralization

One great thing about blockchain is that it doesn't claim ownership of data, which means that it is decentralized (Shuaib et al., 2023b). It implies that users may access data according to the roles that have been assigned to them. With a distributed ledger and linked chains that store hashed information about prior blocks, no one entity can access or manipulate the data. Here is the mathematical expression of this notion in Eq. 9:

$$\int_{i=0}^{\infty} \text{Chain} = \sum_{i=1,g=geo}^{i=N} \left(B_{1g} + B_{2g} + \ldots + B_{Ng}\right)$$

3.7 Interoperability

Aside from physicians, hospitals, and pharmacies, there are a plethora of vendors offering healthcare services due to the vastness of the healthcare area. With so many moving parts, it's no surprise that different individuals and technologies approach data collection, storage, and processing in their unique ways. Because of this, integrating data from many sources becomes a major challenge for both humans and machines (Reegu et al., n.d.). The integration of data into a common platform and subsequent processing are the two primary steps necessary to make data interoperable. Time, money, and energy are all wasted as a result. Therefore, healthcare spending and quality of treatment might be enhanced by facilitating the free flow of data between various devices and IT systems. The same is seen in Equation 10.

$$\text{Healthcare}_{\text{Data}} \propto \text{Interoperability}_{\text{PatientCare}}$$

Coding for interoperability reads datasets and sends cloud-based data that has been standardized. One way to make huge data more comprehensible is to normalize it. Any processing method may now take this data.

3.8 Smart Contract

A digital contract is known as a smart contract—an electronic protocol for the purpose of digitally easing, enforcing, and verifying contract negotiation and performance. Without the need for a middleman, a smart contract enables the execution of a legitimate transaction. The most advantageous aspect of blockchain technology is its decentralized nature; as a result, it eliminates the requirement to pay intermediates or mediators, which in turn reduces the likelihood of dispute and saves time. Secrecy and security are other features that smart contracts include. These contracts guarantee that miners, along with blockchain users, will face severe consequences for any infraction.

3.8.1 Mathematical Model

Since blocks are the building blocks of a blockchain, we must first define them before we can create our blockchain. A blockchain's primary data structure is a block. The fundamental purpose of the blockchain is the safe storage of blocks. The acronym BI stands for a generic block. A transaction between two entities forms a block. The following is one possible definition of block Bl_f, given that it contains multiple entries (D) of size M:

$$\text{Bl}_{\text{f}} = (\text{D1}, \ldots, \text{DN})$$

D represents the entries included inside the block. By solving a mathematical puzzle called the proof of labor, a connection may be made between two blocks. You may find this link in the second block's header. Anyone seeking tangible results from their endeavors is called a miner. Imagine a quantity represented by the letter t, together with two blocks, Bprev and Bnew, that is, bits. The value of t, which indicates the difficulty of the proof of work, may be used directly to construct a target number. A 64-digit hexadecimal number, with mostly zeroes in the last two positions, such as:

Figure 2. Smart Contract Model

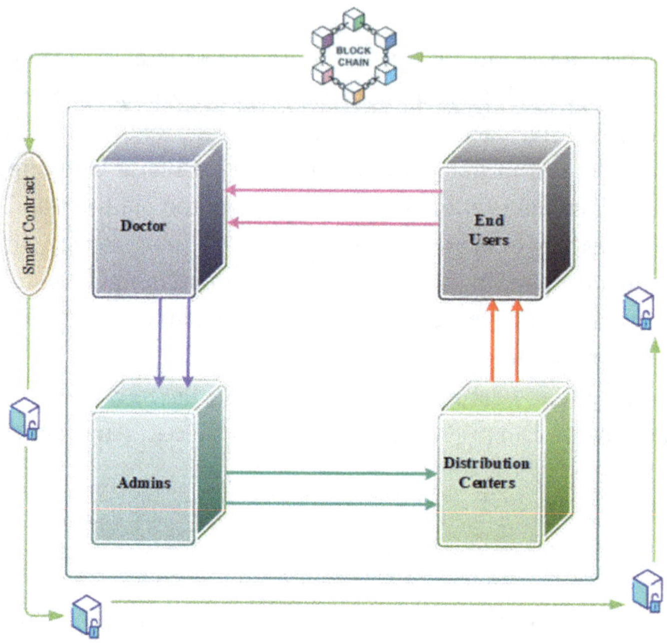

On the blockchain, we use the Sha-256 hashing method. We shall determine the hash of a particular block after supposing that we know the hash of the previous block, $\mathrm{SHA}(BI_t)$. To get the hash value of the new block, we apply the formula:

$$\mathrm{SHA}(Bl_{new}) = \mathrm{SHA}(\mathrm{SHA}(BI_t) \oplus \mathrm{stamp}(t) \oplus t \oplus \mathrm{nonce}) \leq \mathrm{target}$$

where the current time is represented by stamp(t) and the concatenation operation is denoted by $\oplus$. Following the proof working for blocks, we may provide the header for the block / using the notations discussed before (Bl_j, BI) has been resolved:

$$\mathrm{Heading}(\mathrm{Bnew}) = (i_m, SHA(B_p), \mathrm{stamp}(t), t, \mathrm{nonce}, \mathrm{SHA}(Bl_{mew}))$$

where i_m is the transaction information.

3.8.2 Blockchain Consensus Algorithms

A consensus algorithm is used to reach an agreement on the state of the system for blockchains and distributed ledger systems. Its primary function is to ensure that all nodes in the network agree on a single version of the ledger or blockchain, regardless of any errors or malicious actors. We zero down on the five most popular consensus algorithms, while there are many others.

Figure 3. Blockchain Network Model

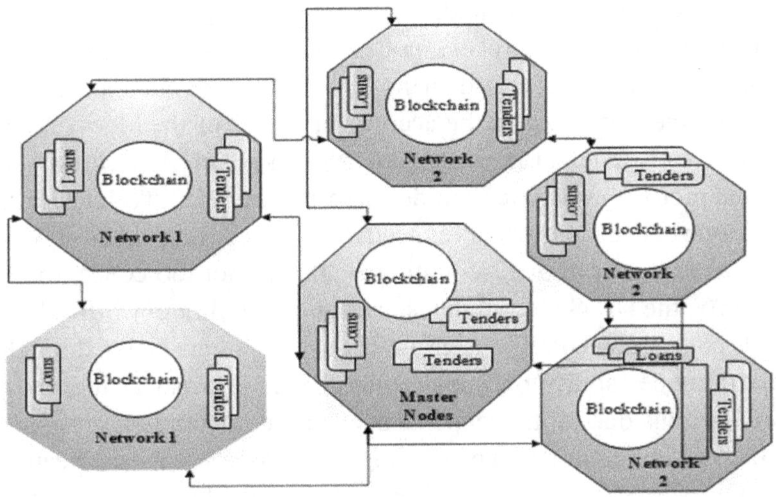

Proof of Work (PoW)

Prior to sending transactions, users spend computing effort into solving a mathematical equation. The original intent of the Proof of Work (PoW) method was to thwart spam assaults. With the introduction of proof of work (PoW) by Satoshi Nakamoto into the Bitcoin system, the first public blockchain network to adopt a Byzantine fault-tolerant consensus technique was Bitcoin. In Proof-of-Work (PoW), nodes on the blockchain compete to solve a mathematical issue; the node that completes the task first gets to reward itself and add a block to the chain. In order to accomplish a purpose as a network, nodes use certain methods to determine nonce values. If everything checks out, the node will broadcast the block for others to check. Although PoW is one of the most reliable consensus algorithms, it does have a few drawbacks, like high computational costs, long consensus periods, and limited transaction throughput (Alam, 2023b).

Proof of Stake (PoS)

To address the inefficiencies and high computational costs of the proof of work (PoW) technique, the Proof of Stake (PoS) approach was introduced in 2011 as an alternative. Its first implementation was in the cryptocurrency Peercoin. Proof of stake (PoS) selects accounting nodes based on the amount and age of tokens they own, as opposed to proof of work (PoW), which relies on processing power to validate transactions. An increase in a node's stake makes it more likely that it will validate transactions and collect rewards; this simplifies the "mining" process, speeds up the processing of blocks and transactions, and improves consensus efficiency. One of its drawbacks is that it has the potential to reduce user participation by giving nodes larger stakes, which in turn may reduce blockchain activity.

Delegated Proof of Stake (DPoS)

There is little difference between the Delegated Proof of Stake Algorithm and the representative election technique. Based on its currency holdings, each node in the framework is allocated a certain number of votes. During the consensus process, nodes are selected to act as decision-makers based on their perceived level of trustworthiness. Based on the number of votes obtained, several decision-makers are appointed. When it comes time to gain the accounting rights of the block, decision-makers rotate. The ability to make choices is inherent in every node in the system. Any current decision-maker who breaches the blockchain protocol will have their decision-making identity deleted. The system will add more members to the group of decision-makers as needed. Thanks to the multi-decision-maker technique, which may limit over-centralization, the accounting rights are not too concentrated on one node. By combining PoS with PoW, the DPoS algorithm achieves the best of both worlds. Faster communication between nodes is made possible by DPoS consensus. The system's transaction throughput is significantly enhanced as a result of the nodes' ability to complete block packing, broadcasting, and verification swiftly. DPoS achieves power savings due to its independence from computational resources. After decision-makers are elected, the system's transaction processing speed rises significantly, and transaction latency drops. It also makes it easy for a lot of nodes to join and leave the blockchain system at the same time. Its performance is quite robust and unaffected by changes in node size, demonstrating great scalability (M. Khubrani & Alam, 2023).

Proof of Authority (PoA)

The Proof of Authority (PoA) method for blockchain consensus relies on a set of trustworthy validators rather than computational power or stake to ensure the network's security [64]. Proof of authority (PoA) is an alternative to proof of work (PoW), while proof of stake (PoS), which relies on competing techniques, authenticates transactions while generating new blocks. PoW and PoS rely on large, trustworthy organizations to do this. A proof-of-authority network expedites the consensus process and boosts transaction throughput by selecting validators based on their dependability and identification. Since the network's security and integrity depend on the designated authorities' credibility, PoA may potentially raise the danger of centralization. Despite these cautions, PoA works well with consortium or private blockchains where members have established confidence and are trying to find a middle ground between security and efficiency (M. M. Khubrani & Alam, 2021b).

Practical Byzantine Fault Tolerance (BFT)

More than two-thirds of the nodes must have a good view of the block for this strategy to achieve consensus. Voting for the addition of the next block is something that every node must do. The PBFT is unaffected by one-third of the usual platform activity. Compared to proof of work, this makes consensus-building faster and cheaper. Additionally, unlike proof of stake, this method does not need the staking of any asset during the consensus process.

3.9 Validation

The procedure involves masking and unmasking, which is why validation is essential. To summarize, Eq. 11 shows that before adding a block to a blockchain, it must be validated to ensure its integrity. The block would be inserted into the chain in the event that the result is 1, and it would be removed in the event that the result is 0.

$$\Pi_{\text{Data Block}} = \begin{cases} 1, & \text{Valid block would be added to chain} \\ 0, & \text{Invalid Blocks would be dropped} \end{cases}$$

Figure 4. Blockchain Model

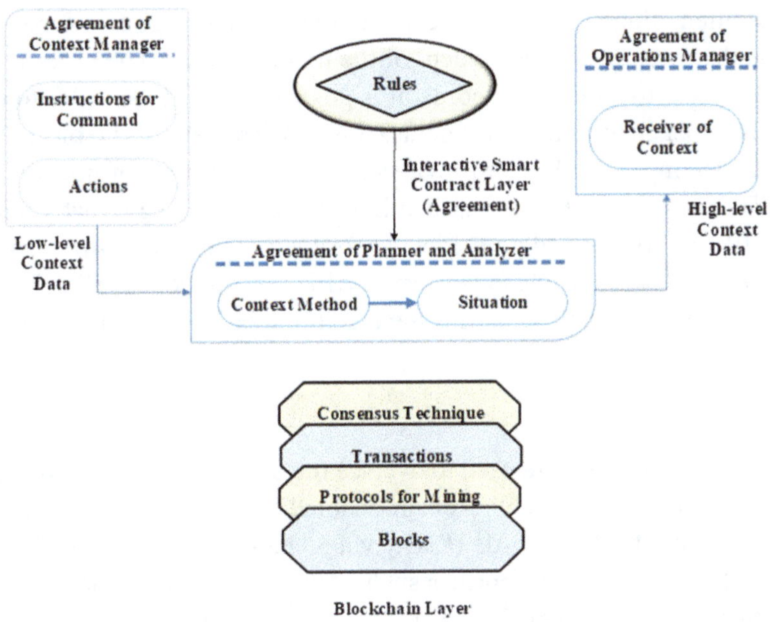

4. IMPLEMENTATION AND WORK FLOW

At its heart, the blockchain is essential for putting this concept into action. Although there are several blockchains, Hyperledger is used for testing and development purposes because of its simplicity, as stated in Section 2. We may build our private blockchain for research and testing using Hyperledger Fabric, another permissioned private blockchain with its own features and block parameters. The hospital-developed and -used front-end client application is the means by which a patient's electronic health record (EHR) may be viewed inside the network. The patient is identified on the blockchain network, and administrative rights are immediately added to their account when the EHR is created. When EHRs are created, the hospital changes the network settings so that patients may access and manage their information. It happens because the ordering serves as the administrative point that grants all entities regulated access to the system (Fig. 4). There is now parity between the patient and the hospital in terms of control over the network's setup.

Assuming it can connect to the network, the patient shares administrative rights over EHRs, even though the ordering function is hosted by the hospital. Third parties are, therefore, granted restricted access to this information despite the fact that the hospital is administering the ordering service and the patient has complete administrative rights over EHR. The patient, as the record owner, must provide their consent before the hospital, acting as the network administrator, may grant access to their EHR via requests from third parties. The network configuration stores the regulations and configurations for distribution access. In this paper, the network configuration specifies the distribution configuration, which includes the entities that patients, pharmaceutical companies, family doctors, physicians, and other third-party companies like insurance and interested government bodies can be part of in order to share EHRs on the blockchain. A channel is established for a specific entity to access EHRs after the patient grants access. However, the patient alone may permit access to their EHRs since this access is controlled by a channel configuration that is entirely independent of the main network. The ordering service monitors the nodes that provide access to all ledger records. It is possible to use index files to store metadata before storing data on the blockchain. The smart contract is a component of the blockchain that specifies usual procedures for accessing the ledger; it provides a clear framework for how the node may change or query the ledger. The data from EHRs or hashed information from them that points to the core data kept on individual EHR servers is saved on the ledger for the sake of distribution simplicity. By establishing a connection between our blockchain platform's API and the client applications running on all of the nodes in the network, we were able to access the electronic health record server in our experiment.

4.1 Experiments

Various methods and technologies are used to oversee the block transactions in the suggested cyber-physical EHR sharing architecture that is blockchain-enabled. Members of the blockchain network may access the system's electronic health records (EHR) via a shared public key and symmetric key. The suggested system, which includes several entities such as the blockchain, patient, doctor, and others, is shown in Fig. 7 by a basic step-by-step method. Sensors and other Internet of Things (IoT) gadgets gather patient health information and transmit it instantly to processing devices in the network's periphery. Developed apps save all patient data records at edge devices. In order to upload prescriptions for patients based on their healthcare records, the registered doctor must first submit a request to access this data. Only authentic physicians will have their requests approved. Also, without patients' consent, physicians can't provide any personal information. Blockchain technology is crucial in this context to ensure the data's security while being sent over the Internet. Authorizing authorized entities and validating transaction data utilizing protocols are the responsibilities of the blockchain. A concise overview of the primary features of various technologies and tools used in the execution of EHR based on blockchain is provided.

A. **The Interplanetary File System (IPFS)** is a distributed database that uses a P2P architecture for data storage and sharing. Every piece of content that makes it into IPFS is given its unique hash. You may make a single edit, but the hash will still be unique. The data's name cannot be changed, and IPFS may use the file's content instead of a domain name to find it. Data reference tables based on Kademlia are used. In addition to assisting in the discovery of sought-after data, routing entails broadcasting new data to the network. The DHT is immediately combined with a variety of tiny data values, each around 1 KB in size. The DHT keeps track of which nodes have the block information as it grows in size.
B. **BigchainDB:** Built on top of features like built-in asset support, immutable data storage, decentralized control, low latency, and high throughput, it has powerful query capabilities. The software's open-source nature means it's compatible with Docker and other programming languages, including Java, Python, and Javascript. A database that is updated in real time defines these transactions. Users may add new database records using the first CREATE transactions. To change one user's ownership of a record to another, you may utilize the second transaction, the TRANSFER transaction. The fact that BigchainDB transaction blocks include three main components—Asset, Metadata, and Transaction ID—is another crucial feature.
C. **Tendermint:** A program may be safely and reliably replicated on several machines using this piece of software. Even if a random failure might affect one-third of PCs, Tendermint will keep running. Each malfunctioning machine always calculates a unique state, and they never see the same transaction log. System fault tolerance relies on consistent and dependable replication, which is a fundamental problem in distributed systems. This problem arises in various contexts, including financial transactions, voting, and infrastructure management. What we term "Byzantine fault tolerance" (BFT) is the ability of a system to withstand failures, even when malicious ones happen.
D. **MongoDB:** While authentication systems may store usernames and passwords, doing so on the user interface of blockchain or IPFS incurs costs. It led to the relocation of all extra local data to a new storage facility and the assignment of a cryptographically secure public key to every account. So, it was only natural to use MongoDB.
E. **Cryptographic Algorithm:** It is essential to use an encryption method in order to limit data access to authorized individuals. Documents may be rendered unintelligible by the use of a key and symmetric encryption. Recovering the original document requires decryption using the same key. Because of its symmetric encryption and decryption capabilities, Advanced Encryption Standard (AES) has been chosen to build the blockchain-enabled healthcare system architecture that has been presented.

4.2 Results

An address is associated with every wallet on the blockchain. Here, we'll pretend that our blockchain has three wallets. The four features that make a blockchain resilient are its decentralized nature, the fact that its hashing code is ineffective, the need to link blocks together, and the existence of a consensus method. We demonstrated that our suggested solution used an improved SHA-256 hash function technique. This function generates an immutable hash code. Additionally, we demonstrated that the hash function combined the hash code of the previous block with the transaction data, thereby connecting the blocks in our blockchain. The suggested system was built on top of the Ethereum blockchain, which by default uses Proof of Stake for consensus. Because it relies on a distributed ledger, the proposed blockchain is decentralized. Because of this, the blockchain approach that has been suggested is superior. A party-authentication mechanism was used in the suggested method to verify the identities of persons prior to granting them access to the data. Additionally, we prove that updating any block information is very challenging. Thus, the suggested approach may be trusted.

We used the LZ4 technique to compress data and tweak the hashing mechanism. That is why our suggested approach has a temporal complexity of O(n), where n is the size of the hash function, supposing the hashing code does not start with repeated zeros. Implementing LZ4 data compression shortens the time. The O(1) time complexity is a reflection of how little time is required to construct a smart contract (1).

In Table 1, we can see how our suggested solution stacks up against previous research, other blockchain implementations, and adjacent fields. All blockchain versions required a longer time than the proposed method to produce a new block, as seen in Table 1. The table further demonstrates that the suggested method may be easily expanded due to the usage of a decentralized database.

Table 1. Comparison between related work and proposed method

Measurements	BLOCKCHAIN 1.0	BLOCKCHAIN 2.0	BLOCKCHAIN 3.0	Proposed System
Data that secure	Cryptocurrency	financial	financial	Medical data
Scalability				✓
Interoperability			✓	✓
Address can be read		✓		✓
Transaction time	2–4 (min)	14 (s)	14 (s)	1.5 (s)
Time complexity	O(n22)	$n$log$n$log	O(n + d)	O(n)
Party authentication				✓

5. CONCLUSION AND FUTURE WORK

Our study presents a novel approach to using blockchain technology in a healthcare cloud. A healthcare cloud is an idea for a consolidated cloud that stores data related to healthcare. This strategy calls for the creation of a central report housing all healthcare data, with the usage of blockchain technology to provide decentralization and security. A safe and efficient strategy was developed by combining healthcare cloud computing with blockchain technology for healthcare data. Our next step is to create a commercially viable version of our prototype setup that might be used in the actual world. It is also possible to reduce the time and money needed for execution. The healthcare cloud has to be developed further. Additionally, blockchain implementation is limited to private blockchain, with the possibility of expanding to public blockchain. An enhanced data masking method is possible to provide data anonymity against data miners. Putting this structure up in a way that abides by all applicable regulations and laws is part of the next effort. Making sure there's an established procedure for healthcare cloud setup is also important. Additionally, there are plans to integrate blockchain security with healthcare cloud machine learning in order to derive useful information.

REFERENCES

Abdellatif, A. A., Samara, L., Mohamed, A., Erbad, A., Chiasserini, C. F., Guizani, M., O'Connor, M. D., & Laughton, J. (2021). MEdge-Chain: Leveraging Edge Computing and Blockchain for Efficient Medical Data Exchange. *IEEE Internet of Things Journal, 8*(21), 15762–15775. DOI: 10.1109/JIOT.2021.3052910

Alam, S. (2023a). Security concerns in smart agriculture and blockchain-based solution. *2022 OPJU International Technology Conference on Emerging Technologies for Sustainable Development (OTCON)*, 1–6. DOI: 10.1109/OTCON56053.2023.10113953

Alam, S. (2023b). The current state of blockchain consensus mechanism: Issues and future works. *International Journal of Advanced Computer Science and Applications, 14*(8). Advance online publication. DOI: 10.14569/IJACSA.2023.0140810

Alam, S., Bhatia, S., Shuaib, M., Khubrani, M. M., Alfayez, F., Malibari, A. A. A., & Ahmad, S. (2023). An Overview of Blockchain and IoT Integration for Secure and Reliable Health Records Monitoring. *Sustainability (Basel), 15*(7), 5660. DOI: 10.3390/su15075660

Alsharif, A., & Nabil, M. (2020). A Blockchain-based Medical Data Marketplace with Trustless Fair Exchange and Access Control. *GLOBECOM 2020 - 2020 IEEE Global Communications Conference*, 1–6. DOI: 10.1109/GLOBECOM42002.2020.9348192

Aqeel, I., Khormi, I. M., Khan, S. B., Shuaib, M., Almusharraf, A., Alam, S., & Alkhaldi, N. A. (2023). Load Balancing Using Artificial Intelligence for Cloud-Enabled Internet of Everything in Healthcare Domain. *Sensors (Basel), 23*(11), 5349. DOI: 10.3390/s23115349 PMID: 37300076

Aruna, E., & Sahayadhas, A. (2024). Blockchain-Inspired Lightweight Dynamic Encryption Schemes for a Secure Health Care Information Exchange System. *Engineering, Technology & Applied Science Research, 14*(4 SE-), 15050–15055. DOI: 10.48084/etasr.7390

Bhan, R., Pamula, R., Faruki, P., & Gajrani, J. (2023). Blockchain-enabled secure and efficient data sharing scheme for trust management in healthcare smartphone network. *The Journal of Supercomputing, 79*(14), 16233–16274. DOI: 10.1007/s11227-023-05272-6 PMID: 37359328

Colace, F., De Santo, M., Marongiu, F., Santaniello, D., & Troiano, A. (2022). In Gupta, B. B., & Mourelle, L. M. (Eds.), *Secure Medical Data Sharing Through Blockchain and Decentralized Models BT - Robotics and AI for Cybersecurity and Critical Infrastructure in Smart Cities (N. Nedjah, A. A. Abd El-Latif* (pp. 249–262). Springer International Publishing., DOI: 10.1007/978-3-030-96737-6_13

Hoang, H. D., Duy, P. T., Tien, N. T., Hien, D. T. T., & Pham, V.-H. (2022). A Blockchain-based approach and Attribute-based Encryption for Healthcare Record Data Exchange. *2022 RIVF International Conference on Computing and Communication Technologies (RIVF)*, 65–70. DOI: 10.1109/RIVF55975.2022.10013886

Khubrani, M., & Alam, S. (2023). Blockchain-Based Microgrid for Safe and Reliable Power Generation and Distribution: A Case Study of Saudi Arabia. *Energies, 16*(16), 5963. DOI: 10.3390/en16165963

Khubrani, M. M., & Alam, S. (2021). A detailed review of blockchain-based applications for protection against pandemic like COVID-19. *Telkomnika, 19*(4), 1185–1196. DOI: 10.12928/telkomnika.v19i4.18465

Merhej, J., Harb, H., Abouaissa, A., & Idoumghar, L. (2024). Toward a New Era of Smart and Secure Healthcare Information Exchange Systems: Combining Blockchain and Artificial Intelligence. In *Applied Sciences* (Vol. 14, Issue 19). DOI: 10.3390/app14198808

Ozturk, B. A., Tayyeh, H. K., Namiq, H. E., Mahajan, H. B., Junnarkar, A. A., Uke, N., Shamaileh, A. A., Deshpande, S. D., Futane, P. R., & Rane, M. (2024). The Blockchain for Healthcare 4.0 Apply in Standard Secure Medical Data Processing Architecture. *Internet Technology Letters, n/a*(n/a), e614. https://doi.org/https://doi.org/10.1002/itl2.614

Reegu, F., Daud, S. M., & Alam, S. (n.d.). BLOCKCHAIN AND INTEROPERABLE STANDARDS FOR EHR-A COMPREHENSIVE REVIEW. *Turkish Journal of Physiotherapy and Rehabilitation, 32*(2).

Rosa, B. M. G., Anastasova, S., & Yang, G. Z. (2023). NFC-Powered Implantable Device for On-Body Parameters Monitoring With Secure Data Exchange Link to a Medical Blockchain Type of Network. *IEEE Transactions on Cybernetics, 53*(1), 31–43. DOI: 10.1109/TCYB.2021.3088711 PMID: 34197334

Shuaib, M., Alam, S., & Reegu, F. A. F. A. (2023a). Blockchain-based self-sovereign identity for COVID-19 medical passports and immunity certificates. *AIP Conference Proceedings, 2587*(1), 070003. Advance online publication. DOI: 10.1063/5.0150394

Shuaib, M., Alam, S., & Reegu, F. A. F. A. (2023b). Blockchain-based self-sovereign identity for COVID-19 medical passports and immunity certificates. *AIP Conference Proceedings, 2587*(1), 070003. Advance online publication. DOI: 10.1063/5.0150394

Singh, A., Nagabhooshanam, N., Kumar, R., Verma, R., Mohanasundaram, S., Manjith, R., & Rajaram, A. (2025). Deep learning based coronary artery disease detection and segmentation using ultrasound imaging with adaptive gated SCNN models. *Biomedical Signal Processing and Control, 105*, 107637. DOI: 10.1016/j.bspc.2025.107637

Venkatesh, R. (2024). A Lightweight Quantum Blockchain-Based Framework to Protect Patients Private Medical Information. *IEEE Transactions on Network Science and Engineering, 11*(4), 3577–3584. DOI: 10.1109/TNSE.2024.3378922

Vidhya, S., Siva Raja, P. M., & Sumithra, R. P. (2024). Blockchain-Enabled Decentralized Healthcare Data Exchange: Leveraging Novel Encryption Scheme, Smart Contracts, and Ring Signatures for Enhanced Data Security and Patient Privacy. *International Journal of Network Management, 34*(5), e2289. https://doi.org/https://doi.org/10.1002/nem.2289. DOI: 10.1002/nem.2289

Xia, Q., Gao, J., & Amofa, S. (2021). Blockchain Medical Data Sharing. In *Wireless Blockchain* (pp. 245–268). https://doi.org/https://doi.org/10.1002/9781119790839.ch11

Chapter 13
Achieving Seamless Interoperability of Health Data Across Digital Healthcare Systems

Umesha Raddy
https://orcid.org/0009-0001-1089-7830
East West Institute of Technology, India

A. Divya
Sathyabama Institute of Science and Technology, India

Manjunath G. Asuti
BNM Institute of Technology, India

M. Manickam
SRM Institute of Science and Technology, India

G. Michael
Saveetha University, India

A. Rajaram
E.G.S. Pillay Engineering College, India

ABSTRACT

The evolving demands of healthcare, driven by demographic shifts and the digital economy, necessitate efficient data exchange and service interoperability. These capabilities are fundamental to coordinated care, regulatory oversight, clinical and health economics research, and enhancing service quality and patient satisfaction. Effective interoperability is critical for electronic health records, facilitating improved medical delivery and system integration. However, existing frameworks often fall short in data exchange, security, and privacy. Healthcare organizations deploy numerous information systems and IoMT technologies, generating diverse data types that require swift, secure interoperability. Inadequate interoperability raises costs and complicates patient data analysis. This chapter examines key obstacles and underscores the need for robust inter- and intra-entity data exchange to elevate healthcare outcomes and operational efficiency.

DOI: 10.4018/979-8-3373-1022-0.ch013

1. INTRODUCTION

When two or more programs can exchange and use data and information with one another, we say that they are interoperable (Amos et al., 2024). When healthcare practitioners are able to exchange electronic health information across various systems securely, they can access and share patient data effectively; It is called interoperability (Thantharate & Thantharate, 2023). Care coordination, patient outcomes, and the quality of healthcare services as a whole are all enhanced by interoperability, which also allows for better decision-making (Hendawi & Li, 2024) (Timme et al., 2020). The interoperability of EHRs presents substantial obstacles in areas such as data interchange, privacy, and security, notwithstanding the many advantages.

In an effort to promote digital health as a science-based subject, the World Health Organization (WHO) has provided support for the field for more than 20 years (Sayeed et al., 2020). This dedication to the long term highlights the need to develop strong frameworks to handle issues with the interoperability of EHRs and EMRs. While EHRs and EMRs relate to electronic health records and medical records, respectively, they serve quite distinct practical purposes and have similar qualities (Alam et al., 2021) Therefore, in this study, the names are used interchangeably. This article begins by reviewing current EHR/EMR interoperability frameworks, pointing out their shortcomings, and establishing the need for a new framework. When it comes to healthcare, "interoperability" means that electronic health records can be accessed, integrated, and utilized in a timely and secure manner to improve the health of both individuals and communities (F. Reegu et al., n.d.). Accessing and securely sharing health data has always been a challenge. Despite its importance, health data is paradoxical: Sharing it is challenging because of its sensitive nature and the high degree of privacy and security it demands; nonetheless, being unable to access it when necessary might result in substantial damage. Bad results and increased expenses might emerge from not fully comprehending a population's or an individual's health demands due to a lack of interoperability. Interoperability and data exchange will be more important for providing good healthcare as the world's populations age and individuals live longer. An estimated 63 percent of American seniors suffer from two or more chronic mental or physical health issues, according to the Agency for Healthcare Research and Quality. Entities in the medical field share vast quantities of diverse data across numerous platforms. Interoperability is often assured within the same medical entity; however, issues with connecting different medical entities are common. A backlog of patients requiring additional exams due to incompatibilities puts a strain on healthcare institutions and drives up associated expenses.

The capacity to transfer data across different sources, such as emails and PDFs, is the first and most fundamental need. Second, structural data types include established data formats, syntaxes, and structures like codes, IDs, and plain text, which allow for data to be read **and utilized on many platforms.** Semantic: A common ground for data entry may be achieved by using standardized language and vocabulary. International Statistical Classification of Diseases and Related Health Problems (ICD) 10 codes and the Medical Dictionary for Medical Regulatory Activiti**es (MeDRA)1 are two examples.** Organizational: This category includes things like policies, supervision, governance, and compliance with legal and regulatory requirements.

Conversely, healthcare capabilities are gradually becoming overwhelmed by the ever-increasing global population. The elimination of superfluous inspections is now critical to raising the availability and operating expenses of these buildings. Also, with the rise of telemedicine, there's no longer any need to transport patients to hospitals routinely. System interoperability and data interchange standard efficiency improvements are necessary for cost savings and improved efficiency.

1.1 Data Interoperability

The capacity to efficiently store, transmit, and retrieve data from many sources is what we mean when we talk about interoperability. There are many categories into which it falls: When two objects are technically interoperable, it means they are physically connected such that they may interchange data bits and bytes. With an emphasis on information comprehension as an integration object rather than its actual use, not only can data but also contexts and information be exchanged. When it comes to infrastructure and governance, electronic health records (EHR) are the way to go at this level of interoperability (Siddiqui et al., 2020). As for semantic interoperability, ontologies from the European Interoperability Framework (EIF) are the way to go for describing the explicit representation of clinical concepts. This level also pertains to health professionals, data protection authorities, individuals, and patient associations. For semantic interoperability in the European Health Data Space (EHDS), the ISO 23903 standard is a good place to start. With dynamic interoperability, objects for integration are changes in context, and information, its use, and its applicability (knowledge) can be exchanged. Health Level Seven (HL7) Fast Healthcare Interoperability Resources (FHIR) is the most used format for exchanging health data; syntactic interoperability allows for the standardization of data exchange protocols. When all parties involved are using the same protocols and formats, as is the case when health records are saved in XML or Rest format according to the European Interoperability Framework (EIF), we have service interoperability, wherein two programs trade services and communication interoperability, wherein data is treated as an integration object apart from context. At the most fundamental level, interoperability is achieved at the organizational level via the harmonization and precise definition of processes, user roles, and access rights; at the second level, there is the capacity to interchange data and use information as an integration object, which pertains to data format and syntax (Singh et al., 2022).

1.2 Challenges of Healthcare Interoperability

While there are obstacles to overcome, advances in interoperability have great potential to improve healthcare efficiency, efficacy, and cost-effectiveness. In order to overcome these obstacles and make health information more accessible, everyone from health technology vendors and providers to payers and consumers, as well as government lawmakers and regulators, must work together. Improved healthcare interoperability will lead to improved patient outcomes. Still, experts are up against a mountain of obstacles in their quest to link diverse systems that store massive quantities of data (Adeniyi et al., 2023; Alam et al., 2022). Find out more by reading on.

- Limitations on Funds and Resources: When healthcare organizations are already short on funds and human resources, the prospect of investing in a state-of-the-art, interoperable health system might seem overwhelming. Putting off digital modernization efforts may be tempting. Still, healthcare organizations that do so will pay the price in the end due to security vulnerabilities, a lack of data for decision-making, and clinicians burdened with tedious data entry.
- Concerns Over Data Security and Privacy: With the increased accessibility of patient data, companies need to establish protocols to safeguard this data, whether it's stored in their own data centers or with their cloud service providers. The Journal of Medical Internet Research released an article outlining the methods by which healthcare clearinghouses, health insurers, and providers may exchange data in accordance with HIPAA, specifically on the sharing of data with patients.

Due to the elimination of human mistakes and potential security holes brought about by manual data entry, the advent of autonomous digital health systems will aid in protecting patient privacy and data integrity.

- Inadequate Standardization: HL7 FHIR paves the way for the next generation of internet-based, standards-based data exchange. Even while adoption is picking up steam, additional businesses in the sector, such as healthcare providers, government agencies, and health IT suppliers, still need to join forces (Saripalle et al., 2019).
- Data silos and fragmented systems: Disclosure of patient information to research institutions may be seen by some doctors as an unfair advantage. Even within a single healthcare company, data silos may occur. It happens, for instance, when one department utilizes a specialist electronic health record system that is not linked to another department's system. Government authorities must commit to establishing and enforcing standards, and healthcare providers and researchers must commit to sharing data in order to improve interoperability. Some medical facilities have yet to implement electronic health record systems; for instance, mental health facilities are behind the curve when it comes to the adoption of EHRs due to antiquated privacy regulations that mandate data segregation.
- Difficulty with Technology and Interoperability: The use of several incompatible EHR systems is a major obstacle to interoperability since it may lead to data silos, duplicate patient records (some of which are erroneous or incomplete), and other problems. Adverse effects on patient treatment and financial losses from rejected claims are the results of these identification mistakes. When data transport is one-way only, interoperability becomes much more of a problem—according to studies conducted by the US Office of the National Coordinator for Health Information Technology (ONC), over half of the hospitals surveyed reported exchanging data with other entities without receiving any data in return. Legacy technology that prevents providers from communicating with one another and an absence of standards for healthcare data formats are further obstacles to interoperability.
- Policies and Governance for Interoperability: "Information blocking" refers to practices that hinder the access, sharing, or use of digital patient data. It is becoming more of a worry as interoperability grows at a national level. As a result, the 21st Century Cures Act was passed with the goals of enhancing privacy protections for study participants and facilitating more data exchange among researchers funded by the National Institutes of Health. The legislation specifies eight scenarios in which it is acceptable to prohibit access to some information, such as when there are legitimate concerns about privacy or system security. The US Department of Health and Human Services (HHS) Office of Inspector General started fining firms that deny access to information with fines of up to $1 million per infraction towards the end of 2023. Complaints that endanger patients, disrupt healthcare delivery, or drain funds from federal healthcare programs or other organizations will be given top priority by the HHS.
- Ensuring Data Integrity, Quality, and Completeness: By allowing physicians to pin important patient data (such as allergies, current medications, and critical illnesses) to the top of the screen in the form of alert bars, new interoperability capabilities are reducing data overload. In the future, digital assistants with voice recognition will make it easier for doctors and nurses to update patient records, and some will even use decision-support tools based on artificial intelligence to listen in on doctors' appointments, suggest contextual next steps, and update the patient's electronic health record automatically. With organizations sharing records using different systems and patient data

collected from multiple locations, it becomes more complicated to assign information about patients to the correct person. It is an additional challenge as patient data flows among health providers. Numerous healthcare organizations have voiced their support for the Match IT Act of 2024. This legislation aims to standardize patient matching and use the match rate as a clinical quality evaluation. The Lown Institute found that over 20% of Medicare stents implanted between 2019 and 2021 were superfluous, costing an estimated $2.44 billion. The National Library of Medicine also released research that found that superfluous bloodwork was done on 76% of patients with simple acute surgical problems.

Finding the problems and developing solutions requires research into and comparisons of data standards and system interoperability standards. Finding solutions to problems with real-world interoperability models and developing a data interoperability proposal are the primary objectives.

This paper's key contributions are as follows:

- A synopsis of the most critical medical data standards
- An analysis of the various interoperability models, including their advantages and disadvantages
- A list of the characteristics that must be included in a medical interoperability reference model

2. RELATED WORK

The methods and technology described in (Bossenko et al., 2024) make it possible for domain experts with little technical knowledge to build and test transformation rules and maps with reusable visual transformation components, thereby establishing semantic interoperability in health data. Methods Design Science is a popular approach for producing software artifacts, including tools and methods, and it was used to design and evaluate the tools and processes for health data semantic interoperability. Final Product: In order to make EHRs more interoperable, their methods and tools allow for the real-time, seamless unification of different health data formats, eliminating the need for laborious physical data transfers. By using these technologies, domain experts may more easily define and test elaborate data transformation rules and maps, simplifying complex health data transformations. It is general enough to be used for other data transformation needs, including the European Health Data Space ecosystem. Still, it is currently being implemented to facilitate the ongoing transition of the Estonian National Health Information System from Clinical Document Architecture to Fast Healthcare Interoperability Resources.

Several parts of guaranteeing health data interoperability are included in the proposal's paragraphs (Stellmach et al., 2022). Every Member State must establish a digital health authority and a national point of contact, and a standardized format for exchanging electronic health records, including electronic prescriptions and patient summaries, must be developed. Additionally, a centralized platform must be established to facilitate cross-border digital infrastructure. Medical equipment and electronic health record systems will also be required to fulfill common standards defined by the Commission in order to be interoperable. The present version of the proposal does not provide any globally accepted standards for semantic and syntactical compatibility. Existing standards, such as the International Patient Summary, will need to give these parameters since many datasets are neither standardized nor globally harmonized.

To investigate the encoding requirements for uploading SDoH screening tool results from a big safety-net hospital to the National Covid Cohort Collaborative OMOP dataset, a realistic design and methodology are detailed in (Phuong et al., n.d.). They review the screening findings and provide a detailed overview of the steps used to build the data mapping with ingestion for patient-level SDoH. Their method proves that it is possible to share these crucial data, which are usually kept as non-standard, vendor-specific codes for electronic health records. That research outlines a method that might be applied to additional screening devices to enhance the interoperability of vital data, which could be useful as SDoH screening becomes more widely utilized throughout the country.

In (Kwon et al., 2024), they want to shed light on the history of Korea's health data standardization policy, the work of the Health Data Standardization Taskforce, and the plans for the future of that important initiative. In December 2022, the public and commercial sectors worked together to form the Health Data Standardization Taskforce, whose goal was to guarantee the interoperability of health data. The task force ran three different work groups. It outlined its goals, objectives, and strategies, conducted short-term standardization efforts, studied worldwide trends in interoperability standards, evaluated the present state of health data standardization, and finally, set up a governance mechanism for standardization. A comprehensive revision of the Korean notice of "Health Data Terminology and Transmission Standards" was made on September 15, 2023, with the goal of enhancing the interoperability of health information exchanges across information systems. The results of the work of the task force, including the Korea Core Transfer of Data Standard (HL7 FHIR KR Core) and the Korea Core Data for Interoperability (KR CDI), are included in that announcement. A Health-Data Standardization Promotion Committee was also formed to fortify the uniform system of governance. The development and broad implementation of standards for health data in Korea need the active involvement and assistance of medical informatics specialists (Shen et al., 2025).

The purpose of the study reported in (Costa et al., 2024)was to offer a bibliometric review of the literature on the topic of health data governance and interoperability. They gathered the data by searching Google Scholar, PubMed, and the Web of Science with specific queries (Hakim et al., 2024). After that, they imported the bibliometric data to Endnote and made sure there weren't any duplicates. To generate the final sample, the refined information was exported to Excel and subjected to multiple levels of filtering. The following software was used for data analysis: VOSviewer (Leiden University, Leiden, Netherlands), Excel (USA, Microsoft Corporation, Washington), and WORDSTAT (Provalis Research, Montreal, Canada). Findings: A total of 3,799 distinct findings were used to compile the literature sample, which included 63 papers from 45 separate periodicals. These publications were assessed using two distinct internal global impact rankings. I. Stakeholder demands in e-health information, (ii) trends in e-health information technology governance, and (iii) evaluation of e-health information quality were the three primary clusters found using VOSviewer. There was also a residual association in the sample between linkage studies and interoperability. In sum, In order to build a health information system that works, it is essential to evaluate the demands of the stakeholders.

The effects of current designs on semantics interoperability as it pertains to the incorporation of healthcare data into Big Data analytics are investigated in the research. The research shows how difficult it is to combine medical records from disparate sources that use different vocabularies, data models, and formats. Data integration initiatives run the risk of compromising patient care and research results due to misunderstandings, inconsistencies, and mistakes in the absence of a robust focus on semantic interoperability. In order to provide a shared language and framework for medical data integration, data standards, as well as ontologies, are crucial. Also covered is the significance of data mapping and transformation since inconsistencies in data can cause loss of data and erroneous analysis outcomes. Prioritizing semantics interoperability in current infrastructures is crucial for the successful integration of medical information into Big Data analytics. To harness the revolutionary powers of medical information analysis for better healthcare outcomes, a well-designed architecture must manage data heterogeneity, promote semantic consistency, and enable data standardization.

In (Alam et al., 2023), the research analyzes the influence of current designs on semantics interoperability in the context of integrating medical information into Big Data analytics. The study shows how difficult it is to combine medical records from disparate sources that use different vocabularies, data models, and formats. Data integration initiatives run the risk of compromising patient care and research results due to misunderstandings, inconsistencies, and mistakes in the absence of a robust focus on semantic interoperability. In order to provide a shared language and framework for medical data integration, data standards, as well as ontologies, are crucial. Also covered is the significance of data mapping and transformation since inconsistencies in data can cause loss of data and erroneous analysis outcomes. Prioritizing semantics interoperability in current infrastructures is crucial for the successful integration of healthcare information into Big Data analytics. To harness the revolutionary powers of medical statistical analysis for better healthcare outcomes, a well-designed architecture must manage data heterogeneity, promote semantic consistency, and enable data standardization.

The work done in (Gaudet-Blavignac et al., 2021)was part of a larger Swiss Federal drive to create a national infrastructure for exploiting consented data obtained from the healthcare and research system. That will allow Switzerland to do research in customized medicine. The Swiss Personalized Health Network is the campaign behind that. Funding for that effort is going toward encouraging the sharing and use of health data for scientific purposes. The project included the development and implementation of a national policy to facilitate the creation of a semantically compatible environment for clinical data. Methods In order to identify obstacles and evaluate sustainability, a thorough examination of different approaches to interoperability was conducted initially. That included large healthcare frameworks like Health Level Seven while Integrating Healthcare Enterprise, as well as approaches from regulatory agencies and research communities. A method with three main components was developed from that study. It caters to the demands of different communities with its robust multi-dimensional semantics, a descriptive formal language for exchanges, and an unlimited number of data models.

By cataloging their features and mapping data items used by each application, researchers in (Lazuardi et al., 2021)evaluated the possible interoperability of MCH systems in both government and private primary health care, hospitals, health offices, and the community. The difficulties of digital system interoperability were the subject of the online focus groups held with different application vendors. The corporate sector, health institutions, and both the federal and state governments have collaborated to create eighteen different health information systems pertaining to mothers and children. So far, system-to-system communication has just begun to facilitate routine reporting between health offices and the Ministry of Health. With the goal of facilitating the digitalization of services while routine reporting, it was necessary to enhance IT facilities and infrastructure, establish health data standards, fortify governance and regulation, and make better use of data in order to monitor, evaluate, and maintain interoperability between systems. Final thoughts and the digitalization of MCH services in Indonesia offer the possibility of assisting the continuum of care via an interoperable system.

In (Satti et al., 2020), authors published the Ubiquitous Health Profile, a multi-dimensional information storage approach in a semi-structured data curation engine, which offers fundamental support for archiving heterogeneous medical data and enabling partial data interoperability in the healthcare arena.

They also provide the results of the examination of the suggested platform's correctness, scalability, and timeliness. With a good scalability ratio between the amount of information stored and its retrieval speed, their results show that the UHPr can retrieve an error-free comprehensive medical record for a single patient from an ensemble of slightly over 116.5 million recorded medical parts for 390,101 patients.

3. INTEROPERABILITY IMPORTANCE IN HEALTHCARE

All healthcare and medical records must be fully accessible. All the right people, including patients, doctors, laboratories, researchers, insurance companies, and public health officials, may then make educated choices.

- The inaccessibility of all healthcare data is a result of the fact that several systems save different versions of patients' information. Because of this, there is a chance that data may be missing, duplicated, or inconsistent when accessed from several EHR and EMR systems, among others. Possible problems that may arise as a result of this include unnecessary test repetition, which may lead to delays in patient care and mistakes in diagnosis or treatment. Patients compelled to live with illnesses that alter or endanger their lives are profoundly affected by delays.
- Now, we are also gathering information on people's genetic tendencies, lifestyle choices, dietary habits, smoking habits, and other behavioral patterns. Care providers and public health administrators can use this supplemental data to conduct in-depth analyses of healthcare trends and needs, improve therapies, drive new developments, change or create policies, identify gaps in medical histories, and enhance the quality of care. They can also make decisions about every part of the system.
- The need for interoperability in healthcare data is recognized by the healthcare industry, regulatory agencies, and governments as a result of the crucial importance of key stakeholders having secure, appropriate, and timely access to data needed to make healthcare decisions.

4. MATERIALS AND METHODS

In Figure 1, we can see the schematic of the system that was created to accomplish data quality evaluation and data interoperability. To be more precise, the steps that make up the mechanism are (i) Data Collection, (ii) Data Cleaning, (iii) Data Quality Estimation, and (iv) Data Interoperability.

Data Collection

As shown in Figure 2, the first step of the process involves locating and connecting all of the available heterogeneous IoT medical devices, after which data is collected from them. After that, we used the method from our earlier work to find all the devices that were already on the market and link them to the mechanism. It includes things like activity trackers and body weight scales. For further specifics, this system can interact with Bluetooth-only devices since it employs a Bluetooth interface based on Bluetooth Low-Energy (BLE). As soon as the devices are linked, the mechanism finds all the methods in the connected devices' Application Programming Interface (API), extracts them, and uses the ones that collect data from the various devices, according to the procedure. Because private devices do not publicly disclose information about their methods, this mechanism can only connect to public devices with open APIs that allow access to their methods. The nature of these devices, whether known or unknown, determines the type of device they are. Not only that, but the suggested technique can distinguish between medical-grade and consumer-grade IoT medical devices; thus, it can be used for both types.

Data Cleaning

Cleaning up the acquired data occurs in the second step of the process. To get into further depth, the data cleansing mechanism that was designed follows a multi-step approach. In particular, the following steps are involved: (i) data validation, which checks for errors related to conformance to specific constraints; this ensures that the collected data measures meet the defined business rules and constraints, such as specific data types, value representation, range constraints, pre-defined values, and cross-field validity. (ii) data cleaning, which removes the errors found during validation by fixing the incorrect records of data. (iii) data completion, which deals with missing data, checks for completeness and compliance with mandatory fields, such as required fields that are filled in. It should be mentioned that in order to identify errors and clean them up, the data validation and cleaning steps consider well-defined rules that the manufacturers of IoT devices can set. However, they don't necessarily need advanced machine-learning business logic.

So, to provide the completeness step of the process of cleaning, finishing, and correctly verifying data, the data cleaning process considers the stated business rules in addition to the available current and historical data. As a consequence, we can see the final cleaning findings, which detail all of the fixes applied to the original datasets and their respective derivatives. To be more specific, using the cleaning results as a basis, the accuracy (i.e., Data_Accuracy) of each dataset is determined using Equation (1). Here, Total_Records represents the number of records in each dataset derived from each connected device, and Total_Actions is the number of total errors (i.e., erroneous data, missing data, dropped records) encountered in each dataset throughout the cleaning process.

Data Quality Estimation

The third step of the process involves estimating the quality of the cleaned data from the linked devices. Much of the obtained data may have come from unreliable devices or from reliable equipment that is defective and error-prone, so it is not enough to retain all of it and utilize it for further analysis. This step is crucial. Therefore, it is important to test and assess the data quality of all outputs before deciding which ones to retain. It will ensure that only trustworthy data from trustworthy sources is retained. As mentioned in our earlier work on data quality levels, it is more effective to evaluate the quality of the devices and the data they create in order to do this. As can be seen in Figure 4, there are three distinct processes involved in this stage of the mechanism.

Long Short-Term Memory

An LSTM-based classification method was used to compare the performance of the suggested technique further. One subset of recurrent neural networks (RNNs) used for deep learning is the long short-term memory (LSTM) RNN, which uses backpropagation to learn about input variables' relationships and long-term dependencies from time-series information. Time series while sequence prediction issues seem to favor it. Its use in healthcare prognostics and other forms of systems, along with rotating machinery health monitoring, has recently been the subject of much research. A few healthcare diagnostics initiatives also sought to use LSTM.

An input layer, an LSTM layer, and a conventional feedforward output layer make up a common LSTM architecture for classification. Using its memory unit or cell, the LSTM layer encodes the incoming information in a time series or sequence. A long short-term memory (LSTM) unit's three gates—the forget gate, the input gate, and the output gate—are shown in the figure. Values are stored by the cell for indefinite periods, and the flow of information into and out of the cell is controlled by both the input and output gates, respectively.

Figure 9 shows the connections that may be utilized to build mathematical statements for the gates and LSTM cell outputs, such as:

$$f_t = \sigma\left(w_f^h \cdot h_{t-1} + w_f^x \cdot x_t + b_f\right)$$
$$i_t = \sigma\left(w_t^h \cdot h_{t-1} + w_t^x \cdot x_t + b_t\right)$$
$$g_t = \tanh\left(w_g^{h_g} \cdot h_{t-1} + w_g^x \cdot x_t + b_g\right)$$
$$C_t = \Psi + \varphi$$
$$\Theta_t = \sigma\left(w_\Theta^h \cdot h_{t-1} + w_\Theta^x \cdot x_t + b_\Theta\right)$$
$$h_t = \tanh\left(C_t\right) \times \Theta_t$$

The current input is represented by x_t, the sigmoid activation function is denoted by σ, the prior hidden state is represented by h_{t-1} and the cell state is represented by C_(t-1). f_t, i_t, Θ_t, C_t, and h_t on time step t, are the following states: forget, input, output, cell, and hidden. w_f^h and w_f^x signifies the input forget gate weight and the hidden state forget gate weight, respectively. w_t^h and w_t^x look up the hidden state's input gate weights and the input gate weights. w_Θ^h and w_Θ^x represent the hidden state's output gate weights and the input's weights, respectively. In the input gate that updates the cell state, g_f is one of the potential cells w_g^h and w_Ω^x stand for the input weights and the hidden state weights, respectively. b_f, b_i, b_g, and b_Θ stand for the forget gate, the input gate, the cell candidate, and the bias of the output gate in that order.

Figure 1. CNN with Bi-LSTM Model

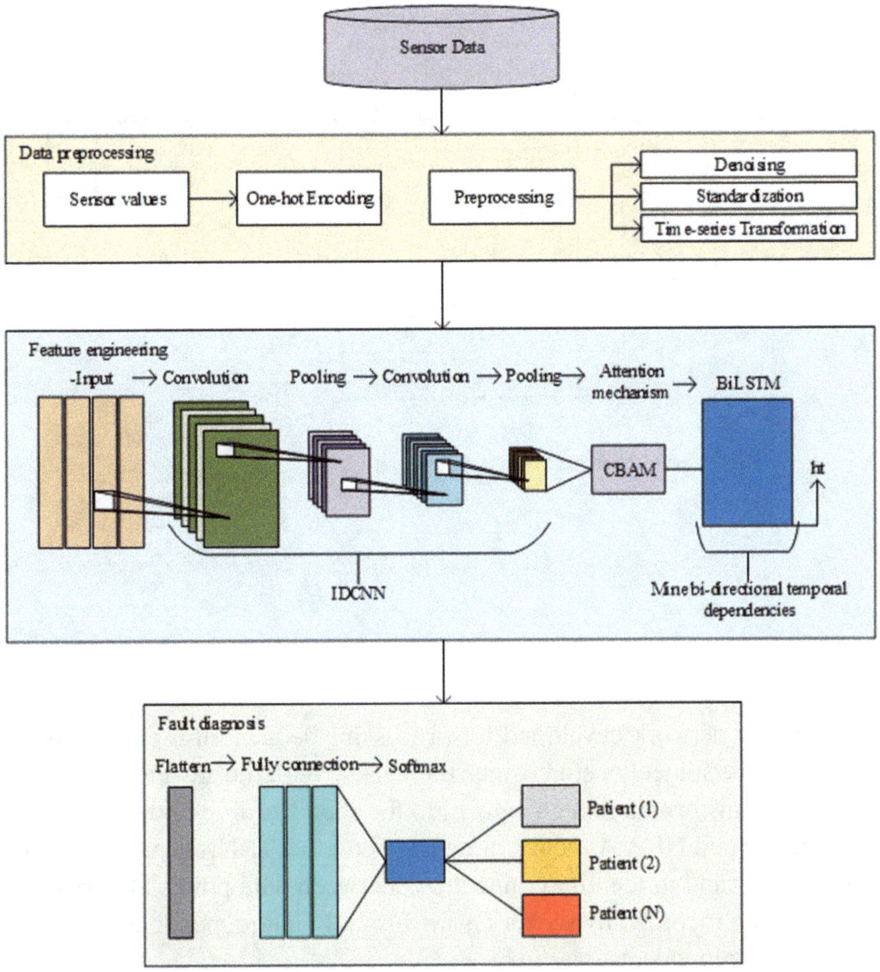

Bidirectional LSTM (BiLSTM) is superior to LSTM because it can better capture both backward and forward dependencies; LSTM, on the other hand, can only capture forward dependencies. In a BiLSTM architecture, a single layer consists of a pair of LSTMs, with one layer processing the input sequence in a left-to-right fashion and the other in a right-to-left fashion. Once finished, the outputs of both LSTMs are combined and sent to the subsequent network layer.

Figure 2. Convolutional Model

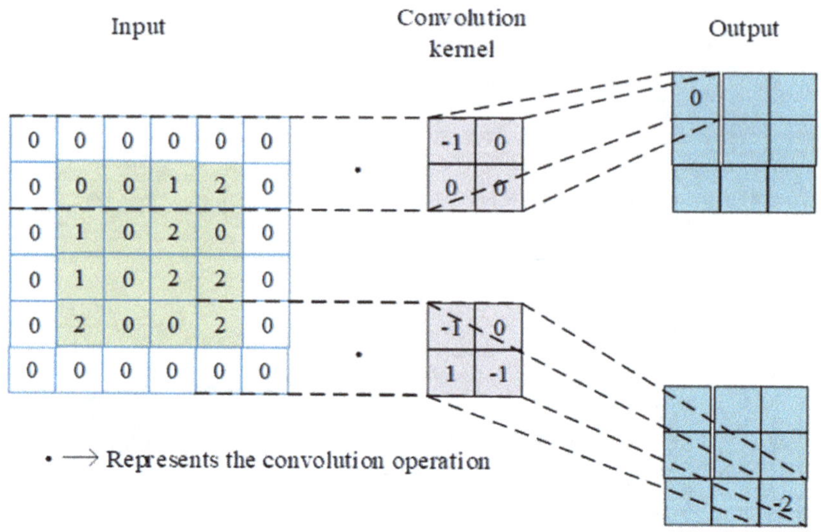

BiLSTM

An early kind of neural network developed for processing sequential input, Recurrent Neural Networks (RNNs) have been the subject of study since the 1980s. With the advancement of both theory and computing power, RNN transformed into an algorithm for deep learning in the early 2000s; since then, it has found widespread use in NLP. A recurrent neural network's (RNN) capacity to recall previously presented data sequentially and to identify connections between data points at various time steps is its fundamental property. Data recorded by sensors is intrinsically interdependent due to the deteriorating health state of equipment components over time.

However, RNN has problems during training, namely long-term data dependencies and the possibility of ballooning or disappearing gradients when backpropagating mistakes. To tackle these issues, a subset of RNNs called Long Short-Term Memory (LSTM) networks handle long-term dependencies in time series information and help with the vanishing gradient problem. The BiLSTM network can process input patterns in both ways because of its bidirectional topology. Because it can receive input in both directions, the network can learn more about the data's temporal linkages and better collect information from earlier and later time steps. When it comes to fault detection, being able to capture significant information that may show trends in either direction of time is a huge plus.

5. CONCLUSION

When healthcare data is fully accessible across all systems, it benefits patients, the healthcare ecosystem, R&D, government policy, and quality of treatment. Health results, public health, and safety are all affected by the need for interoperability, which also has a significant monetary effect on everyone. Both the quantity and velocity of data produced continue to grow dramatically year-on-year due to the evolution of healthcare practices and technology. Establishing data-sharing agreements and trust frameworks, providing a technical mechanism that enables efficient data communication, and tackling the ambiguity and flexibility in data standards are all necessary steps toward achieving interoperability goals. In order to improve healthcare outcomes, healthcare technology must take advantage of this unprecedented degree of interoperability. In the future, similar to what Medidata has accomplished, technology solution providers will continue to revolutionize various aspects of healthcare and clinical trials. These areas will include patient-centered care, personalized medicine, data management, AI-driven decision support, simplified workflows, reduced resource burdens, and the ability to share data in real time among systems and participants. Most importantly, patients' lives will be improved or perhaps saved, and financial and resource burdens will be significantly reduced.

REFERENCES

Adeniyi, A. E., Awokola, J. A., Alam, S., Bharany, S., Agboola, P., Shuaib, M., & Ahmed, R. (2023). A Hybrid Framework of Blockchain and IoT Technology in the Pharmaceutical Industry: A Comprehensive Study. In *Mobile Information Systems* (Vol. 2023). DOI: 10.1155/2023/3265310

Alam, S., Ahmad Reegu, F., Daud, S. M., & Shuaib, M. (2021). *Blockchain-Based Electronic Health Record System for Efficient Covid-19 Pandemic Management. Preprints*. DOI: 10.20944/preprints202104.0771.v1

Alam, S., Bhatia, S., Shuaib, M., Khubrani, M. M., Alfayez, F., Malibari, A. A. A., & Ahmad, S. (2023). An Overview of Blockchain and IoT Integration for Secure and Reliable Health Records Monitoring. *Sustainability (Basel)*, *15*(7), 5660. DOI: 10.3390/su15075660

Alam, S., Shuaib, M., Ahmad, S., Jayakody, D. N. K., Muthanna, A. S., Bharany, S., & Elgendy, I. A. (2022). Blockchain-Based Solutions Supporting Reliable Healthcare for Fog Computing and Internet of Medical Things (IoMT) Integration. In *Sustainability (Switzerland)* (Vol. 14, Issue 22). DOI: 10.3390/su142215312

Amos, J. D., Zhang, Z., Tian, Y., Lowry, G. V., Wiesner, M. R., & Hendren, C. O. (2024). Knowledge and Instance Mapping: Architecture for premeditated interoperability of disparate data for materials. *Scientific Data*, *11*(1), 173. DOI: 10.1038/s41597-024-03006-8 PMID: 38321063

Bossenko, I., Randmaa, R., Piho, G., & Ross, P. (2024). Interoperability of health data using FHIR Mapping Language: transforming HL7 CDA to FHIR with reusable visual components. *Frontiers in Digital Health, Volume 6-*. https://www.frontiersin.org/journals/digital-health/articles/10.3389/fdgth.2024.1480600

Costa, T., Borges-Tiago, T., Martins, F., & Tiago, F. (2024). System interoperability and data linkage in the era of health information management: A bibliometric analysis. *The HIM Journal, 18333583241277950*, 18333583241277952. Advance online publication. DOI: 10.1177/18333583241277952 PMID: 39282893

Gaudet-Blavignac, C., Raisaro, J. L., Touré, V., Österle, S., Crameri, K., & Lovis, C. (2021). A National, Semantic-Driven, Three-Pillar Strategy to Enable Health Data Secondary Usage Interoperability for Research Within the Swiss Personalized Health Network: Methodological Study. *JMIR Medical Informatics*, *9*(6), e27591. DOI: 10.2196/27591 PMID: 34185008

Hakim, T., Ahmi, A., & Alam, S. (2024). A Decade in Blockchain: A Bibliometric Reflection on the Growth and Interdisciplinary Reach of a Disruptive Technology. *Journal of Information and Communication Technology*, *23*(4), 627–665. DOI: 10.32890/jict2024.23.4.3

Hendawi, R., & Li, J. (2024). Comprehensive Personal Health Knowledge Graph for Effective Management and Utilization of Personal Health Data. *2024 IEEE First International Conference on Artificial Intelligence for Medicine, Health and Care (AIMHC)*, 92–100. DOI: 10.1109/AIMHC59811.2024.00026

Kwon, A., Lee, H.-Y., Shin, S.-Y., Yang, K., Sung, Y., Lee, K., Byeon, N.-S., Lim, T.-H., & Lee, J.-H. (2024). Current Health Data Standardization Project and Future Directions to Ensure Interoperability in Korea. *Healthcare Informatics Research*, *30*(2), 93–102. DOI: 10.4258/hir.2024.30.2.93 PMID: 38755100

Lazuardi, L., Sanjaya, G. Y., Ali, P. B., Siahaan, R. G. M., Achmad, L., & Wulandari, H. (2021). Interoperability of Health Digitalization: Case Study on Use of Information Technology for Maternal and Child Health Services in Indonesia. *Business Information Systems, 1*(SE-Applications), 317–327. DOI: 10.52825/bis.v1i.53

Phuong, J., Hong, S., Palchuk, M. B., Espinoza, J., Meeker, D., Dorr, D. A., & Adams, W. G. (2022). Advancing interoperability of patient-level social determinants of health data to support COVID-19 research. *AMIA Joint Summits on Translational Science Proceedings AMIA Summit on Translational Science*, *2022*, 396.

Reegu, F., Daud, S. M., & Alam, S. (n.d.). BLOCKCHAIN AND INTEROPERABLE STANDARDS FOR EHR-A COMPREHENSIVE REVIEW. *Turkish Journal of Physiotherapy and Rehabilitation, 32*(2).

Saripalle, R., Runyan, C., & Russell, M. (2019). Using HL7 FHIR to achieve interoperability in patient health record. *Journal of Biomedical Informatics*, *94*, 103188. https://doi.org/https://doi.org/10.1016/j.jbi.2019.103188. DOI: 10.1016/j.jbi.2019.103188 PMID: 31063828

Satti, F. A., Ali, T., Hussain, J., Khan, W. A., Khattak, A. M., & Lee, S. (2020). Ubiquitous Health Profile (UHPr): A big data curation platform for supporting health data interoperability. *Computing*, *102*(11), 2409–2444. DOI: 10.1007/s00607-020-00837-2

Sayeed, R., Gottlieb, D., & Mandl, K. D. (2020). SMART Markers: Collecting patient-generated health data as a standardized property of health information technology. *NPJ Digital Medicine*, *3*(1), 9. DOI: 10.1038/s41746-020-0218-6 PMID: 31993507

Shen, Y., Yu, J., Zhou, J., & Hu, G. (2025). Twenty-Five Years of Evolution and Hurdles in Electronic Health Records and Interoperability in Medical Research: Comprehensive Review. *Journal of Medical Internet Research*, *27*, e59024. https://doi.org/https://doi.org/10.2196/59024. DOI: 10.2196/59024 PMID: 39787599

Siddiqui, S. T., Shuaib, M., Gupta, A. K., & Alam, S. (2020). Implementing Blockchain Technology: Way to Avoid Evasive Threats to Information Security on Cloud. In *2020 International Conference on Computing and Information Technology, ICCIT 2020*. DOI: 10.1109/ICCIT-144147971.2020.9213798

Singh, A., Joshi, K., Alam, S., Bharany, S., Shuaib, M., & Ahmad, S. (2022). Internet of Things-based Integrated Remote Electronic Health Surveillance and Alert System: A Review. *2022 IEEE International Conference on Current Development in Engineering and Technology (CCET)*, 1–6. DOI: 10.1109/CCET56606.2022.10080629

Stellmach, C., Muzoora, M. R., & Thun, S. (2022). Digitalization of Health Data: Interoperability of the Proposed European Health Data Space. In *Studies in health technology and informatics* (Vol. 298, pp. 132–136). DOI: 10.3233/SHTI220922

Thantharate, P., & Thantharate, A. (2023). ZeroTrustBlock: Enhancing Security, Privacy, and Interoperability of Sensitive Data through ZeroTrust Permissioned Blockchain. In *Big Data and Cognitive Computing* (Vol. 7, Issue 4). DOI: 10.3390/bdcc7040165

Timme, R. E., Wolfgang, W. J., Balkey, M., Venkata, S. L. G., Randolph, R., Allard, M., & Strain, E. (2020). Optimizing open data to support one health: Best practices to ensure interoperability of genomic data from bacterial pathogens. *One Health Outlook*, *2*(1), 20. DOI: 10.1186/s42522-020-00026-3 PMID: 33103064

Chapter 14
Advancements in Remote Health Monitoring Systems Technologies:
Applications and Future Trends

Madiha Munawar
https://orcid.org/0009-0001-7211-9022
Stanley College of Engineering and Technology for Women, India

Thakur Monika Singh
https://orcid.org/0009-0006-8534-9130
Stanley College of Engineering and Technology for Women, India

R. Madana Mohana
Stanley College of Engineering and Technology for Women, India

ABSTRACT

Remote health monitoring systems are transforming healthcare by leveraging IoT, AI, and wearable devices for continuous monitoring and real-time data collection, improving diagnosis and treatment. These systems enhance chronic disease management, elderly care, and post-operative support through IoT-driven sensors and mobile connectivity. With hardware, software, and wireless networks as their foundation, they support applications like vital sign monitoring and emergency response. While benefits include reduced hospital readmissions and improved outcomes, challenges such as data security and regulatory issues persist. Advances in AI, blockchain, and wearable technologies address these hurdles, enabling predictive monitoring and secure data sharing. Applications in rural healthcare and chronic disease management showcase their potential, with future trends promising AI-driven analytics, blockchain for data integrity, and advanced wearables, paving the way for proactive, patient-centered care.

DOI: 10.4018/979-8-3373-1022-0.ch014

1. INTRODUCTION TO REMOTE HEALTH MONITORING SYSTEMS

1.1 Definition and Importance

Remote Health Monitoring Systems (RHMS) refer to systems through which patient measures will be ceaselessly obtained, analyzed, and communicated ultimately outside the conventional clinical in-door setting (Priya et al., 2009). Such systems would include devices such as wearables, smartphones, or connected hubs that measure vital biological functions, chronic health status, or rehabilitation status in near real-time (Ghosh et al., 2016). This feature is increasingly becoming a requisite in health care to counter the problem of busy hospitals and uneven access points.

Figure 1. Remote Health Monitoring System

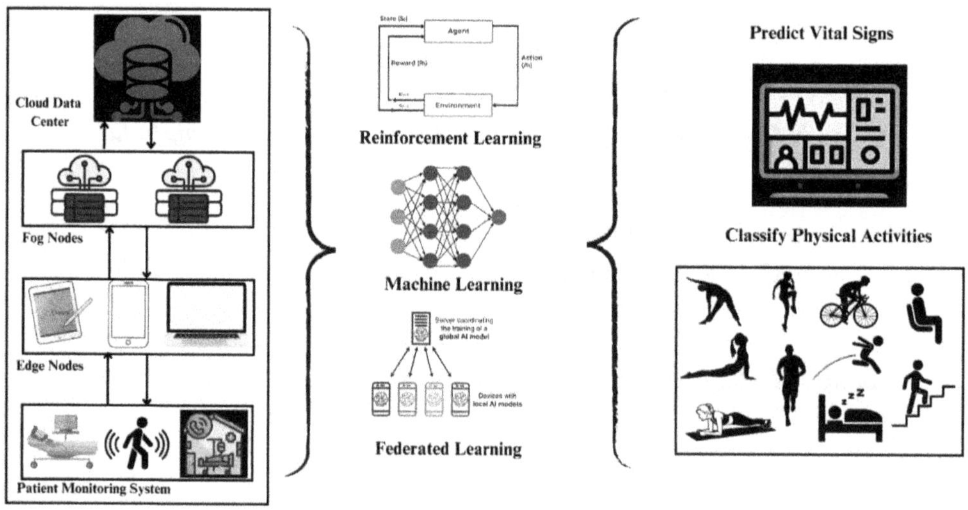

Figure 1 demonstrates how AI-enabled remote health monitoring works, Advancing modern patient care through advanced technology. The patient data fed into monitoring systems (for example, IoT sensors) is shown here as a hierarchical system on the left hand (edge nodes, fog nodes, and then the cloud data center for storage and advanced analysis). The middle focuses on how predictive insights are fortified with optimization in decision making and privacy-preserving AI model training using Reinforcement Learning, Machine Learning and Federated Learning on the set-up. It's all applications as seen on the right-hand view - vital signs prediction (for example, heart rate) and classifying physical activities (for example, walking, exercise, sleeping) - where AI can be seen in action in real-time health monitoring and activity recognition.

It will transform the whole idea of health management from reactive to proactive management (Baig & Gholamhosseini, 2013). One would expect it to detect some abnormal changes in heart rate or blood pressure earlier(Albahri et al., 2018) . It can thus save lives and also save the health system from spending huge amounts on treating the complications of such conditions (Sathya & Kumar, 2017). These systems also empower the patients with creating awareness towards their health and making them involved in their health care strategies. This will be a huge jump in terms of democratizing the health access around the world (Bansal et al., 2015). In times of resource restrictions, remote monitoring closes some amazing distances in health care access (Benhaddou et al., 2008). Rural and under-served populations have greatly benefited from these systems since they do not have immediate access to quality medical facilities (Nurshod et al., 2021). DHIS, together with advanced data collection and real-time communication, can remotely diagnose, treat, and follow up patients without the need for an expensive and lengthy in-person visit (Mohammed et al., 2019).

Significance:

- Ensures continuous surveillance for chronic disease upkeep.
- Lessens hospital and clinic burdens by enabling care within the home.
- Increases empowerment around decision making regarding personal health.
- Gives immediate warnings of serious conditions that might reduce emergency response times.
- It bridges healthcare access gaps, especially in rural or underprivileged sections.

1.2 Evolution of Remote Monitoring Technologies

The progression of remote monitoring technologies has made itself felt from telehealth services, like telephone auscultations and primitive telemetry devices, which used to transmit simple ECG data via phone line only (Salah & Zneid, 2019). Those facilities now transformed into all-inclusive platforms that enable real-time, high-definition, continuous health monitoring as a result of the internet, wireless communication, and IoT(Ng et al., 2020) .

Remote Patient Monitoring (RPM): It is where electronic devices are used to gather real-time medical data for the remote analysis of healthcare practitioners.

Machine learning and artificial intelligence integration have granted many more powers to these systems (Sivani & Mishra, 2022). Nowadays, one can use modern RHMS or remote health-monitoring solutions that apply predictive analytics to detect health risks, suggest interventions, and empty into cloud storage-where bulk data is managed and analyzed. The introduction of consumer wearable devices such as the Fitbit (Landolina et al., 2012), Apple Watch, and smart medical patches has democratized self-monitoring by ensuring clinical-grade functionality fits well while the user interface remains simple (Atreja et al., 2019). Edgeless computing and 5G promise the most in future remote health monitoring (Krapivin & Shutko, 2012). These advancements are designed to heighten speed, lessen the latency, and enhance real-time capabilities of health data transmission and monitoring (Lightsey et al., 2021). Such limitations are also being breached with the positive developments in these technologies: connectivity challenges would be easy to solve, and there would also be scalability limitations that would be easily addressed with these technologies (Loupian et al., 2018).

1.3 Key Applications in Modern Healthcare

Remote health monitoring systems have many applications in modern health care. These include applications in chronic disease management, rehabilitation, and preventive health. For example, diabetic patients can use continuous glucose monitoring devices, which will alert them to changes in blood glucose levels, and patients with heart diseases can use wearable ECG monitors to monitor irregularities and intervene at the earliest.

Post-operative care and management of older patients are two other critical applications of RHMS where much impact has been witnessed (Chronaki & Vardas, 2013). Various systems equipped with sensors can detect falls or remind users to take their medications, allowing older people to live alone while being safe. Such systems also provide caregivers with the updates they require regarding the patient's health and enables healthcare provider consultations from remote locations. So much impact has also been felt in the post-operative care and elderly management areas using RHMS systems. The devices which have these features like fall detection or medication reminder can assist older people to have all privacy while living alone but in safety (Farias et al., 2020). Moreover, these systems are also designed for caregivers such that they also get real-time updates on the patient health status and facilitate their remote consultations with health providers.

The COVID-19 pandemic threw a glaring light on the usefulness of remote monitoring in the management of infectious diseases (Safavi et al., 2019). These systems enabled the continued monitoring of patients suffering from mild symptoms during periods of isolation, taking some pressure off the healthcare system. RHMS also serve as critical tools during health emergencies in tracking vitals such as oxygen saturation and body temperature.

Table 1 provides a comparison between traditional health monitoring systems and the other hand, remote health monitoring systems. The statements actually describe the parameters of features, cost and effectiveness by which these two systems may be differentiated. The first one describes how traditional systems rely on in-person visitations for collecting data and diagnosis over some periods, whereas the same term remote describes real-time monitoring via wearable devices or IoT technology. The differences between these two systems are also highlighted by some costs and efficiency savings possible using remote monitoring in reducing hospital visits and providing time interventions, also noting possible challenges, such as technological dependence and privacy concerns.

Table 1. Comparative Analysis of Traditional vs. Remote Health Monitoring Systems

Aspect	Traditional Health Monitoring	Remote Health Monitoring
Features	Requires in-person visits for diagnosis and monitoring.	Real-time monitoring using IoT and wearable devices.
Accessibility	Limited to hospital or clinic visits.	Accessible from home or remote locations.
Cost	Higher due to frequent visits and hospital stays.	Lower due to reduced travel and hospitalization costs.
Efficiency	Time-consuming with delayed feedback.	Faster data collection and immediate alerts.
Technology Use	Minimal use of technology; manual processes.	Leverages IoT, AI, and cloud technologies.
Patient Engagement	Limited interaction outside appointments.	Continuous engagement through mobile apps and devices.
Data Collection	Periodic, based on scheduled visits.	Continuous, real-time data collection.
Scalability	Difficult to scale for large populations.	Easily scalable through connected devices.
Emergency Response	Delayed response to critical health events.	Immediate alerts for emergencies.

2. TECHNOLOGICAL FOUNDATIONS

2.1 Role of IoT in Remote Health Monitoring

Their Intermittent Access and speed of function of devices through networks allow cell poles, patients, and providers to communicate with each other: this is a characteristic of the Internet of Things (Guntur et al., 2018). IoT connects active sensors, wearable devices, and gateways that gather and relay real-time health data (Khoi et al., 2015). Their continuous monitoring of critical parameters such as heart rates, blood glucose levels, and blood pressure provides the overall health profile of a patient (Alshamrani, 2022).

The Internet of Things is an automating process and thus reduces the need for collecting and analyzing the data manually (Singh et al., 2024). It is also an automatic updating in contact with the cloud through the user's mobile application's account concerning data collected by a wearable fitness tracker or medical-grade IoT-sensored device-the flow of data into cloud servers with respect to accuracy and efficiency. The provider is, thus, able to keep tabs on the patient remotely, hence informing him of potential risks and timely interventions if and when needed (Sehar et al.).

Figure 2. IoT Driven Remote Health Monitoring System for COVID-19 Patients

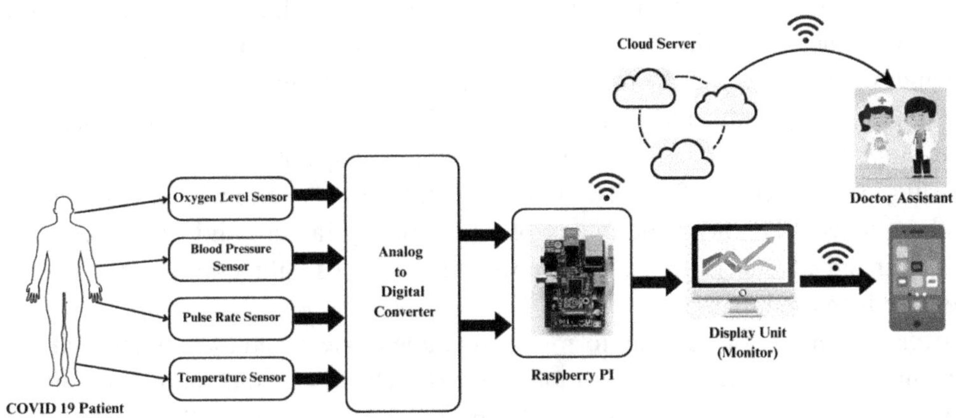

Figure 2 illustrates a remote health monitoring system intended for the tracing of vital signs of even such patients that are infected by a virus called COVID-19. Mainly, the system consists of some sensors, including, but not limited to, those used to measure breath oxygen level, blood pressure, pulse rate, as well as temperature; all of which later relay real-time patient data collated by means of the system. The classified signals are converted to digital form using an analog-to-digital converter, and the processed data relayed would be sent to the Raspberry Pi unit in charge of further transmission from both units. That data will hence be displayed in a monitor for the purposes of visualization and uploaded simultaneously to a cloud server, thus allowing for remote access by a doctor assistant. The system also provides a wireless connection with mobile devices as a means of ensuring that real-time monitoring and prompt medical intervention are possible.

IoT technology paves the way for extending and democratizing the remote health monitoring system (Singh et al., 2025). With the inclusion of IoT-facilitated devices with different wireless communication technologies like Wi-Fi, Bluetooth, and 5G, healthcare can find its way into the most remote or neglected population (Reddy & Satvika, 2023). These systems can be helpful in tackling underserved health systems to accomplish realtime decision-making and preventive care approaches altogether to improve overall health efficiency (Reddy, 2023).

2.2 Integration with Mobile and Wearable Devices

Mobile devices and wearable devices are the important remote health monitoring components (Castillejo et al., 2013). These devices provide the most user-friendly interface with patients as well as their healthcare providers. The most important device among those present is the smartphone, which connects all those devices, serves as the platform through which health data will be viewed, stored, and shared, and serves as a reminder through mobile apps, tracks the progress, and delivers real-time feedback. The use of wearable technology like smartwatches, smart patches, movement bands, and fitness bands has made remote health monitoring personal and reachable. These devices measure different metrics, such as fitness activity levels, bodily biological cycles, patterns of sleep, and vital signs like recordings of continuous glucose monitoring, which mean that an increasing proportion of these devices will give people feedback-actionable recommendations concerning their health and well-being. Some of these advanced wearables such as continuous glucose monitors are even regarded as medical-grade because they have been designed to help in the medical management of chronic diseases.

Wearable devices are greatly enhanced in functionality by the mobile apps. For instance, gathering and analyzing such data by AI enabled app to start giving the specific recommendations or detecting abnormal readings (Zhang et al., 2024). These devices and apps also allow health practitioners to communicate with patients at any hour and in any place for timely inquiry and assistance (Naddeo et al., 2017). Such continued advancements in making wearable devices light, comfortable, battery-efficient, and accurate have increased their acceptance.

Table 2 gives a summary of different forms of wearable devices and their functional application in health monitoring and fitness tracking. Wearable devices such as heart rate monitors, glucose monitors, and fitness bands perform important roles in real-time physiological data collection for efficient health management and general well-being.These contemporary devices have advanced sensors for measuring other specific metrics like heart rate, blood glucose levels, levels of activity, and sleep patterns. They may be accessible either from mobile applications or from cloud platforms. In this way, individuals and their healthcare providers can view health conditions and abnormalities and make well-informed decisions for future preventive care and medical interventions.

Table 2. Types of Wearable Devices and Their Primary Functions

Wearable Device	Primary Function	Description
Heart Rate Monitor	Measures heart rate and heart rhythm.	Tracks heartbeats continuously to identify arrhythmias and monitor heart health.
Continuous Glucose Monitor	Monitors blood glucose levels in real time.	Helps diabetic patients maintain stable blood sugar levels throughout the day.
Blood Pressure Monitor	Measures blood pressure remotely.	Provides real-time blood pressure readings, useful for hypertension management.
Oxygen Saturation Monitor	Tracks blood oxygen levels (SpO2).	Monitors oxygen levels to assess respiratory health and detect conditions like COPD.
Sleep Tracker	Monitors sleep patterns and quality.	Helps users understand sleep stages and quality, identifying issues like apnea.
Fitness Tracker	Tracks steps, calories burned, heart rate, and sleep patterns.	A multi-function device for general physical activity monitoring and health insights.
Heart Rate Variability Monitor	Analyzes variability in heart rate intervals.	Provides insights into stress levels and autonomic nervous system health.
Activity Tracker	Monitors physical activity, including steps, distance, and intensity.	Provides feedback for exercise, weight loss, and overall fitness improvement.

2.3 Sensor Technologies for Health Data Collection

The onboard sensors are very small yet highly advanced devices, qualified to collect health data like temperature, pulse rate, or oxygen saturation in a remote monitoring system. The area of concern with them goes across a range of platforms such as wearables, implantable devices, or home diagnostic tools.

The functions of optical sensors depend on light-based techniques used to measure or detect heart rates and oxygen levels. A biosensor is also available that can measure or sense chemical changes in blood, including glucose levels (Majumder et al., 2017). Activity monitoring through activity trackers may also incorporate accelerometers and gyroscopes to sense motion and trigger fall detection processes. Therefore, all those combined would often prove helpful in elderly care. Advances in nanotechnology further miniaturize the performance of such sensors for a better ability to carry them around because of increased portability and use within daily life.

However, it is more than the hardware innovations. The major software innovation has become adaptive and intelligent health monitoring with this kind of hardware. Artificial intelligence algorithms, such as signal processing algorithms, can filter noise and detect anomalies in recorded signals and ensure high-quality data collection (Vijayan et al., 2021). So, as sensor technology progresses into the parameters of remote health monitoring, it has made the empowerment of patients along with transformation in the delivery of health services.

3. CORE COMPONENTS OF REMOTE HEALTH MONITORING SYSTEMS

3.1 Hardware: Devices and Sensors

They are sensors and health devices that collect vital health data and form important hardware components in the remote health monitoring systems. They would include devices like fitness trackers, smartwatches, or some biosensors as their user-helpful elements, and specialized equipment such as blood pressure monitors and ECG machines. All the devices are compact, portable, and user-friendly, allowing easy accommodation in the daily lives of patients. Precise health metrics are captured high-performance sensors within the devices, establishing the ground for very accurate analyses. One main category of wearables is devoted to the patient and their monitoring of health. Examples: Fitbit devices that track steps, heart rate, and sleep while advanced smartwatches like Apple Watch and others create new dimensions, such as ECG and blood oxygen (Magrupov et al., 2021). Most of these devices have options for wireless connectivity, such as Bluetooth and Wi-Fi, to maintain the automatic transfer of collected data to a smartphone or a cloud platform. When the fabrication of miniaturized hardware components started, implantable devices have continued their development offering quality continuous monitoring without pain.

The efficiency of these remote health monitoring systems depends on reliability and accuracy of hardware. Robust hardware collects data even in some of the worst environments without interruption (Ahmed et al., 2016). This adds to the development of flexible and biocompatible sensors that can keep the patient comfortable by recent developments in materials science. Moreover, with future developments in hardware technologies, one can envisage that remote health monitoring systems will be have much wider scope and new applications.

3.2 Software: Platforms and Applications

These are the softwarehouses underpinning the infrastructure of remote healthmonitor-ing systems, which convert the data collected into practical insights. These include mobile apps, cloud infrastructures, and already machine learning algorithms. The platforms incorporate, process, analyze, and visualize health data. They ensure that data to be gathered through monitors and sensors gets enhanced and construed into meaningful insights from the patient and the healthcare provider's views. Key functions of such applications are data storing, analysis, trend visualization, and personalized recommendations.

Mobile and web-based applications have uses that can communicate with a patient in how the app registers and allows the patient to follow their health metrics in real-time. For instance, they serve as a reminder for taking medicine, encourage the user to meet daily activity goals, and even send emergency alerts. These embedded features enable interactive health-tracking applications. Noteworthy examples include MyFitnessPal, which monitors various vital signs while at the same time gives health tips based on the inputs of the user data. They are heavily dependent on specialized platforms to analyze the pooled patient data on the lookouts for potential risks to health (Xu et al., 2017). These advanced systems run artificial intelligence and predictive analytics algorithms to alert anomalies to enable timely intervention.

Cloud-based platforms are capitalizing on the enhancement and security of remote health monitoring systems. The cloud infrastructures host plenty of patient data and give real-time access integrated with healthcare structures. Encrypted communication alongside multi-factor authentication guarantees safety and privacy patient data (Zhang et al., 2014). The software platforms are evolving to complement cutting-edge technologies such as blockchain and generative AI to make future remote health monitoring systems more reliable, transparent, and predictive.

3.3 Communication Technologies: Wireless Protocols and Networks

Communication technology is a backbone in ensuring data transfer in distant medical monitoring systems. Such technologies are the ones that allow access to information in-between devices, hubs, cloud platforms, and health providers. The most recognized wireless protocols including Bluetooth, Wi-Fi, and Zigbee have their differentiated plays depending on system requirements (Fotouhi et al., 2016). Bluetooth, for example, could be used to connect short distance communication gadgets, such as wearables, to smartphones, while Wi-Fi and mobile network technologies including 3G, 4G, and 5G would provide long-range data transfer from one point to another.

Figure 3. Flow Diagram of Remote Health Systems Data Collection and Transmission

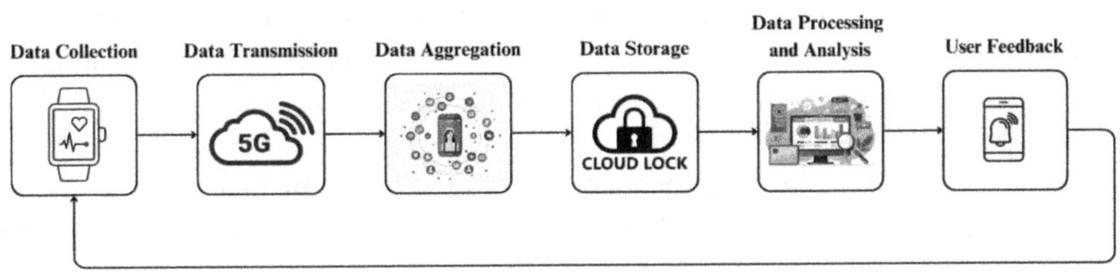

Figure 3 describes how remote health systems collect and send medical information from patients using several sensors and digital network connectors. This includes sensors such as oxygen level sensors, blood pressure sensors, pulse rate sensors, and temperature sensors, which sense real-time health parameters from the patient. The output signals from these sensors are converted from analog to digital form from the outputs through an Analog to Digital Converter (ADC) and forwarded to the Raspberry Pi microcontroller. The data are further processed and sent wirelessly to a cloud server for access and analysis. This would allow the medical official to see the data through the display unit or mobile devices, making real-time decision-making possible (Verma et al., 2022). The system is meant for continuous monitoring of health parameters; it enables care given distance, more so in high-risk cases, for example, a COVID-19 patient.

It has been prophesied that 5G would give a new dimension to remote health monitoring. 5G has remarkable low latencies in combination with a very high range of bandwidth availability.. This will allow instant transfer of crucial health data such as ECG readings and alert signals from any destination to another within seconds because there will not be any delay. Other comparative reference protocols like Zigbee and LoRaWAN can be applied in home-based monitoring systems to efficiently interconnect many devices but within a small area. They use a low-current optimization ideal for battery-driven devices. Data integrity and confidentiality are the most critical elements in communication technologies. Information about patients is secured by high protocols to secure the data under transmission. Also, Edge Computing technologies enable the processing of data right at the local end, thus reducing their dependency on cloud networks for quicker responses. In the future of communication technologies, remote health monitoring systems will change towards achieving much greater scalability, accessibility, and efficiency.

4. APPLICATIONS AND USE CASES

4.1 Chronic Disease Management

The remote health monitoring system is significant for chronic disease management in such cases as diabetes, hypertension, and asthma today. The continuous monitoring systems allow measurement and assessment of health parameters, availing timely data needed to symptom control and avoidance of complications. For example, a blood sugar monitor can be used to automatically track blood glucose trends and inform patients whether or not to adjust their insulin dosage (Peyroteo et al., 2021). In a similar manner, a hypertension monitor provides real-time feedback and alerts for optimally managing blood pressure levels for people with hypertension.

Healthcare providers will benefit since the entire patient record is collected to help create a personalized evolving treatment plan. As changes occur in a patient's condition, doctors can quickly adjust medication or therapies because most of the time, routine monitoring is done. Hence, the quality of life for patients improves since they do not have to visit the hospital as often. With remote monitoring, patients also take a more active role in the management of their health by facilitating compliance to the treatment scheme. Collectively or individually, these systems enable population health management, by being able to analyze trends and patterns among large groups of patients. Such predictive analytic tools embedded in remote monitoring systems may also easily forecast a community outbreak and/or peaks of chronic disease cases and suggest preventive control programs at the community level. The improvement in technology will push the chronic disease management through remote monitoring forward in effectiveness and accessibility.

4.2 Elderly and Post-Surgery Care

Elderly and post-operatory patients require constant observation to prevent complications and assist in recovery. Remote health monitoring systems offer safe, non-invasive, and efficient options for monitoring their health without the need to visit a clinic. Such systems, for instance, can be configured to monitor heart rates, oxygen levels, and blood pressure, minimizing the amount of time they would have otherwise spent making multiple visits to a hospital. For the elderly, the fall detection sensor and emergency alert system act as additional safety mechanisms (Zhang et al., 2022). After surgery, monitoring for infection, arrhythmia, or any other complications is usually carried out by health care providers. Remote systems with wearables help in early detection of such complications for timely interventions. Healthcare providers may also remotely access substantial patient information and make more personal recommendations for fast recovery. Virtual consultations on telemedicine platforms associated with the system enable patients to receive advice without having to travel, especially in cases of mobility problems.

Caregivers thus benefit from their beloved using remote monitoring systems. Real-time updates on the said patient's condition will make it easier for caregivers to feel assured. Alerts and notifications will enhance immediate proper actions upon detection of any critical changes evident with the monitoring systems. Technology keeps changing, and features like AI predictive analytics will continuously improve the capability and advantage that these systems will provide for elderly and post-surgery patients.

4.3 Real-Time Vital Sign Monitoring

As further development in the health monitoring system at home, real-time monitoring of the vital signs ranks among the very first. Wearable devices containing sophisticated sensors keep a close watch on heart rate, respiratory rate, oxygen levels, and temperature, among other parameters (Swaroop et al., 2019). Such information gets transmitted in real-time to health personnel for immediate alert and response to health-related emergencies. For example, patients can monitor their ECG online while programing alarms at pre-defined limits to advise them of arrhythmias or other heart abnormalities in time for intervention. It makes this feature particularly suitable for patients with cardiovascular diseases or respiratory conditions that put them at increased risk. If monitored in this way, they would probably get picked up even with the slightest changes, reducing the chances for complication development. Real-time data equips the health profession for more refined decisional inputs, such as narrowing down prescription dosages or providing lifestyle advice. During emergencies, these systems can directly alert healthcare teams or emergency services to save lives.

It gives patients more leverage regarding their health. By checking their data regularly on a mobile app, they can see the real-time data, identify trends, and change their lifestyles before being forced to by events. This revolutionizes the efficiency of health systems as possible admissions to hospitals are averted and interventions are executed just in time. Real-time actual monitoring could undoubtedly be made still more accurate and responsive through advances in AI and edge computing.

Table 3 classifies the applications of wearables according to different health conditions, indicating their potential role in personalized health monitoring. For example, diabetes management apps use glucose trackers that automatically monitor blood sugar levels throughout the day, hypertension apps use blood pressure monitors for occasional readings to prevent emergencies for patients-thereby allowing for aftercare in regard to surgery to monitor heart rate, oxygen saturation levels, and temperature for ongoing recovery. Again, these particular applications sum up the varieties of performance available with wearable technology for chronic disease management as well as improvements in patient outcomes and proactive healthcare interventions.

Table 3. Applications of Wearable Devices Categorized by Health Conditions

Health Condition	Application	Description
Diabetes	Continuous Glucose Monitoring (CGM) Devices	Tracks blood glucose levels in real time, reducing the need for manual checks.
Hypertension	Remote Blood Pressure Monitoring	Allows patients to monitor blood pressure at home with lo T-enabled devices.
Post-Surgery Care	Remote Rehabilitation Programs	Monitors patient recovery progress and provides virtual physiotherapy sessions.
Cardiac Conditions	Remote Heart Monitoring (ECG)	Tracks heart rate and detects abnormalities like arrhythmias.
Chronic Respiratory	Remote Spirometry and Oxygen Level Monitoring	Helps manage COPD and asthma by monitoring lung function and oxygen saturation.

continued on following page

Table 3. Continued

Health Condition	Application	Description
Mental Health	Virtual Counseling and Stress Monitoring	Tracks stress levels and provides online therapy or meditation guidance.
Pediatrics	Remote Pediatric Monitoring	Monitors growth metrics and childhood diseases remotely.

4.4 Emergency Response Systems

Emergency performances systems combined with remote technical health monitoring methods play a very vital role in the lifesaving missions. Such systems are configured to detect when health emergencies-like heart attack, stroke, falls-are occurring and then activate prompt alerts to health care providers or even call for emergency services. Some examples include wearables like smartwatches or just any devices like medical alert systems that have sensors detecting irregularities in the vital sign readings or sudden movements and taking that as a sign for immediate action. Such responsiveness turns out to provide a layer of security for patients who have ongoing ailments or just the aged. At such points in moments the system sends alerts to the different contact people and shares the location data in real time with emergency response services. This largely lessens the time before access to medical service under the emergency condition (Antevski et al., 2021). A few of those existing systems are also coupled with telemedicine facilities, where telehealth professionals can view the situation and even give further instructions before the arrival of the first responders.

Almost all advanced systems in emergency response are under constant improvement to ensure their increased reliability and efficiency. Artificial intelligence integration enables such systems to tell the difference between real and snags to minimize unnecessary interventions. Furthermore, they will also send important information-from-source to avoid hanging because of the advance in communication technologies like 5G. The most spread use of such systems will be important in many ways to improve patient safety, especially under high-risk circumstances.

5. BENEFITS AND OPPORTUNITIES

5.1 Enhanced Patient Engagement and Outcomes

The idea behind Remote Health Monitoring systems is to actively engage the patient in a more participative healthcare journey. This system enables an individual to assess vital health metrics like blood pressure, heart rate, and glucose levels via mobile apps or wearable devices and thus, through continuous feedback, improve the lifestyle and treatment compliance among patients. As an example, consider wearable fitness trackers encouraging activity goals to help improve cardiovascular health.

Patient engagement may also expand into better engagement with meaningful health care providers. Real-time connection from monitoring systems allows patients to contribute their data for immediate response and guidance (Agali et al., 2024). The two-way interaction creates a trusting environment and increased quality of care. Other features, such as personalized recommendations in health and interactive dashboards, help customers better understand their health status and take corrective action. More engaging surely translates into better output. Studies have shown that monitoring one's health actively can lead to improved clinical results-in this case, lower blood sugar and less hypertension. Ones observed via remote systems are less likely to be readmitted since most early warning signals will be caught by the system and acted upon at the right time (Kunbi et al., 2024). Thus, technology has changed how personalized care is given by incorporating it into remote patient health monitoring. The 21st century proves to be very promising in providing patient experiences and care-related efficiency for all.

Table 4 gives the most significant advantages of using wearables for health and the impact that these benefits have been shown to have when expressed as a percentage. It shows that the most significant benefit is reduced readmissions to hospitals (30%), which corresponds to less stress on health care systems. Closely behind are the cost savings, 25%, which are further made apparent by how wearable technology reduces costs for the patient and the provider. An improvement in patient outcomes (20%) as well as real-time monitoring with early detection (15%) demonstrate just how effective these devices can be in promoting changes in the quality of care. Other areas that need improvement include accessing services (10%), providing personal treatment plans (5%), preventing complications (5%), and increasing patient involvement in care (5%). These effects can be pooled into increasing patient-centered care delivery.

Table 4. Benefits of Wearable Health Devices with Corresponding Percentages

Benefit	Percentage
Reduced Hospital Readmissions	30
Cost Savings	25
Enhanced Patient Outcomes	20
Real-Time Monitoring and Early Detection	15
Improved Access to Healthcare	10
Personalized Treatment Plans	5
Prevention of Complications	5
Better Patient Engagement	5

Figure 4. Distribution of Key Benefits of Wearable Health Devices

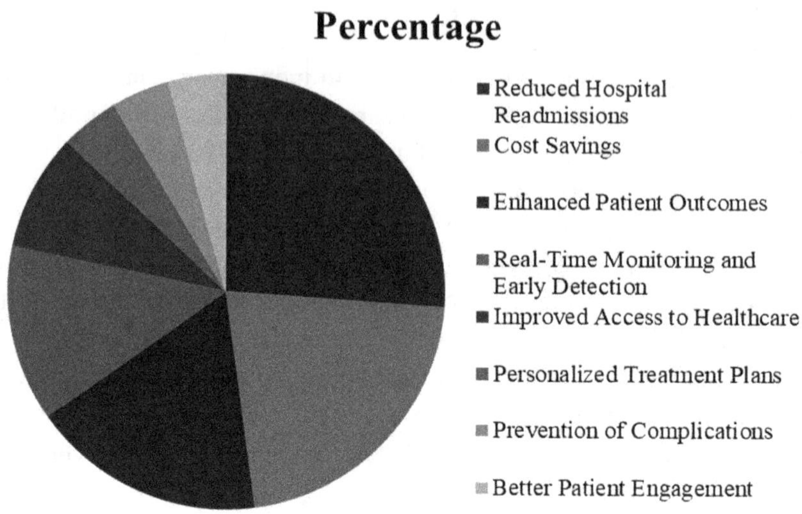

Figure 4 represents the sum total of all the aforementioned benefits graphically in the form of a pie chart that actually depicts and indicates the benefits of wearable health devices as a whole. The maximum pie-slice display refers to reduced hospital readmissions at 30 percent, revealing the true significance attached to the reduced hospital admissions due to the use of wearable health devices. The cost savings on hospital admission accounts for 25% while the rest contributes to enhanced patient outcomes with a 20% claim, real-time monitoring with early detection at 15%, and improved management and interventions. These are some of the small-sized yet important benefits such as improved access to health care by 10%, personalized treatment plans of about 5 percent, prevention of complications by about 5 percent, and engagement of patients being 5 percent to show the variety of benefits attracted by wearable technology in the modern health setting.

5.2 Cost-Effectiveness for Healthcare Providers

The remote health monitoring systems are nearly heaven to the health costs of the health care providers as they are able to save by reducing operational costs and optimizing resource allocation. Continuous monitoring of patients makes it easy for health professionals to focus on severe cases, as well as avoid unnecessary hospital visits and admissions. For instance, the appointments with stable patients can be spanned while focusing on those whose health changes are alarming.

It is a great way to improve cost-effectiveness as telemedicine and virtual consultation decrease the requirement for actual infrastructure and medical staff on-site. It also provides preventive care, which is less costly than treating extended medical conditions (Niu et al., 2022). Such problems can be prevented through early detection of health issues, which would save them from complications in the future and reduce the cost incurred by healthcare systems. For example, irregular heart rhythms can be detected early and treated, thereby preventing expensive hospitalizations for emergency cases of cardiac problems. Such systems have also made healthcare services scalable; that is, a health provider can reach more people without much increase in costs. Automating normal functions such as data collection and analysis permits healthcare workers to concentrate on other complex clinical responsibilities. Well, the healthcare industry is going to save a lot of their money towards better quality health services in the near future as it is embracing this remote health monitoring.

5.3 Reduced Hospital Readmissions

Readmissions are one of the difficulties that healthcare services have because they leverage a lot of resources while failing to achieve satisfaction from patients hence the involvement of continuous remote health monitoring systems that can allow patients to be monitored outside of the hospitals. Patients recovering from surgery or suffering from any chronic illness can now be closely monitored at home, with the realization of early recognition and intervention in any pregnant complications. For instance, remote tracking of wounds of post-surgical patients can alert patients about an impending infection.

Healthcare providers have also been made to keep close contact with patients through teleconsultations and routine reviews of their data. There are also automated alerts for anomalies, such as high blood pressure or irregular heart rate, flagged to inform medical teams about any urgent intervention. This reduction of deaths practically reduces the chances of readmissions because it enhances health outcomes for patients besides using up several resources by readmitting them.

Not only do patients benefit when there are fewer readmissions, but so also healthcare institutions stand to reap in terms of avoiding penalties associated with high readmission rates under specific regulatory frameworks. It places hospitals in a better position to show continuity of care and satisfaction to patients with these online monitoring systems. With continuous advancements in these systems, the role they play in the reduction of readmissions will just gain more prominence, thereby developing a more sustainable environment for healthcare.

Table 5 represents different potential opportunities with respect to remote health monitoring technologies as well as their effects. The highest opportunity is possibly for improved patient engagement, accessed through adherence improvement to treatment plans and proactive health management action. Improved diagnostics far lead to the provision of early detection and intervention of medical conditions and, thus, complication prevention. Personalized treatment plans are tailor-made care and therefore individualized outcomes in health. They include easy remote visits to healthcare professionals, regardless of geographical limitations, reduced hospital visits, and lower costs. Real-time monitoring provides continuous monitoring of vital signs, thus enabling timely action in case of health change. The above opportunities highlighted in this table bear institute-the revolution from remote health monitors in current health services delivery.

Table 5. Opportunities and Their Impact in Remote Health Monitoring

Opportunity	Impact	Description
Enhanced Patient Engagement	Improved adherence to treatment plans and regular monitoring.	Patients can actively participate in their health management through mobile apps and wearable devices, leading to better outcomes.
Real-Time Health Monitoring	Early detection of health issues and immediate response.	Enables timely intervention for conditions like hypertension, diabetes, and heart diseases.
Cost Savings	Reduced hospital readmissions and emergency visits.	Cuts down on healthcare costs by minimizing the need for frequent doctor visits and hospitalization.
Better Health Outcomes	More personalized care through detailed patient data analysis.	Tailored treatment plans based on real-time data, leading to better health management and recovery.
Improved Diagnostics	Early identification and intervention of diseases.	Utilizes data from remote monitoring devices to detect anomalies and prevent serious health issues.

6. CHALLENGES IN IMPLEMENTATION

6.1 Data Security and Privacy Concerns

The adoption of health monitoring systems at a distance raises valid safety issues concerning data and privacy of the patient. They collect sensitive health information, which now is very much open to cyber-intrusion. Hacking patient data and illegally substituting them might include identity theft and fraud, as well as manipulative health records (Ianculescu et al., 2020). To prevent these security issues, there would be robust encryption protocols, with multi-factor verification processes, to protect the data while in their transmission and storage. Strict control measures are instituted under authorities such as HIPAA-the Health Insurance Portability and Accountability Act, which is applicable in the United States, and Europe under the General Data Protection Regulation- for full protection of patient information. Compliance with these standards eases the process of ensuring that the institution practices data privacy and data security best standards.

Figure 5. Venn Diagram of Overlapping Issues in Remote Health Monitoring

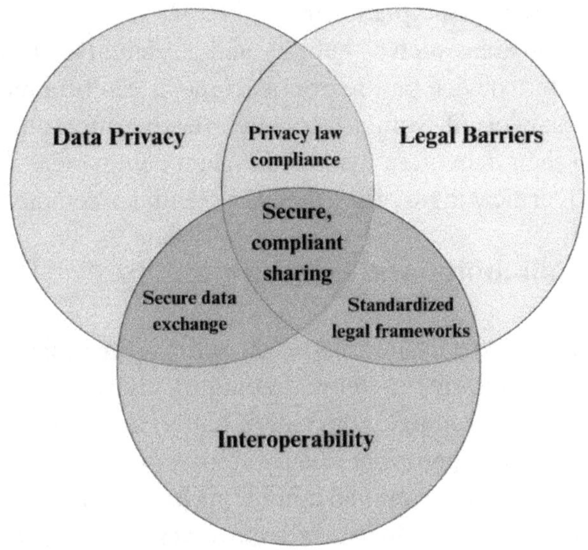

Figure 5 shows the losing components that can be related to remote health monitoring-it shows data privacy, legal barriers, and interoperability. The circle bears the intersection of the overlapping circles marking the key concerns that create a mesh of patient consent, data security regulations, and cross-system compatibility. Each circle represents a separate issue-challenges in bringing forth issues such as privacy of data where the main concern is ensuring patient data protection, legal barriers defined in terms of regulatory compliance for health, and interoperability denoting needs for devices and platforms to freely transmit and receive information. The area showing the circle overlap notes the interrelation between the problems, thus producing a very complicated environment concerning remote health management that will need delicate solutions put together for coordination.

Despite the security, issues abound primarily when it comes to integrating IoT devices with cloud-based platforms. Such collaborative systems usually encompass many stakeholders in the integration efforts, which further complicates data flow security. New solutions such as blockchain technology have bright prospects concerning contributing to data integrity and transparency. A balance between the usability and security of the remote monitoring systems is, and will remain a significant priority.

6.2 Regulatory and Legal Barriers

There are issues related to complex regulatory and legal system which hamper the implementation of remote health monitoring systems. These systems are normally at the crossroad of health and technology systems and are subjected to compliance with laws on medical devices and data privacy, as well as telemedicine practice. The diverse regulations at different levels then further complicate the global adoption of such technologies. Key among these challenges lies in the classification of remote monitoring devices as medical devices that generally require such devices to pass through more tests and certification procedures than are applied to other categories. Delayed entry into the market as well as restricted innovation are consequences of not having a clear and coherent standard for approving the devices. Rules about telemedicine also vary significantly affecting even the cross-border deployment of remote monitoring systems. For instance, some countries cut off cross-border flows of data and, thus, limit the scalable capacity of cloud-based platforms.

Legal challenges also arise in areas such as liability and consent. Determining who may be deemed liable during an investigation into device failure or misdiagnosis can become very complicated, particularly if there are many parties involved. Similarly, communicative efforts to ensure patients understand the collection and sharing of their data often make the system deployment suspend. Overcoming these regulatory and legal barriers is critical to revealing the full potential of remote health monitoring systems.

6.3 Technical Issues: Reliability and Interoperability

Apart from this, mismatches in device configuration and malfunctions can significantly affect the effectiveness of remote health monitoring systems, leading to failure to meet patient's needs in proper time. Present side effects of malfunctioning of devices or batteries or inaccurate functioning of sensors lead to loss of quality and eventually inappropriate diagnosis or slow intervention with treatment. Assuring consistent performance under various operational conditions is a critical requirement for these systems.

The interoperability problem remains, since it often involves devices and application software from different vendors. Even a slight misalignment in data formats or communication protocols can wreck havoc to the information flow across the very system setup. For instance, an end-user possibly cannot get measurement from his/her handheld device that may sync seamlessly with that of his/her healthcare provider. To overcome these problems, important standardization processes are happening because common protocols can then be used to communicate and share data with the devices. Examples include FHIR (Fast Healthcare Interoperability Resources), which encourage interoperability between systems. The use of emerging artificial intelligence and machine learning would also altogether help in improving data accuracy because noise and anomaly are filtered out from sensor readings. All these hurdles must be crossed so that the remote health monitoring architecture meets most and reliable and uninterrupted care.

7. CASE STUDIES AND REAL-WORLD APPLICATIONS

7.1 Remote Health Monitoring in Rural Areas

In fact, a lot of remote medical monitoring systems are very helpful in rural and underprivileged countries. These would be some of the most important barriers to accessing health care services (Banbury et al., 2014). There is an acute shortage of medically trained personnel; infrastructure is poor; and long distances can require a patient hours or even days of travel before reaching a doctor. Now with such technology, no one should travel thousands of miles to receive treatment for their ailments (Nedungadi et al., 2018). For instance, IoTs can provide equipment that's handy when individuals need to monitor their vital signs and share that information in real-time with their networks of healthcare providers for early detection of possible health problems.

Through telemedicine, such systems complement each other to give virtual appointments and consultations even for patients. This brings some burden-off to patients and health care workers. This, for agency in rural areas, can provide a direct link to an urban center specialist for advice, diagnosis, or even prescriptions. Such a structure of remote monitoring and telemedicine ensures that the quality of deliverance of care in rural areas is not that different from that in urban settings (Minoi & Yeo, 2014). Sometimes, community health workers may be used to get portable monitoring devices to collect data from remote field locations and relay the information he gathered to a health facility.

Remote health monitoring technologies touch more areas than just those that directly translate into an improvement in health outcomes for patients. The cost of providing healthcare in rural areas is expected to drop by remote systems that would decrease physical visits. Hence, investment is increasingly attracting governments and NGOs into these portfolios to bridge equality in improving healthcare access and limiting disparity between urban and rural populations. Remote health monitoring systems look forward to establishing an even more inclusive and comprehensive health system, especially covering areas that currently exist in isolation.

7.2 Success Stories in Chronic Disease Care

Chronic ailments like diabetes, mild to severe hypertension, and cardiac problems require close monitoring and management for the prevention of complications. Remote health monitoring systems are proven methods of improving the quality of life in patients who have such conditions. For example, the patients can use glucose monitoring devices connected to smartphone apps for blood glucose level monitoring, abnormal readings alarms, and medication changes or diet adjustment.

One interesting application of remote monitoring technologies was when it started being heightened with regard to the management of hypertensive patients. People can now be seen wearing blood pressure monitors, and the data they take in are sent straight to their health practitioner, who in response gives personalized advice. In this way, timely intervention reduces the prevalence of stroke or heart failure. The same principle applies to cardiac monitoring devices, which have been put into practice in remote detection of arrhythmias and other heart-related issues that warrant hospitalization during emergencies. An example illustrating technology success with the hospitals has been given by several organizations that provide health care. It included distance monitoring of chronic obstructive pulmonary disease (COPD) patients, which prevented them from having to visit the hospital and positively influenced the respiratory health of patients. These successes illustrate how remote monitoring of healthcare systems has an impact for chronic conditions on improving care. They demonstrate how remote monitoring systems can be successfully used: yielding healthier outcomes in a cost-efficient manner.

8. FUTURE TRENDS IN REMOTE HEALTH MONITORING

8.1 AI-Powered Predictive Monitoring

Artificial Intelligence (AI) has been an important factor in remote health monitoring, especially in the way it has enabled a predictive capacity level of health issues. The predictive monitoring aspect uses an AI algorithm capable of studying a huge number of health data especially from IoT wearables and electronic health records. With the ability to observe patterns and anomalies, such AI algorithms make predictions regarding events such as heart attacks or diabetic crises that may occur in a certain time period, promising early intervention.

Most of the applications of predictive monitoring are in the arena of chronic disease management. In fact, such models powered by AI can detect minute changes in a patient that a human would not be able to observe before. An early sign of fluid retention might be detected through its AI-based monitoring quite early, for instance, in a patient with heart failure; this could then be used to adjust treatment guidelines quickly. In this sense, fewer admissions to hospitals are achieved while optimizing patient outcomes. Another domain where monitoring by AI features concerns patients with mental health disorders, in which analysis through algorithms is used on speech patterns, activities, and sleeping data to draw indications of early signs of depression and anxiety. And as these systems further advance, it will radically alter how health care is delivered in the near future through an emphasis on preventive management rather than reactive care with applications currently using these systems coupled to remote health monitoring technologies.

8.2 Blockchain for Secure Data Sharing

Blockchain technology has entirely changed how secure data are shared for remote patient monitoring. This decentralized, immutable ledger grants sensitive health data a level of security and transparency that traditional data-sharing methods, by their very nature, cannot provide and are subject to breaches, unauthorized access, and sometimes outright tampering. Blockchain could address all these problems by providing end-to-end encryption and secure authentication protocols, where every transaction or data exchange is dubbed as a block in the chain that is almost impossible to modify. This guarantees that the entire network must reach a mutual agreement before that happens. Thus, blockchain has proven to be an outstanding solution in sharing health data among many players such as the patient, hospitals, and insurers.

This is because, with the advent of blockchain technology, patients will now have the ability to access their health data and decide who else can have access to that data, thereby protecting their privacy. Their modalities of sharing health-related data become facilitated with smart contracts, which are part and parcel of the blockchain. Smart contracts enable agreements set out for the sharing of health data without third parties, thus cutting down operational costs.

It also promotes interconnectedness between diverse health monitoring systems-kinds of devices and platforms that generally work alone and cannot share data with each other. Fill this gap with the universal, transparent architectures of systems such as blockchain and allow real-time data exchange between their different applications. Movement of heart rates from wearable devices to hospitals or research institutions can hence be improved by methods deriving from diagnostics accuracy and medical innovation. The more health care-apt and theoretically strong it becomes, the more it will abolish longstanding busy troubles related to health data sharing.

8.3 Advances in Wearable Technologies

Wearable devices are at the vanguard of innovation in telehealth with real-time face-to-face monitoring during patient health care and providing proactive care. Modern wearables have far surpassed simple activity tracking via advanced sensors and algorithms that measure critical health parameters, including blood oxygen levels, electrocardiograms (ECG), and even stress levels. Smartwatches, fitness bands, biosensors will increasingly become vital tools for patients and healthcare providers as they allow continuous monitoring without having to go through hospital visits. Thus, it is revolutionizing preventive care by flagging possible health issues before they blossom full-blown. One serious development in wearable technology is an artificial intelligence implementation in wearables. For instance, intelligent wearables employ real-time data analysis to derive personalized health recommendations for the users. An AI-based wearable gadget can sense an irregular heart rhythm and notify the user to consult a doctor. AI-enabled glucose monitors can predict blood sugar trends and even give food or medicine prescriptions. These smart specks offer a richly improved experience for the end-user as they result in a more positive outcome regarding health through their timely interventions.

Little by little, the other glaring trend is downsizing and multi-functionality of wearables. Manufacturers are already developing smaller, lighter devices that can integrate multi-functional capabilities for monitoring health in a single device. For example, now there are wearables that can do heart rate monitoring and at the same time sleep tracking with the measurement of hydration levels in one miniature device. Further battery innovations mean that these devices will be capable of going long periods without frequent recharging for greater user comfort. Advanced wearable technologies will probably influence consumer-oriented healthcare by directly linking patients and providers and lead to a more connected and informed health care ecosystem.

CONCLUSION

They are transforming into some of the most significant revolutions in the healthcare scenario, offering novel approaches toward some of the most important issues today-the very healthcare systems. This is one area where the most admirable powers of the latest and cutting-edge technologies, such as IoT, AI, and advanced wearable devices, provide patients and health professionals, tools to implement real-time continuous health management systems. It has once again proved its potential by showing a significant lot against chronic disease care or the rural accessibility of healthcare. Adverse elements for the post-adoption use of remote health monitoring systems: data security, regulatory compliance, and technical reliability are not insignificant startups problems. It is going to take the cooperation of technical developers with the providers and the policy makers in order to protect patient privacy and facilitate interoperability across devices and platforms. Such kind of focused investment in R&D would also be needed for making such systems more affordable, accurate, and user-friendly.

Opportunities for remote health monitoring will continue to grow in breadth, as should the march of innovations such as AI and blockchain. All of these should provide greater efficiency, reliability, security, and scalability to such systems. Opening new avenues and overcoming barriers is the way to a better future for the health system, and its transformation will occur, as the system becomes even more inclusive, patient-centric, and proactive in care: Its embrace of high technology. Indeed, remote health monitoring systems transcend technological innovations- it is a leap toward a healthier world.

REFERENCES

Agali, K., Masrom, M., Abdul Rahim, F., & Yahya, Y. (2024). IoT-based remote monitoring system: A new era for patient engagement. *Healthcare Technology Letters, 11*(6), 437–446. DOI: 10.1049/htl2.12089 PMID: 39720747

Ahmed, S. S. T., Thanuja, K., Guptha, N. S., & Narasimha, S. (2016, January). Telemedicine approach for remote patient monitoring system using smart phones with an economical hardware kit. In 2016 international conference on computing technologies and intelligent data engineering (ICCTIDE'16) (pp. 1-4). IEEE.

Albahri, O. S., Zaidan, A. A., Zaidan, B. B., Hashim, M., Albahri, A. S., & Alsalem, M. A. (2018). Real-time remote health-monitoring Systems in a Medical Centre: A review of the provision of healthcare services-based body sensor information, open challenges and methodological aspects. *Journal of Medical Systems, 42*(9), 1–47. DOI: 10.1007/s10916-018-1006-6 PMID: 30043085

Alshamrani, M. (2022). IoT and artificial intelligence implementations for remote healthcare monitoring systems: A survey. *Journal of King Saud University. Computer and Information Sciences, 34*(8), 4687–4701. DOI: 10.1016/j.jksuci.2021.06.005

Antevski, K., Girletti, L., Bernardos, C. J., de la Oliva, A., Baranda, J., & Mangues-Bafalluy, J. (2021). A 5G-based eHealth monitoring and emergency response system: Experience and lessons learned. *IEEE Access : Practical Innovations, Open Solutions, 9*, 131420–131429. DOI: 10.1109/ACCESS.2021.3114593

Atreja, A., Francis, S., Kurra, S., & Kabra, R. (2019). Digital medicine and evolution of remote patient monitoring in cardiac electrophysiology: A state-of-the-art perspective. *Current Treatment Options in Cardiovascular Medicine, 21*(12), 1–10. DOI: 10.1007/s11936-019-0787-3 PMID: 31832887

Baig, M. M., & Gholamhosseini, H. (2013). Smart health monitoring systems: An overview of design and modeling. *Journal of Medical Systems, 37*(2), 1–14. DOI: 10.1007/s10916-012-9898-z PMID: 23321968

Banbury, A., Roots, A., & Nancarrow, S. (2014). Rapid review of applications of e-health and remote monitoring for rural residents. *The Australian Journal of Rural Health, 22*(5), 211–222. DOI: 10.1111/ajr.12127 PMID: 25303412

Bansal, A., Kumar, S., Bajpai, A., Tiwari, V. N., Nayak, M., Venkatesan, S., & Narayanan, R. (2015). Remote health monitoring system for detecting cardiac disorders. *IET Systems Biology, 9*(6), 309–314. DOI: 10.1049/iet-syb.2015.0012 PMID: 26577166

Benhaddou, D., Balakrishnan, M., & Yuan, X. (2008, April). Remote healthcare monitoring system architecture using sensor networks. In 2008 IEEE Region 5 Conference (pp. 1-6). IEEE.

Castillejo, P., Martinez, J. F., Rodriguez-Molina, J., & Cuerva, A. (2013). Integration of wearable devices in a wireless sensor network for an E-health application. *IEEE Wireless Communications, 20*(4), 38–49. DOI: 10.1109/MWC.2013.6590049

Chronaki, C. E., & Vardas, P. (2013). Remote monitoring costs, benefits, and reimbursement: A European perspective. *Europace : European Pacing, Arrhythmias, and Cardiac Electrophysiology : Journal of the Working Groups on Cardiac Pacing, Arrhythmias, and Cardiac Cellular Electrophysiology of the European Society of Cardiology, 15*(suppl_1), i59–i64. DOI: 10.1093/europace/eut110 PMID: 23737233

Farias, F. A. C. D., Dagostini, C. M., Bicca, Y. D. A., Falavigna, V. F., & Falavigna, A. (2020). Remote patient monitoring: A systematic review. *Telemedicine Journal and e-Health, 26*(5), 576–583. DOI: 10.1089/tmj.2019.0066 PMID: 31314689

Fotouhi, H., Causevic, A., Lundqvist, K., & Björkman, M. (2016, June). Communication and Security in Health Monitoring Systems--A Review. In 2016 IEEE 40th annual computer software and applications conference (COMPSAC) (Vol. 1, pp. 545-554). IEEE.

Ghosh, A. M., Halder, D., & Hossain, S. A. (2016, May). Remote health monitoring system through IoT. In 2016 5th International Conference on Informatics, Electronics and Vision (ICIEV) (pp. 921-926). IEEE.

Guntur, S. R., Gorrepati, R. R., & Dirisala, V. R. (2018). Internet of Medical things: Remote healthcare and health monitoring perspective. In *Medical big data and internet of medical things* (pp. 271–297). CRC Press. DOI: 10.1201/9781351030380-11

Ianculescu, M., Coardo , D., Bica, O., & Vevera, V. (2020, October). Security and privacy risks for remote healthcare monitoring systems. In 2020 International Conference on e-Health and Bioengineering (EHB) (pp. 1-4). IEEE. DOI: 10.1109/EHB50910.2020.9280103

Khoi, N. M., Saguna, S., Mitra, K., & Åhlund, C. (2015, October). IReHMo: An efficient IoT-based remote health monitoring system for smart regions. In 2015 17th international conference on e-health networking, application & services (HealthCom) (pp. 563-568). IEEE.

Krapivin, V., & Shutko, A. M. (2012). *Information technologies for remote monitoring of the environment*. Springer Science & Business Media. DOI: 10.1007/978-3-642-20567-5

Kunbi, A., Silver Cross, D. P., & Oladele, S. (2024). Increased Patient Engagement with Wireless Monitoring Systems.

Landolina, M., Perego, G. B., Lunati, M., Curnis, A., Guenzati, G., Vicentini, A., Parati, G., Borghi, G., Zanaboni, P., Valsecchi, S., & Marzegalli, M. (2012). Remote monitoring reduces healthcare use and improves quality of care in heart failure patients with implantable defibrillators: The evolution of management strategies of heart failure patients with implantable defibrillators (EVOLVO) study. *Circulation, 125*(24), 2985–2992. DOI: 10.1161/CIRCULATIONAHA.111.088971 PMID: 22626743

Lightsey, H. M.IV, Yeung, C. M., Samartzis, D., & Makhni, M. C. (2021). The past, present, and future of remote patient monitoring in spine care: An overview. *European Spine Journal : Official Publication of the European Spine Society, the European Spinal Deformity Society, and the European Section of the Cervical Spine Research Society, 30*(8), 2102–2108. DOI: 10.1007/s00586-021-06921-1 PMID: 34241698

Loupian, E. A., Bourtsev, M. A., Proshin, A. A., & Kobets, D. A. (2018). Evolution of remote monitoring information systems development concepts. Sovremennye problemy distantsionnogo zondirovaniya Zemli iz kosmosa, 15(3), 53-66.

Magrupov, T. M., Yuldashev, Z. M., & Abdihalikov, S. P. (2021). A Medical Hardware-Software System for Remote Monitoring of Heart Diseases., 24(2), 78-86.

Majumder, S., Mondal, T., & Deen, M. J. (2017). Wearable sensors for remote health monitoring. *Sensors (Basel)*, *17*(1), 130. DOI: 10.3390/s17010130 PMID: 28085085

Minoi, J. L., & Yeo, A. W. (2014, December). Remote health monitoring system in a rural population: Challenges and opportunities. In *2014 IEEE Conference on Biomedical Engineering and Sciences (IECBES)* (pp. 895-900). IEEE. DOI: 10.1109/IECBES.2014.7047641

Mohammed, K. I., Zaidan, A. A., Zaidan, B. B., Albahri, O. S., Alsalem, M. A., Albahri, A. S., Hadi, A., & Hashim, M. (2019). Real-time remote-health monitoring systems: A review on patients prioritisation for multiple-chronic diseases, taxonomy analysis, concerns and solution procedure. *Journal of Medical Systems*, *43*(7), 1–21. DOI: 10.1007/s10916-019-1362-x PMID: 31187288

Monika Singh, T., Kishor Kumar Reddy, C., Ramana Murthy, B. V., Nag, A., & Doss, S. (2025). AI and Education: Bridging the Gap to Personalized, Efficient, and Accessible Learning. In M. Ouaissa, M. Ouaissa, H. Lamaazi, M. El Hamlaoui, & K. Reddy C. (Eds.), Internet of Behavior-Based Computational Intelligence for Smart Education Systems (pp. 131-160). IGI Global. DOI: 10.4018/979-8-3693-8151-9.ch005

Naddeo, S., Verde, L., Forastiere, M., De Pietro, G., & Sannino, G. (2017, February). A real-time m-health monitoring system: An integrated solution combining the use of several wearable sensors and mobile devices. In Special Session on Smart Medical Devices-From Lab to Clinical Practice (Vol. 6, pp. 545-552). SciTePress.

Nedungadi, P., Jayakumar, A., & Raman, R. (2018). Personalized health monitoring system for managing well-being in rural areas. *Journal of Medical Systems*, *42*(1), 1–11. DOI: 10.1007/s10916-017-0854-9 PMID: 29242996

Ng, M., Borst, E., Garrity, A., Hirschfeld, E., & Lee, J. (2020). Evolution of do-it-yourself remote monitoring technology for type 1 diabetes. *Journal of Diabetes Science and Technology*, *14*(5), 854–859. DOI: 10.1177/1932296819895537 PMID: 31893941

Niu, B., Mukhtarova, N., Alagoz, O., & Hoppe, K. (2022). Cost-effectiveness of telehealth with remote patient monitoring for postpartum hypertension. *The Journal of Maternal-Fetal & Neonatal Medicine*, *35*(25), 7555–7561. DOI: 10.1080/14767058.2021.1956456 PMID: 34470135

Nurshod, A., Khujamatov, K., & Lazarev, A. (2021, November). Remote monitoring system architectures in healthcare. In 2021 International Conference on Information Science and Communications Technologies (ICISCT) (pp. 01-05). IEEE. DOI: 10.1109/ICISCT52966.2021.9670405

Peyroteo, M., Ferreira, I. A., Elvas, L. B., Ferreira, J. C., & Lapão, L. V. (2021). Remote monitoring systems for patients with chronic diseases in primary health care: Systematic review. *JMIR mHealth and uHealth*, *9*(12), e28285. DOI: 10.2196/28285 PMID: 34932000

Priya, B., Rajendran, S., Bala, R., & Gobbi, R. (2009, July). Remote wireless health monitoring systems. In 2009 Innovative Technologies in Intelligent Systems and Industrial Applications (pp. 383-388). IEEE

Reddy, C. K. K. (2023). An Efficient Early Diagnosis and Healthcare Monitoring System for Mental Disorders Using Machine Learning. In *Sustainable Science and Intelligent Technologies for Societal Development* (pp. 22–43). IGI Global.

Reddy, C. K. K., & Satvika, P. (2023). An Efficient Early Diagnosis and Healthcare Monitoring System for Mental Disorder using Machine learning Approach.

Safavi, K. C., Driscoll, W., & Wiener-Kronish, J. P. (2019). Remote surveillance technologies: Realizing the aim of right patient, right data, right time. *Anesthesia and Analgesia*, *129*(3), 726–734. DOI: 10.1213/ANE.0000000000003948 PMID: 31425213

Salah, W. A., & Zneid, B. A. (2019). Evolution of microcontroller-based remote monitoring system applications. *International Journal of Electrical and Computer Engineering*, *9*(4), 2354. DOI: 10.11591/ijece.v9i4.pp2354-2364

Sathya, D., & Ganesh Kumar, P. (2017). Secured remote health monitoring system. *Healthcare Technology Letters*, *4*(6), 228–232. DOI: 10.1049/htl.2017.0033 PMID: 29383257

Singh, T. M., Reddy, C. K. K., & Lippert, K. (2024). Advancing Human-Centric Solutions: The Future Trajectory of Soft Computing in Modern Society. In Kumar, N., Pal, S., Agarwal, P., Rosak-Szyrocka, J., & Jain, V. (Eds.), *Human-Machine Collaboration and Emotional Intelligence in Industry 5.0* (pp. 1–18). IGI Global., DOI: 10.4018/979-8-3693-6806-0.ch001

Sivani, T., & Mishra, S. (2022). Wearable devices: evolution and usage in remote patient monitoring system. In *Connected e-Health: Integrated IoT and Cloud Computing* (pp. 311–332). Springer International Publishing. DOI: 10.1007/978-3-030-97929-4_14

Swaroop, K. N., Chandu, K., Gorrepotu, R., & Deb, S. (2019). A health monitoring system for vital signs using IoT. *Internet of Things : Engineering Cyber Physical Human Systems*, *5*, 116–129. DOI: 10.1016/j.iot.2019.01.004

Verma, N., Singh, S., & Prasad, D. (2022). A review on existing IoT architecture and communication protocols used in healthcare monitoring system. Journal of The Institution of Engineers (India): Series B, 103(1), 245-257.

Vijayan, V., Connolly, J. P., Condell, J., McKelvey, N., & Gardiner, P. (2021). Review of wearable devices and data collection considerations for connected health. *Sensors (Basel)*, *21*(16), 5589. DOI: 10.3390/s21165589 PMID: 34451032

Xu, B., Xu, L., Cai, H., Jiang, L., Luo, Y., & Gu, Y. (2017). The design of an m-Health monitoring system based on a cloud computing platform. *Enterprise Information Systems*, *11*(1), 17–36. DOI: 10.1080/17517575.2015.1053416

Zhang, J., Yang, M., Ge, Y., Ivers, R., Webster, R., & Tian, M. (2022). The role of digital health for post-surgery care of older patients with hip fracture: A scoping review. *International Journal of Medical Informatics*, *160*, 104709. DOI: 10.1016/j.ijmedinf.2022.104709 PMID: 35144101

Zhang, W., Thurow, K., & Stoll, R. (2014). A knowledge-based telemonitoring platform for application in remote healthcare. *International Journal of Computers, Communications & Control*, *9*(5), 644–654. DOI: 10.15837/ijccc.2014.5.661

Zhang, Y., Zheng, X. T., Zhang, X., Pan, J., & Thean, A. V. Y. (2024). Hybrid integration of wearable devices for physiological monitoring. *Chemical Reviews*, *124*(18), 10386–10434. DOI: 10.1021/acs.chemrev.3c00471 PMID: 39189683

Chapter 15

Advancing Smart Healthcare Through 5G and Innovative Technologies

P. Ashok
https://orcid.org/0000-0002-5859-6041
Symbiosis Institute of Digital and Telecom Management, India

A. Pon Bharati
https://orcid.org/0000-0003-1217-449X
Amrita College of Engineering and Technology, India

A. Rajasekar
Sri Sairam Institute of Technology, India

D. Vedha Vinodha
https://orcid.org/0000-0001-9753-8189
JCT College of Engineering and Technology, India

T. Cowsalya
Nehru Institute of Engineering and Technology, India

Ravi Gorli
https://orcid.org/0000-0002-4381-3250
GITAM University, India

K. S. Shreenidhi
https://orcid.org/0000-0002-6844-0454
Rajalakshmi Engineering College, India

Harishchander Anandaram
https://orcid.org/0000-0003-2993-5304
Amrita Vishwa Vidyapeetam, India

Khushal Vashishth
Symbiosis Institute of Digital and Telecom Management, India

ABSTRACT

The healthcare industry is currently experiencing a significant and groundbreaking change as a result of the integration of fifth-generation (5G) mobile communication technologies, Artificial Intelligence (AI), Machine Learning, Deep Learning, and Internet of Things (IoT). This research paper explores the complex interaction of various technologies, with a specific focus on the crucial role of 5G in enabling and improving healthcare applications. The study examines the potential of 5G-enabled IoT technologies in the field of smart healthcare, focusing on their ability to bring about significant changes in terms of network performance, device density, energy efficiency, and security. The paper addresses necessary prerequisites for the effective implementation of 5G scenarios in healthcare settings as it evolves. The technical requirements, analyzed key performance indicators (KPIs), and deployment circumstances

DOI: 10.4018/979-8-3373-1022-0.ch015

together provide a roadmap for the future development and integration of advanced healthcare solutions that utilize the latest technology breakthroughs.

INTRODUCTION

The advent of 5G mobile communication technology heralds a new era in healthcare delivery, leveraging enhanced communication capabilities. 5G brings forth attributes like very-low latency, higher transfer speed, dependability, massive device connection and increased network availability, paving the way for innovative healthcare applications. The versatility of 5G is evident in wearable device scenarios, such as service robotics for assisted living, remote robotic surgery, diagnostic and telephonic consultation, in-ambulance care facilitated by distant physicians, remote diagnosis/teleconsultation, wearable device applications, and medical big data management as in Fig. 1.

Figure 1. 5G Based Latest Technologies

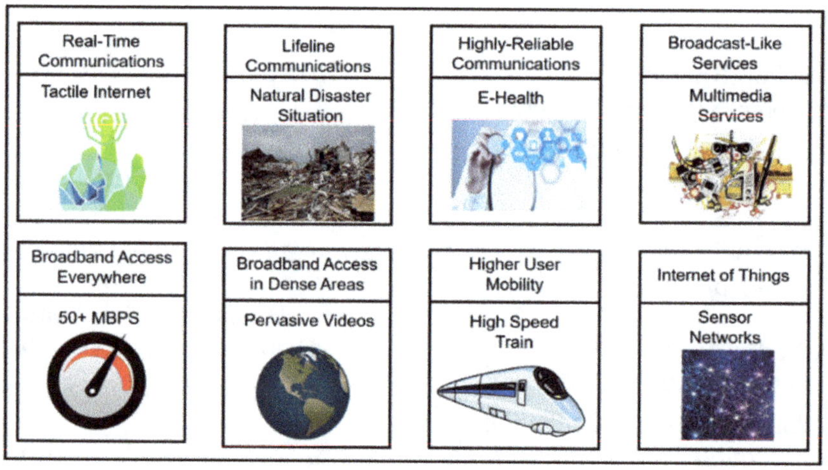

Using 5G technology in healthcare will improve service delivery and patient care. This study explores how 5G's ultra-low latency, increased mobile broadband, and large machine-type communications boost smart healthcare systems. 5G networks enable real-time remote patient monitoring, high-definition telemedicine, and seamless IoMT device integration by analysing current implementations and theoretical frameworks. AI-powered medical imaging and fast transfer of enormous medical files improve diagnosis accuracy due to the technology's capacity to manage vast volumes of data. 5G's network slicing prioritizes important medical services, assuring emergency communication. The report also discusses how 5G provides low latency and great dependability for precise control in remote robotic surgical systems. Implementation issues including infrastructure and cybersecurity are addressed. The results indicate that 5G technology is essential for the future generation of healthcare services, possibly lowering prices and boosting quality and accessibility in urban and rural areas. 6G technology will transform smart healthcare systems based on current research and theoretical estimates. Sub-millimeter waves, terahertz communications, and quantum networking in 6G will improve medical connection and data processing.

6G's predicted peak speeds of 1 Tbps and near-zero latency might allow new healthcare applications including holographic medical imaging, brain-computer interfaces for patient care, and cellular-level precision medicine. 6G's integration with AI and sensor technologies might enable molecular-level health monitoring and instantaneous data processing. The research predicts that 6G networks will allow enhanced biomedical digital twins, providing unparalleled predictive healthcare and individualized treatment planning. 6G's improved capabilities might allow seamless XR integration in surgery and medical training.

AI, ML, and Big Data Analytics have revolutionized smart healthcare systems by allowing data-driven decision-making and individualized patient care. This research analyses how these technologies synergistically improve healthcare delivery, concentrating on predictive diagnosis, treatment optimization, and operational efficiency. Deep learning algorithms used to large-scale electronic health records (EHR) may predict patient outcomes with extraordinary precision and detect health hazards before they appear clinically. The project emphasizes natural language processing for automated medical recording and real-time clinical decision assistance. Big data analytics helps healthcare professionals improve resource allocation, readmission rates, and preventative treatment by analysing several case studies. When trained on varied medical imaging datasets, ML models identify and classify diseases with expert accuracy. Additionally, healthcare data privacy, algorithmic bias, and system integration are addressed. The results show that AI, ML, and Big Data Analytics enhance clinical outcomes, lower healthcare costs, and make healthcare more accessible and equitable for various groups. Due to improved connection and real-time monitoring, IoT and Massive IoT (mIoT) technologies have transformed healthcare delivery. This study analyzes how IoT integration makes healthcare systems intelligent, responsive networks that monitor patients and intervene automatically. IoT-enabled medical devices and wearables provide proactive health monitoring and early intervention by collecting data on vital metrics, medication adherence, and lifestyle variables. mIoT designs link hundreds of medical sensors and equipment to form dense health monitoring networks in hospitals and distant care settings. IoT-driven healthcare solutions enhance patient outcomes via real-time anomaly detection, automated emergency response systems, and precision medicine applications, according to systematic examination. IoT/mIoT integration lowers operating costs and improves healthcare accessibility and quality, according to implementation case studies. The results imply that IoT technologies are essential to building robust, scalable healthcare systems that can fulfil current healthcare delivery expectations and enable individualized patient care at unprecedented sizes.

LITERATURE REVIEW

This literature study emphasizes the diverse array of uses that 5G technology (Schaich et al., 2018; Hamm et al., 2020; Padmashree & Nayak, 2020; Gupta & Ghosh, 2019; Qureshi et al., 2020; Li, 2019)

can have in the healthcare industry, including fields such as big data (Yang et al., 2018; Thuemmler & Bai, 2017; Deloitte, 2015; Krasniqi et al., 2019; 3GPP, 2017; Ojaroudi Parchin et al., 2019), artificial intelligence (AI) (Eid et al., 2010; Marshall et al., 2008; NSF, 2016; Ojaroudiparchin et al., 2016; Alibakhshi-Kenari et al., 2016; Schaeffer et al., 2016), machine learning, and the Internet of Things (IoT) (Ahad et al., 2019; (Qi et al., 2017; Hartmann et al., 2019; Rohokale et al., 2011; Mutlag et al., 2019; Terkelsen et al., 2002). Rural healthcare issues make homecare for older persons and cross-sectoral integrated care for chronically sick and multimorbid patients complicated and expensive. Mobility, logistics, and other difficulties must be addressed. Therefore, new solutions throughout the whole healthcare value chain must be realized to offer patient-focused, value-based healthcare in the future. The project

5G4Healthcare evaluates the feasibility, potential, and constraints of 5G for rural healthcare efficiency and effectiveness improvements to provide suggestions and scalable solutions (Hamm et al., 2020). Despite intense efforts, providing healthcare to an elderly population remains difficult. Recent findings have highlighted worries about rising healthcare expenses, resource imbalance, ineffective healthcare system management, and uncomfortable medical experiences. To overcome these challenges, cutting-edge technologies like IoT, big data, artificial intelligence, and 5G wireless transmission technology are being developed to improve patient experience and healthcare service quality while lowering healthcare costs. In subtle ways, these new technologies are transforming healthcare. Although the technologies above are integrated, this analysis briefly examines 5G wireless transmission instances in healthcare. 5G technology availability issue is also discussed in detail (Li, 2019).

With the rise of the Internet, Internet of Things (IoT) is a growing study issue in several fields, particularly healthcare. With the rise of wearable gadgets and smartphones, the Internet of Things is transforming healthcare from a hub-based system to a personalized one. However, implementing advanced IoT technology in PHS remains challenging due to factors such as limited cost-effective and accurate smart medical sensors, unstandardized system architectures, heterogeneity of connected devices, multi-dimensional data, and high interoperability demands. A rigorous study of sophisticated IoT-enabled PHS can help comprehend its advancement. It will discuss IoT-enabled PHS research, essential enabling technologies, significant applications, and successful healthcare case studies, as well as future research trends and difficulties (Qi et al., 2017). The fast progress of computer and communication technology has made individualized healthcare monitoring popular. Expect new products and services to raise healthcare user expectations. Internet of Things brings the physical world closer to the Internet. From 6LoWPAN sensor nodes to the Internet online user interface, the system communicates via IP connection and the Internet. The Gateway algorithm multithreads medical signals to convert them to actual data, extract features, and display them wirelessly. Mobile and portable devices may access and see medical data via the server user interface. A ubiquitous system is studying ways to link Internet to products and people for health services (Chung et al., 2008; Castillejo et al., 2013; Espinoza et al., 2016; Kamal et al., 2020; Rasid et al., 2014).

By minimizing adverse events and hospital readmissions, big data may save health care expenditures. This research examined the rise of big data in the US health care market, assessed hospitals' abilities to exploit complicated information, and predicted their potential advantages if they succeed. The study found that hospitals anticipated cost reductions and business insight from big data analytics. Many hospitals have acknowledged problems in adopting big data, including lack of skills and analytics development costs. Many hospitals will need to hire big data analytics and integration experts. This research suggests that health care professionals will benefit greatly from big data technology acceptance, implementation, and use (Schaeffer et al., 2016). Internet bandwidth is crucial for fast, reliable data transmission. This study analyzes how 5G networks might change healthcare. 5G is expected to have 10 to 100 times more bandwidth than existing health care equipment. Faster internet speed, reduced latency, and larger capacity are projected to improve patient care and telemedicine internationally (Padmashree & Nayak, 2020). This inquiry is upon a deep analysis that predicts a significant change in healthcare (De Brouwer et al., 2018; Kim et al., 2020; Istepanian et al., 2011; Vankadara et al., 2024; Anand et al., 2023; Ravindranathan et al., 2024; Patil et al., 2024), stressing a move from the traditional doctor-controlled model to one that promotes greater patient autonomy and active engagement in the treatment process. The assessment emphasizes the exceptional ability of 5G to manage large amounts of data, which enables patients to establish individualized health ecosystems. The paper underscores the crucial importance of 5G's high reliability and little delay, and explains how these qualities enable patients to participate in secure communication inside their healthcare systems. 5G technology (Krasniqi et al., 2019; 3GPP, 2017; Ojaroudiparchin et al., 2016) enables immediate access to healthcare services, playing a crucial role in transforming the digital integration of healthcare. This fosters an atmosphere where patients actively participate in their own treatment. In addition, the literature analysis thoroughly examines the barriers that impede the full realization of 5G's promise in healthcare (Alibakhshi-Kenari et al., 2016; Ahad et al., 2019; Rasid et al., 2014). In addition to identifying the present obstacles, the analysis offers valuable recommendations for future advancements in 5G technology (Saxena et al., 2024; Sisodiya et al., 2024; Ahad et al., 2019). The literature study aims to offer a progressive perspective in order to surmount challenges and facilitate optimal utilization of 5G technology. This, in turn, will lead to a transformative shift in healthcare delivery that aligns with the evolving needs of patients and the broader healthcare landscape.

5G & Wireless Communication

The advent of the 5G mobile communication technology has ushered in a new era of possibilities, particularly in the realm of healthcare. The enhanced communication capabilities intrinsic to 5G, such as very-low latency, higher transfer speed, dependability, massive device connection and increased network availability hold significant promise for transforming healthcare delivery. Comparison between 4G and 5G technologies is illustrated in Table 1.

Table 1. Performance Comparison of 4G and 5G Technologies (Ahad et al., 2019)

Characteristics	Performance enhancement	
	4G	5G
Data Rate	0.01 - 1 Gbps	0.1 - 20 Gbps
Latency (Control plane)	100 ms	50 ms
Latency (User plane)	10 ms	1 ms
Mobility	Upto 350 km/h	Upto 500 km/h
Spectral efficiency	1.5	4.5
Energy efficiency	0.1 mJ per 100 bits	0.1 μJ per 100 bits
Device density	100k/km^2	1000K/km^2

In the context of healthcare, 5G's advanced features open up novel use cases and enhance existing healthcare scenarios. The technology enables smooth transmission and sharing of data, establishing the basis for novel healthcare applications. Some examples of these applications include wearable devices used in service robotics for assisted living, remote robotic surgery, diagnostic and telephonic consultations, in-ambulance care supplied by distant physicians, remote diagnosis/teleconsultation, and effective administration of medical big data. 5G technology possesses distinct attributes that are tailored to meet particular communication requirements in a wide range of healthcare applications. Collaboration among developers, network operators, and regulatory agencies is essential to ensure the successful adoption of healthcare solutions offered by 5G technology. Collaboration is crucial for effectively managing the unique standards and requirements of many healthcare applications, including wearable devices, in-ambulance therapy, and remote robotic surgery. The incorporation of 5G technology in healthcare extends beyond acute care situations as in Fig. 2. 5G-enabled smart healthcare devices offer real-time monitoring of vital signs and facilitate the use of sophisticated diagnostic tools.

Internet of Things (IoT)

The Internet of Things (IoT) is a revolutionary concept that includes a flexible framework spanning a wide range of intelligent, physical, and virtual things, each with unique identities. This network of networked devices signifies the advent of a new era of efficient and practical automation, where the processes of data gathering, tracking, and transmission effortlessly merge and make their way to either private or public clouds. The defining characteristic of the Internet of Things (IoT) is its innate ability to efficiently utilize energy, CPU, and memory resources as in Fig. 3. This makes it a remarkable technology with versatile applications. This innovative technology demonstrates its capabilities in a wide range of fields, including smart urban planning, control systems, retail, waste treatment, security, emergency services, and transportation logistics. The range of IoT goes beyond traditional applications, as it becomes a crucial factor in the upcoming revolution of healthcare delivery. Within the healthcare industry, the Internet of Things (IoT) (Yang et al., 2018; Deloitte, 2015; Rasid et al., 2014) serves as a powerful force driving innovation and offering new solutions that fundamentally transform the way patient care is delivered. Notable uses of this technology include tele-auscultation, which allows for remote aural examination, chronic disease management, which provides customized solutions for long-term health concerns, and remote health monitoring, which enables real-time surveillance of patients' vital signs. The diagnostic capabilities of IoT enhance its influence by enabling remote diagnostics and autonomous care for the aged, where smart gadgets actively contribute to the welfare of aging populations.

Figure 2. Architecture of Smart healthcare based on 5G (Ahad et al., 2019)

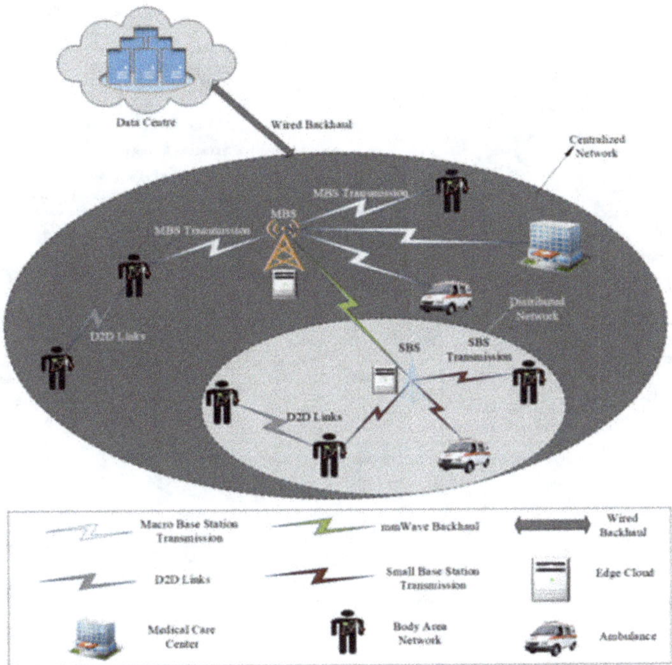

In addition, the Internet of Things (IoT) tackles important obstacles in the healthcare industry by improving patient adherence to prescription schedules through intelligent systems that authenticate drugs, track medical inventory, and optimize resource allocation. This holistic strategy not only leads to measurable cost reductions but also enhances the quality of user experiences, hence raising the overall standard and efficacy of healthcare delivery. The Internet of Things is not just a technological advancement, but a fundamental change in healthcare. It promises a future where connectivity and intelligence come together to create a healthcare system that is efficient, cost-effective, and transformative in its approach to patient well-being.

Figure 3. IoT Based Smart Healthcare Solutions

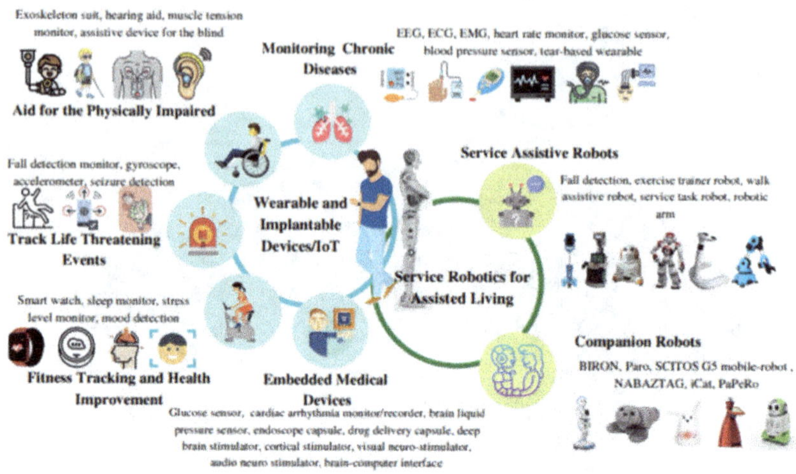

Big Data Analytics

Over the past several years, there has been a widespread shift towards digitalization, leading to a significant increase in health data from many sources such as biological and wearable sensors, ubiquitous mobile phones, and huge electronic health record (EHR) databases. The extensive and varied collection, generally referred to as "big data," has become a powerful resource with significant promise to transform healthcare through evidence-based and patient-centered methods. The progress of digitalization is advancing with innovations that enable the continuous remote monitoring of a wide range of health markers. This range encompasses fundamental measures like as blood pressure, heart rate, and oxygen saturation, as well as more complex markers like glucose levels, body temperature, daily activities, and even emotional states. The incorporation of these technologies signifies a fundamental change in healthcare, introducing a period of proactive and individualized methods that go beyond conventional reactive models. Nevertheless, the ambitious endeavour to achieve individualized treatment through the utilization of big data is not without of its complexities as in Fig. 4. Technological problems involve the need to ensure that different sources of data can be integrated smoothly to enable complete analysis. Legal issues encompass the intricate domains of data privacy, security, and ethical ramifications related to health information (Thuemmler & Bai, 2017; Deloitte, 2015; Schaeffer et al., 2016; Kamal et al., 2020). Furthermore, a comprehensive and inclusive strategy is required to address socioeconomic issues, such as healthcare accessibility, equity, and the digital divide. Notwithstanding these difficult hurdles, the appeal of improved healthcare results, the possibility of early and accurate diagnoses, and the potential for significant cost savings continue to be strong incentives. The healthcare industry is actively incorporating big data solutions to analyse and utilize the vast amount of health data available.

Figure 4. Cloud Computing in Smart Healthcare

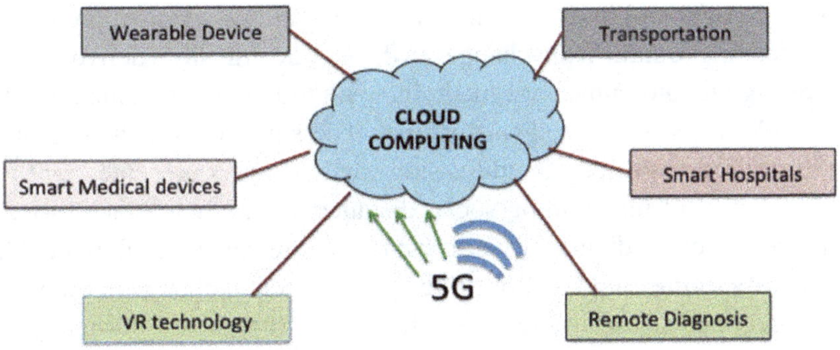

Artificial Intelligence (AI) and Machine Learning (ML)

Artificial intelligence and machine learning are leading a revolutionary transformation in the healthcare sector, namely in the field of smart healthcare. These advanced tools utilize large amounts of patient data, exploring extensive databases that contain medical records, lifestyle traits, and environmental elements. The main goal is to forecast the probability of particular diseases, which is achievable through the complex examination and pattern identification skills inherent in AI and ML systems. The incorporation of AI-driven devices and sensors is a noteworthy achievement, allowing the instantaneous remote observation of crucial measurements. This ongoing monitoring provides healthcare providers with proactive knowledge, enabling them to promptly control and modify patient care plans. AI and ML systems play a crucial role in analyzing medical pictures like CT scans and X-rays, which helps speed up the diagnostic process and improve accuracy. In the age of personalized medicine, these technologies play a role in the creation of customized treatment strategies (Anand et al., 2023; Ravindranathan et al., 2024; Patil et al., 2024; Saxena et al., 2024; Sisodiya et al., 2024). These plans are carefully designed by evaluating individual patient characteristics and medical histories, guaranteeing that healthcare actions are accurately tailored to the specific requirements of each patient. The trend towards individualization ensures timely detection of health problems, the adoption of tailored treatment plans, and the expedited development of new medications. The cornerstone of AI and ML systems relies on the resilience of scientifically and statistically validated data. By utilizing these data-driven insights, these systems aim to establish and improve healthcare procedures to a uniform level. The future we imagine includes ongoing surveillance, focused medical treatments, and an organized and efficient method of providing healthcare. This data-centric approach signifies a shift away from traditional healthcare systems, indicating a move towards a more standardized, evidence-based, and patient-focused paradigm. The range of capabilities provided by AI-based, machine learning-based, and probabilistic models in healthcare systems is extensive. These technologies provide the potential to completely transform the way healthcare is understood and carried out, by offering detailed treatment recommendations, allowing the prediction of outcomes, and generating immediate assessments of risk. With the growing popularity of deep learning techniques, AI and ML are expected to continue expanding and integrating into many aspects of patient care and wellness management in the healthcare industry.

Telemedicine

Telemedicine is a powerful tool in modern healthcare that allows medical professionals to remotely interact with patients, leading to significant changes in the way healthcare is delivered. This novel method effortlessly combines digital communication methods, with videoconferencing and remote monitoring developing as crucial elements of telemedical services. The significant influence of telemedicine has been substantially magnified, especially in addressing various issues presented by the global COVID-19 epidemic. The imperative of maintaining social distance and reducing face-to-face encounters has expedited the acceptance of telemedicine, propelling it to the forefront of modern healthcare procedures. The increase in popularity of this trend demonstrates a fundamental change in the way consumers may easily obtain medical treatment and consultations without the necessity of physically visiting healthcare institutions. Videoconferencing, an essential component of telemedicine, enables healthcare professionals to conduct virtual consultations with patients, bridging the gap created by geographical distances. This live, graphical communication not only guarantees the ongoing provision of medical treatment but also offers a customized and interactive healthcare encounter. Patients now have the ability to interact with their healthcare providers, have conversations about their symptoms, receive medical advice, and even participate in virtual examinations, all without leaving their homes, ensuring their comfort and safety. Remote monitoring, a crucial component of telemedicine, enables healthcare personnel to remotely watch and follow patients' health data without being physically present. It is especially vital for the management of chronic illnesses, surgical care, and regular follow-ups. Home-based monitoring offers convenience for patients and also gives healthcare practitioners with crucial health information, enabling early interventions and adjustments to treatment plans. The rise in telemedicine's popularity reflects a larger movement towards patient-centered and easily accessible healthcare. This initiative not only tackles the current obstacles presented by the epidemic, but also establishes the groundwork for a future in which telemedical services assume a crucial role in providing healthcare that is easy, efficient, and customized to individual requirements. Telemedicine is poised to become an essential and enduring component of the healthcare landscape as technology progresses, offering patients worldwide a blend of in-person and virtual healthcare options as in Fig. 5.

Figure 5. Remote Patient Monitoring System

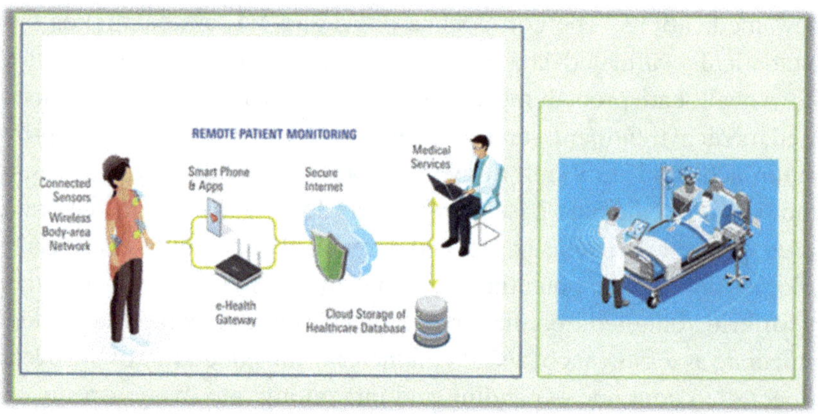

Electronic Health Records (EHRs)

Electronic Health Records (EHRs) are a revolutionary cornerstone in contemporary healthcare, signifying a fundamental change from conventional paper-based records to smoothly integrated digital systems. These digital databases contain all of a patient's medical records, making it easy for healthcare practitioners to access and review the whole medical history. The primary benefit of EHRs is their capacity to streamline data retrieval and guarantee the precision, comprehensiveness, and timeliness of patient information. The ability to access information in real-time enables healthcare practitioners to make well-informed and prompt decisions regarding patient care. Healthcare workers may efficiently get essential data in various healthcare settings, such as hospitals, consultations, or emergency circumstances, enabling a prompter and patient-focused approach. Furthermore, the EHR systems' analytical capabilities enhance the comprehension of patient health. Through the careful examination of extensive datasets, electronic health records (EHRs) reveal patterns and trends that assist doctors in improving their treatment judgments. By utilizing data, this technique improves the delivery of therapy by providing valuable information about areas that may need to be enhanced. This enables a constant process of making improvements and optimizing healthcare operations. Electronic Health Records (EHRs) are crucial in reducing healthcare expenses by improving efficiency and preventing unnecessary duplication of diagnostic procedures. The smooth incorporation of patient data also enables the creation of customized therapy suggestions. Healthcare practitioners can optimize treatment outcomes by utilizing a patient's medical history and pertinent data to create tailored care plans that target specific health requirements. The extensive use of technology into healthcare procedures, as demonstrated by Electronic Health Records (EHRs), represents a wider transition towards a more uniform, evidence-based, and patient-focused approach. This progress is in line with the broader objective of providing healthcare that is not just efficient and cost-effective but also fundamentally sensitive to the distinct requirements and features of each patient. With the ongoing development and widespread adoption of EHR systems, they are positioned to have a greater impact on the future of healthcare delivery as in Fig. 6.

Figure 6. Transformative Impact of EHRs in Healthcare

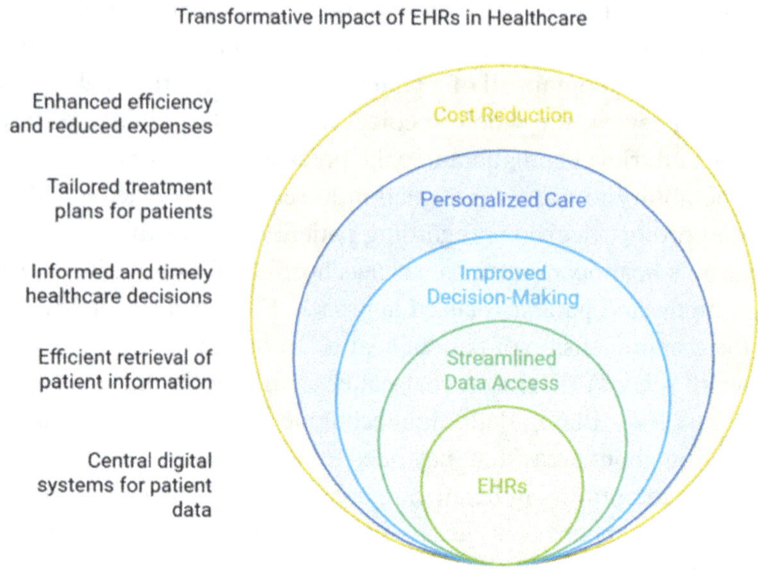

Traditional Healthcare

Conventional healthcare, which is firmly based on historical traditions and established norms, has always been the foundation of medical services. This study project aims to analyze and comprehend existing healthcare systems, investigating their strengths, weaknesses, and the influence of developing technology on these well-established processes. In conventional healthcare environments, patient care is predominantly provided through direct encounters between healthcare practitioners and patients within physical healthcare facilities. These contacts involve a variety of services, such as consultations, diagnoses, and treatments. The conventional paradigm mainly depends on the actual presence of patients in healthcare facilities, frequently necessitating their travel and adherence to rigid appointment schedules. Traditional healthcare excels in delivering individualized and hands-on treatment by highly skilled healthcare personnel. The established rapport between patients and their physicians cultivates a feeling of confidence and uninterrupted provision of medical attention. In addition, the physical examination and hands-on diagnostics are essential aspects of conventional healthcare, enabling a thorough comprehension of a patient's situation. Nevertheless, conventional healthcare is not without of its difficulties. Accessibility continues to be a major issue, especially for people living in distant or underdeveloped regions. The dependence on face-to-face consultations might result in delays in obtaining medical advice and actions. Furthermore, there is frequently a higher demand for healthcare services than there are resources available, resulting in problems such as overcrowding and extended waiting periods. The study project explores both the traditional healthcare landscape and the disruptive effects of new technology. Advanced technologies such as 5G, big data, the Internet of Things (IoT), artificial intelligence (AI), and machine learning (ML) can be used to address some of the limitations in conventional healthcare. For example, the use of telemedicine, made possible by fast and responsive connections such as 5G, enables remote consultations, overcoming geographical limitations and delivering prompt healthcare services to those in faraway places. Furthermore, the utilization of Internet of Things (IoT) devices and wearable technology in combination with conventional healthcare methods can facilitate the continuous monitoring of an individual's health in real-time. This uninterrupted flow of data provides valuable information about the health conditions of patients, enables the early identification of problems, and enables more proactive and tailored therapies as in Fig. 7.

Figure 7. Accessibility Issues in Conventional Healthcare

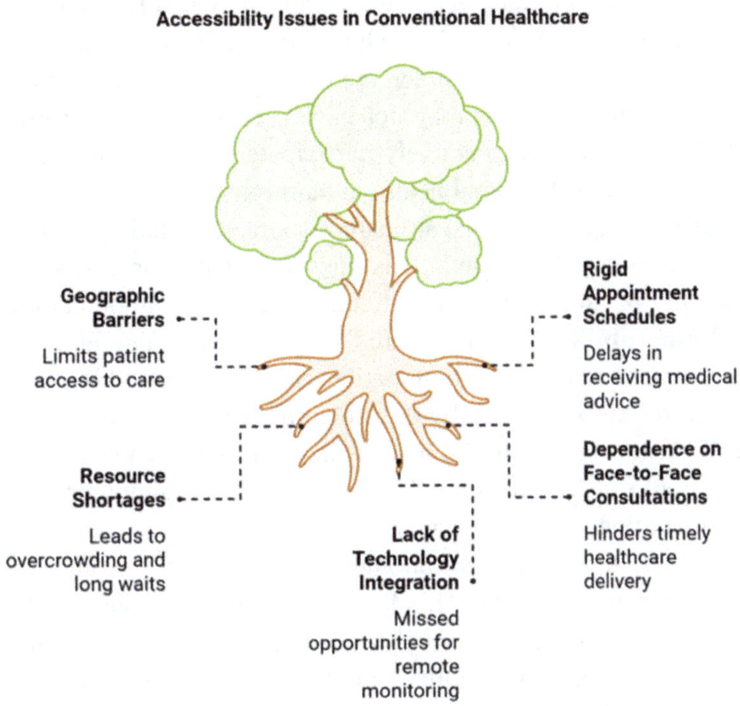

Pain Points in Traditional Healthcare

Traditional healthcare, while serving as a crucial foundation for medical services, faces several pain points that impact its effectiveness and accessibility. Here are some key pain points in traditional healthcare:

- **Geographical Barriers:** Individuals residing in remote or rural areas encounter challenges in accessing healthcare due to the limited availability of medical centers. This creates a significant barrier to timely and essential medical services, impacting health outcomes for these populations.
- **Transportation Issues:** Some individuals face difficulties in reaching healthcare providers due to unreliable transportation. This can lead to delays in seeking necessary medical attention, particularly for emergencies or time-sensitive conditions.

- **Overcrowded Facilities:** The high demand for healthcare services often results in crowded waiting areas and long queues. This overcrowding causes delays in consultations and treatments, negatively affecting the overall efficiency and patient experience.
- **Appointment Scheduling:** Fixed appointment schedules contribute to extended waiting times for patients seeking immediate care. This rigidity can impede timely access to healthcare services, particularly for those with urgent medical needs.
- **Lack of Interoperability:** Limited integration between different healthcare systems and facilities hampers the seamless exchange of patient data. This lack of interoperability can result in fragmented care, as healthcare providers may not have access to comprehensive patient information.
- **Patient Empowerment:** Traditional healthcare models often involve minimal patient engagement in decision-making and treatment planning. This lack of empowerment may lead to reduced patient satisfaction and a potential gap in understanding and managing one's own health.
- **Lack of Health Education:** Patients may not have access to sufficient information about their conditions, hindering their ability to actively participate in their healthcare. This limited health education may contribute to suboptimal health outcomes.
- **Unequal Distribution:** Explanation: Healthcare resources, including medical professionals and facilities, may not be evenly distributed. This uneven distribution can lead to disparities in the quality and availability of care, particularly affecting underserved populations.
- **Paper Records Vulnerability:** Records stored on paper are vulnerable to theft, deterioration, and unwanted access. Concerns concerning patient data security and the possible compromise of private medical records are brought up by this vulnerability.
- **Digital Privacy:** Transitioning to digital records introduces challenges related to the secure storage and transmission of sensitive health information. Ensuring digital privacy becomes crucial in maintaining patient confidentiality and trust.
- **Lack of Coordination:** Insufficient communication and coordination between healthcare providers may result in fragmented care. This lack of coordination can affect treatment outcomes, especially for patients with complex medical needs requiring multidisciplinary care.
- **Slow Adoption of Technology:** Reluctance to embrace modern technologies, such as electronic health records and telemedicine, may hinder the optimization of healthcare delivery. Slow adoption impedes the potential benefits of technological advancements in improving accessibility and efficiency in healthcare services.

Solutions for Smart Healthcare

- **5G Connectivity:** Expand 5G networks to enhance healthcare access. Faster and widespread connectivity facilitates quicker data transfer, enabling remote monitoring, telemedicine, and very efficient communication among healthcare professionals.
- **EHR Implementation:** Integrate Electronic Health Records (EHRs) for seamless data sharing and comprehensive patient records. This approach enhances the efficiency of healthcare delivery by providing real-time access to patient information, reducing delays, and improving overall care coordination.
- **Robot-Assisted Care:** Utilize robots to enhance efficiency in healthcare tasks and patient assistance. Robots can perform routine tasks, assist healthcare professionals, and provide support to patients, thereby optimizing resource utilization and improving the quality of care.

- **Telemedicine Solutions:** Extend telemedicine platforms to enable remote consultations and virtual care. This approach addresses geographical barriers, reduces overcrowded facilities, and provides timely access to healthcare services, especially in situations where physical presence is challenging.
- **AI and Machine Learning:** Implement Artificial Intelligence and Machine Learning for predictive analytics and personalized treatment. These technologies analyze vast datasets to predict health trends, customize treatment plans, and enhance diagnostic accuracy, ultimately improving patient outcomes.
- **IoT Applications:** Leverage Internet of Things (IoT) for real-time vital signs monitoring and patient engagement. IoT devices collect and transmit health data, allowing for continuous monitoring and timely interventions, promoting proactive healthcare management.
- **Data Analytics for Population Health:** Use data analytics to understand population health trends and inform healthcare strategies. Analyzing large datasets helps identify health patterns, assess the effectiveness of interventions, and tailor public health initiatives to specific population needs.
- **Remote Surgery with 5G:** Enable remote robotic surgeries through high-speed 5G networks. This approach allows surgeons to perform procedures from a distance, expanding access to specialized care and expertise, particularly in underserved areas.
- **Chatbots for Healthcare Assistance:** Implement AI-driven chatbots for convenient healthcare information. Chatbots improve accessibility and increase patient engagement by instantly answering questions, helping to schedule appointments, and providing basic healthcare information.
- **AI-Powered Diagnostic Tools:** Deploy AI tools for faster and accurate diagnostics. AI-driven diagnostic tools analyse medical images and data, improving diagnostic precision, reducing waiting times, and facilitating early detection of diseases.
- **Enhanced Patient Experience:** Wearable devices connected to 5G networks enable continuous patient engagement. Patients can actively participate in their health management, receiving real-time feedback and making informed decisions. AI-powered virtual assistants provide patients with health information, medication reminders, and ongoing support. This not only enhances patient education but also fosters a sense of empowerment and control over one's health as in Fig. 8.

Figure 8. 5G for Smart Healthcare Systems

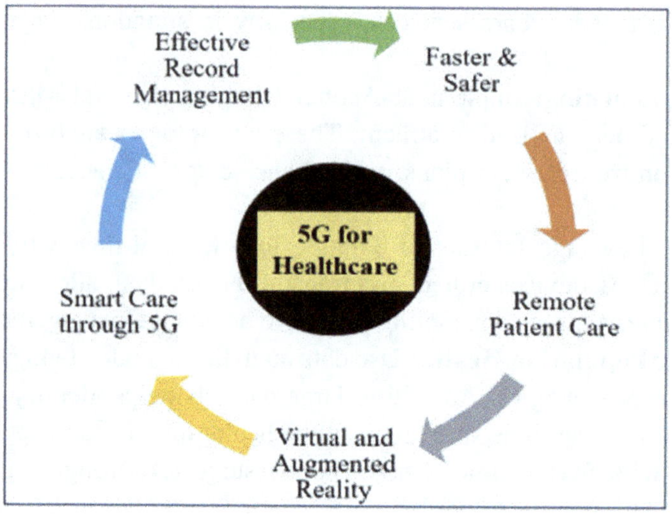

Use Cases of Smart Healthcare (Eid et al., 2010; Marshall et al., 2008; NSF, 2016)

1. Remote Patient Monitoring (RPM):

Remote Patient Monitoring (RPM) is an innovative method of delivering healthcare services that utilizes Internet of Things (IoT) devices and sensors to collect vital patient health information from a remote location. This dataset includes a range of metrics, including vital signs (such as heart rate and blood pressure), medication adherence, and symptom progression. Remote Patient Monitoring (RPM) provides a revolutionary solution in the realm of chronic illnesses such as diabetes or hypertension. Individuals can employ wearable gadgets that are fitted with sensors to continually check their glucose levels or blood pressure throughout the day, eliminating the need for frequent trips to the clinic. These gadgets efficiently communicate live data to healthcare practitioners, allowing for remote monitoring and analysis. Remote access to patient data enables timely intervention and customized therapy modifications based on individual health patterns and variations. Healthcare practitioners have the ability to monitor changes in patients' health indicators from a distance, detect any problems or complications before they worsen, and take proactive measures by implementing personalized treatment plans or making modifications to medicines. The benefits of RPM are significant and diverse. Firstly, it facilitates proactive healthcare management by allowing for timely interventions and early detection of health issues. Remote Patient Monitoring (RPM) assists healthcare practitioners in swiftly addressing possible issues by continually monitoring patients' health data and identifying trends, patterns, and deviations from baseline parameters. Adopting this proactive strategy can effectively avert problems, limit the advancement of chronic illnesses, and enhance overall health outcomes for patients. Furthermore, RPM mitigates the necessity for regular hospital visits or in-person examinations, which can be onerous for patients, particularly those with limited mobility or residing in isolated regions. Remote Patient Monitoring (RPM) improves patient convenience, comfort, and adherence to treatment regimens by offering continuous monitoring and individualized care. In addition, RPM promotes patient involvement in self-care and the management of their health. Remote Patient Monitoring (RPM) encourages patients to actively monitor their health metrics and actively participate in their treatment process, fostering a sense of ownership and responsibility for their own health. Enhanced participation can result in higher compliance with treatment, healthier decisions on lifestyle, and enhanced long-term health results. Finally, RPM provides healthcare systems with the opportunity to save costs by decreasing hospital readmissions, averting problems, and improving resource distribution. Through early intervention and proactive management of health conditions, Remote Patient Monitoring (RPM) can effectively reduce the necessity for costly emergency interventions or hospitalizations, leading to significant cost savings for healthcare providers and payers.

2. Telemedicine and Virtual Consultations:

Telemedicine allows people to engage in video conversations with doctors and other healthcare professionals, primarily for non-emergency medical concerns, follow-up visits, or prescription renewals. This is particularly beneficial for those residing in distant or impoverished regions with restricted availability of medical infrastructure. Instead of suffering long travel times to see a doctor, individuals may conveniently schedule a virtual consultation and receive medical advise or treatment from the comfort of their own homes. Telemedicine provides several benefits for both patients and healthcare practitioners. First and foremost, it greatly enhances the accessibility of healthcare by reducing geographical obstacles and extending the provision of healthcare services to rural or isolated regions. Telemedicine consultations might be advantageous for patients who face challenges in reaching conventional healthcare facilities owing to factors such as distance, transportation limitations, or mobility limits. Furthermore, telemedicine effectively decreases the amount of time and expenses patients incur for traveling, since they are no longer need to journey to healthcare facilities for regular checkups or consultations. This not only improves convenience for patients but also leads to cost savings and resource optimization in the healthcare system. Moreover, telemedicine facilitates prompt consultations in the event of emergencies or public health crises, such as pandemics. Patients may access medical advice, monitoring, and treatment from a distance, which helps minimize the danger of disease transmission and eases the burden on healthcare institutions. Moreover, telemedicine promotes collaboration among healthcare teams by improving communication and information exchange between doctors. Experts have the ability to provide consultations to primary care doctors from a distance, exchange diagnostic pictures or test results, and work together on treatment plans. This results in improved coordination and complete care for patients. Telemedicine is a significant technology that improves healthcare delivery, increases patient access to treatment, and promotes efficiency and collaboration within the healthcare system. The ongoing advancement of technology and increasing adoption of telemedicine have the potential to revolutionize healthcare delivery and enhance patient outcomes.

3. Predictive Analytics for Disease Prevention:

Predictive analytics is a specialized area within data analytics that use machine learning algorithms and artificial intelligence (AI) to analyze large volumes of medical data and predict patient outcomes. This methodology allows healthcare practitioners to actively detect individuals who are susceptible to acquiring particular illnesses or health conditions, hence facilitating prompt intervention and preventative actions. Healthcare professionals can utilize many data sources, such as electronic health records (EHRs), genetic information, lifestyle data, and social determinants of health, to construct prediction models in a predictive analytics scenario. These models utilize data analysis to detect patterns and trends that can identify individuals who are more likely to acquire specific diseases, such as diabetes, heart disease, or cancer. By examining a patient's medical history, genetic predispositions, lifestyle variables (such as food, exercise, and smoking habits), and demographic information, predictive analytics algorithms can evaluate the individual's probability of getting cardiovascular disease in the future. Healthcare professionals may improve patient outcomes and minimize risk by identifying individuals at high risk and applying personalized interventions such as medication management, lifestyle modifications, or preventative screenings. Predictive analytics has several advantages for both patients and healthcare practitioners. First and foremost, it facilitates preventive and tailored healthcare by identifying individuals who are at risk of acquiring particular diseases prior to the appearance of symptoms. This enables prompt intervention and proactive actions, potentially decreasing the occurrence and intensity of illnesses and enhancing patient results. Furthermore, predictive analytics enhances the efficiency of resource allocation in the healthcare system by prioritizing interventions and distributing money to patients who have the highest likelihood of benefiting. Healthcare practitioners may enhance preventive care techniques, lower healthcare expenses, and enhance population health outcomes by concentrating on high-risk groups. Predictive analytics enhances clinical decision-making by providing medical practitioners with evidence-based recommendations and actionable insights. By utilizing predictive models, physicians may customize treatment regimens, efficiently monitor patients, and forecast future healthcare requirements, resulting in a more individualized and efficient provision of care.

4. Smart Medication Management:
    - Smart medication management solutions are a technologically advanced approach in healthcare that target the intricate issues related to drug adherence and strive to decrease prescription mistakes. These solutions utilize advanced technologies such as Internet of Things (IoT), sensors, data analytics, and connectivity platforms to offer patients, caregivers, and healthcare practitioners' tools and assistance in improving drug management processes. An exemplary instance of intelligent medicine management systems is the deployment of Internet of Things (IoT)-enabled pill dispensers. These gadgets are loaded with sophisticated functions that surpass the fundamental functionality of conventional pill organizers. This is the functioning mechanism:
    - IoT-enabled pill dispensers are programmable devices that may be configured to distribute drugs at precise times according to the patient's recommended dose regimen, serving as reminders and ensuring timely dispensing. those or those responsible for care can configure the dispenser to release the necessary drugs at certain times, guaranteeing that dosages are neither skipped or consumed wrongly.
    - • Adherence Tracking: The dispensers are equipped with sensors and connection features that allow them to monitor medicine adherence in real-time. Whenever a dosage is given, the dispenser keeps a record of the occurrence and sends the information to a central platform or application that may be accessed by patients, caregivers, or healthcare practitioners. This enables the ongoing monitoring of drug adherence and offers valuable insights into patient behavior and patterns of compliance.

- • alarms and Notifications: If a dosage is missed or medication is not taken as prescribed, the pill dispenser with IoT capabilities may produce alarms and notifications to inform the patient, caregiver, or healthcare professional. These signals can be transmitted through many mediums, such as visual indicators on the dispenser, auditory alerts, smartphone notifications, or emails. The dispenser rapidly notifies stakeholders of situations when adherence is not followed, enabling timely intervention and remedial measures to address the root causes of pharmaceutical non-compliance.
- Smart medication management systems provide remote monitoring and intervention, allowing healthcare practitioners to track medication adherence even when patients are not physically present in clinical settings. Healthcare practitioners can obtain real-time adherence data using secure web portals or mobile applications. This enables them to monitor patients' medication-taking behavior, identify possible obstacles to adherence, and intervene when required to promote adherence and enhance treatment results.

5. Health and wellness tracking systems:

Health and wellness tracking systems are a technical breakthrough designed to monitor and manage individuals' lifestyle behaviours and general well-being. By incorporating wearable devices, mobile applications, and sensors, these systems effectively gather and analyse data relevant to several aspects of health, such as physical activity, sleep patterns, dietary intake, and stress levels. One of the most common examples of such systems are fitness trackers, which use wearable devices with sensors to track various measurements related to physical activity, sleep quality, and eating habits. For example, fitness trackers consistently monitor a user's physical activity levels throughout the day, including factors such as the number of steps taken, distance travelled, calories burned, and active minutes. By employing accelerometers and gyroscopes, these devices detect movement patterns and measure the intensity and duration of various sports, including walking, running, cycling, and swimming. In addition, fitness trackers have the ability to monitor sleep patterns and quality by recording the length of sleep, different phases of sleep (such as light, deep, and REM sleep), and disruptions such as awakenings. This functionality frequently depends on a combination of motion sensors and heart rate monitors, which allows for the identification of physiological alterations linked to various sleep phases. Moreover, many sophisticated fitness trackers enable the tracking of nutrition consumption. This may be done either by enabling users to manually input their dietary choices or by scanning barcodes of packaged items. Some wearable gadgets include sensors that can estimate calorie intake by considering parameters such as heart rate variability and metabolic rate. Health and wellness tracking technologies, such as fitness trackers, enable individuals to obtain a deep understanding of their health behaviours, establish wellness objectives, and make well-informed choices to improve their overall well-being.

Implications of the Study

The advent of 5G technology ushers in a new age of highly efficient and flexible connectivity, offering exceptional performance and tailored applications to meet the diverse demands of the economy and consumers. 5G, the successor to 4G and 3G, provides unprecedented connectivity, particularly in the realm of intelligent healthcare. However, the utilization of 5G and other technologies in healthcare presents challenges and unresolved research matters. The widespread use of Internet of Things (IoT) devices in the smart healthcare network presents substantial security risks, since they are susceptible to different assaults that can compromise privacy and security. Ensuring universal connectivity for all devices, regardless of their range, is a significant challenge inside the network, particularly for highly mobile equipment such as moving patients and quick ambulances. It is crucial to have a system that enables users to connect to several devices utilizing various communication protocols in order to ensure smooth operations. Within the realm of intelligent healthcare, the large number of devices that make up the network provide a substantial amount of data, which includes crucial patient information like heart rate and electrocardiograms. To effectively process this extensive volume of data, it is imperative to employ sophisticated algorithms and methodologies that guarantee the optimal performance of intelligent healthcare systems, utilizing 5G and other advanced technologies. The lack of global communication standards is a significant obstacle to the development of 5G and IoT by impeding interoperability between different industries, notwithstanding the potential advantages. To overcome this difficulty, it is necessary to apply a crucial intelligent approach that ensures compatibility at many levels and enables effective communication among the vast number of associated devices in the network. To effectively deal with these challenges, the incorporation of 5G and other technologies in smart healthcare requires a thorough strategy that tackles security, accessibility, and interoperability in order to fully use the capabilities of this revolutionary networking model.

Regulatory Compliances

Regulatory compliance in emerging healthcare technologies represents a complex, multidimensional framework that balances technological innovation with patient safety, data privacy, and ethical considerations. Advanced healthcare technologies must navigate intricate regulatory landscapes including HIPAA in the United States, GDPR in Europe, and emerging global digital health standards that address increasingly sophisticated technological interventions. Blockchain-based verification systems and advanced cryptographic protocols are being developed to ensure robust data integrity, patient consent management, and transparent audit trails for emerging medical technologies like AI diagnostics, genomic analysis, and telemedicine platforms. Regulatory bodies are evolving sophisticated risk assessment methodologies that incorporate machine learning algorithms to evaluate the safety and efficacy of emerging medical technologies, creating dynamic compliance frameworks that can adapt to rapid technological advancements. Cybersecurity standards are becoming increasingly stringent, mandating multi-layered security architectures for medical devices, telemedicine platforms, and health information systems that protect against sophisticated cyber threats while maintaining interoperability. Artificial intelligence and machine learning technologies are subject to emerging ethical guidelines that mandate transparency, explainability, and non-discriminatory algorithmic design. International standardization efforts, led by organizations like ISO and IEEE, are developing comprehensive regulatory frameworks that address the complex technological, ethical, and clinical dimensions of next-generation healthcare innovations, ensuring patient safety and technological accountability.

Ethical Concerns and Data Ownership

The convergence of advanced healthcare technologies introduces profound ethical challenges surrounding data ownership, privacy, and informed consent in increasingly complex technological ecosystems. Blockchain and distributed ledger technologies are emerging as critical infrastructures for establishing transparent, patient-centric data governance models that enable granular control over personal health information. Advanced cryptographic techniques and zero-knowledge proof protocols are being developed to facilitate secure, anonymized data sharing while maintaining individual privacy rights and preventing unauthorized data access. Artificial intelligence and machine learning algorithms raise significant ethical considerations regarding algorithmic bias, decision transparency, and the potential for unintended discriminatory outcomes in diagnostic and treatment recommendations. Sophisticated consent management platforms are being designed to provide patients with comprehensive, real-time control over their medical data, allowing dynamic permissions and granular access controls across interconnected healthcare systems. Quantum encryption and advanced anonymization techniques are being explored to mitigate potential risks of patient data re-identification and ensure robust protection of sensitive medical information. Interdisciplinary ethical frameworks are being developed to address complex challenges, including the potential for predictive health technologies to inadvertently compromise individual autonomy, genetic privacy, and personal medical decision-making. These evolving regulatory and technological approaches aim to balance transformative medical innovation with fundamental principles of patient rights, data sovereignty, and ethical technological development.

Future Research

Edge computing is revolutionizing healthcare technologies by enabling real-time, localized data processing and analysis at the point of data generation, such as medical devices, wearables, and IoT sensors. This distributed computing paradigm significantly reduces latency, enhances data privacy, and supports critical medical applications requiring immediate computational response. In healthcare settings, edge computing facilitates advanced functionalities like instant patient monitoring, predictive diagnostics, and personalized treatment strategies by processing complex medical data closer to the source. Sophisticated machine learning algorithms deployed at the edge can perform rapid analysis of vital signs, detect anomalies in continuous health monitoring, and enable immediate clinical interventions. The integration of 5G networks further amplifies edge computing's potential, allowing seamless transmission of high-resolution medical imaging, real-time telemedicine consultations, and synchronized data exchange between medical devices and centralized healthcare systems. Advanced edge computing architectures leverage containerization, microservices, and secure blockchain-like protocols to ensure data integrity, compliance with healthcare regulations like HIPAA, and robust security measures. By decentralizing computational workloads and enabling intelligent, context-aware medical technologies, edge computing is poised to transform healthcare delivery, making it more responsive, precise, and patient-centric as in Fig. 9.

Figure 9. Transforming healthcare with Edge Computing

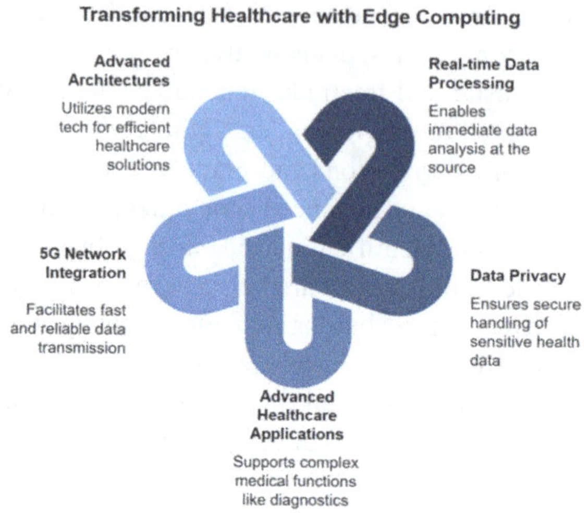

The emerging 6G technology promises to revolutionize healthcare through unprecedented wireless connectivity, characterized by ultra-high frequencies (terahertz spectrum), extreme low latency, and revolutionary computational capabilities. Anticipated to support data transmission rates up to 1 terabyte per second, 6G will enable hyper-realistic holographic telemedicine consultations, allowing physicians to perform remote diagnostics with near-physical interaction precision. Integrated artificial intelligence and machine learning algorithms will leverage 6G's sophisticated network slicing and edge computing capabilities to create adaptive, real-time healthcare ecosystems. Nano-scale communication networks will facilitate advanced biomedical sensing, enabling microscopic medical devices capable of internal patient monitoring, targeted drug delivery, and precise cellular-level interventions. The technology's anticipated sub-millisecond latency will support critical applications like remote robotic surgeries, where instantaneous response times are paramount for patient safety. Quantum computing integration with 6G infrastructure will potentially unlock unprecedented medical data processing capabilities, enabling complex genomic analysis, personalized treatment modelling, and predictive health diagnostics. Advanced security protocols utilizing blockchain and quantum encryption will ensure unprecedented levels of patient data protection, addressing contemporary cybersecurity challenges in medical technology ecosystems. These transformative capabilities position 6G as a fundamental technological catalyst for next-generation precision and personalized healthcare delivery as in Fig. 10.

Figure 10. 6G Technology, A Catalyst for Healthcare Revolution

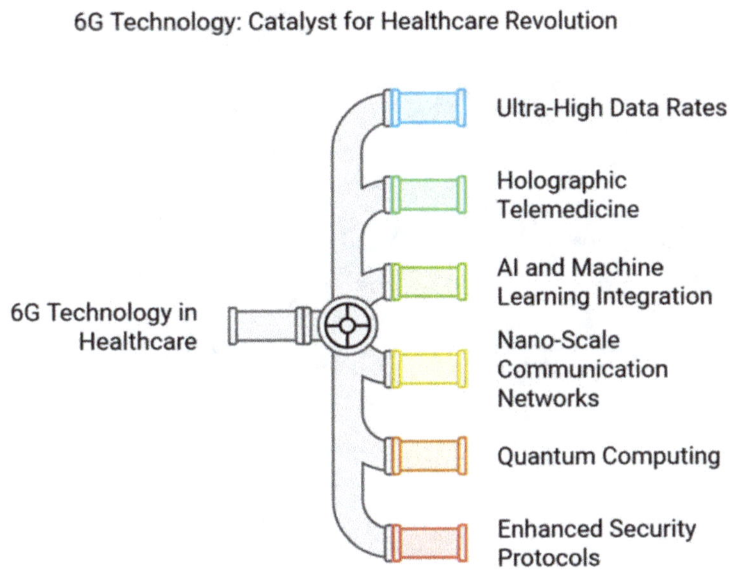

Medical robotics is emerging as a transformative technological domain, integrating advanced artificial intelligence, precision engineering, and adaptive machine learning to revolutionize clinical interventions and patient care. Sophisticated surgical robotic systems, incorporating haptic feedback, microsurgical precision, and real-time imaging integration, enable minimally invasive procedures with unprecedented accuracy and reduced patient trauma. Collaborative robots (cobots) are increasingly designed with advanced sensor technologies and adaptive AI algorithms, capable of performing complex medical tasks ranging from delicate surgical procedures to patient rehabilitation and elderly care support. Nano-robotics represents a cutting-edge frontier, with microscale robotic systems capable of targeted drug delivery, precise cellular-level interventions, and sophisticated diagnostic capabilities within human biological systems. Machine learning algorithms embedded in these robotic platforms enable autonomous decision-making, predictive diagnostics, and adaptive response mechanisms that can dynamically adjust to individual patient physiological parameters. Advanced medical robots are being integrated with augmented reality and computer vision technologies, allowing surgeons to visualize complex anatomical structures with enhanced depth perception and real-time diagnostic overlay. Interconnected through secure 5G and anticipated 6G networks, these robotic systems create intelligent, interconnected healthcare ecosystems that promise personalized, precise, and proactive medical interventions, fundamentally transforming traditional healthcare delivery models as in Fig. 11.

Figure 11. The Future of Medical Robotics

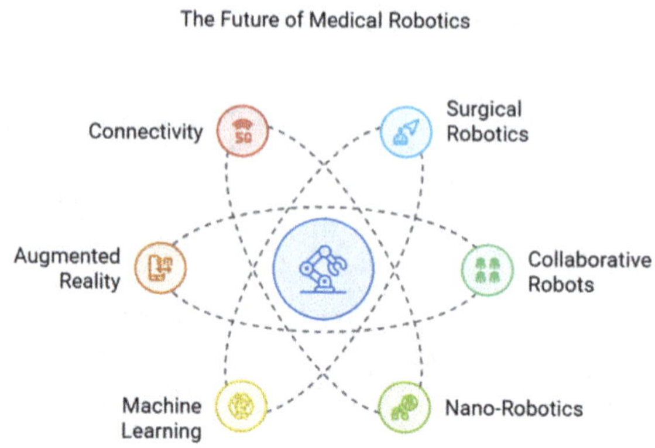

CONCLUSION

Ultimately, the incorporation of 5G networks into applications such as IoT and smart healthcare is leading the way in revolutionary advancements within the healthcare sector. The practical and economic importance of utilizing Internet of Things and smart healthcare in the context of 5G technology is clear. Looking into the future, the implementation of 5G, along with other advanced technologies, is ready to revolutionize the way healthcare is provided, unleashing new possibilities and capacities for both medical professionals and users. The expected ramifications of 5G go beyond simply enhancing internet services; it signifies a fundamental change that will transform the way healthcare services are obtained and provided. 5G is anticipated to empower consumers, healthcare professionals, and social workers due to its improved internet services and widespread accessibility. The introduction of 5G technology directly enables the deployment of efficient and dependable telemedicine services, which in turn facilitates the sharing and collaboration of healthcare expertise. 5G enables the development of a strong and reliable network for smart healthcare, which enhances connection for medical equipment. This advancement is crucial in expanding the functionalities of internet-connected medical equipment, offering enhanced internet access and communication technologies through 5G. The cooperation between regulatory organizations, health app developers, and 5G network operators will play a crucial role in comprehending and enhancing the communication Key Performance Indicators (KPIs) necessary for secure and efficient healthcare services. In the future, the combination of big data, sensing technologies, and Artificial Intelligence/Machine Learning (AI/ML) will enable personalized healthcare in the healthcare system. This movement represents a transition towards personalized and data-driven medical services, offering more efficient and customized treatment to patients. This study report sought to present a thorough examination of the upcoming changes resulting from the integration of 5G technology in smart healthcare. The study aimed to provide significant insights into ongoing research and recent achievements by exploring various technologies and their possible uses in healthcare. The last part emphasized specific topics that require more examination and forthcoming initiatives in the field of intelligent healthcare services on the 5G network. This study provides a basis for scholars to conduct their own research projects, utilizing various methods to investigate the extensive possibilities of 5G-enabled intelligent healthcare. This research establishes the foundation for ongoing inquiry and innovation at the interface of healthcare and advanced technology, as the environment continues to change. This research examines the possible effects of 5G technology on the healthcare industry, specifically in relation to virtual consultations and remote patient monitoring. It aims to meet the current issues presented by an aging population and a rise in the number of people with chronic illnesses. Nevertheless, a significant drawback in the study is the scarcity of source data, mainly due to the continuous growth and expansion of the 5G subject. Although secondary data research provides valuable information, it might limit the depth and legitimacy of the findings made. The existing literature extensively discusses the qualitative handling of communication requirements for healthcare applications. However, there is a lack of understanding of how specific applications might be supported in different scenarios when quantitative demands are identified. This constraint is attributed to the focus on high-level Key Performance Indicators (KPIs). Moreover, the report identifies a deficiency in the assessment of 5G network scenarios, which is marked by a scarcity of experiments, a limited number of infrastructure configurations, restricted coverage regions, and a dearth of diversity in trials done in controlled laboratory settings. The limitations affect the capacity to apply and generalize the results. In order to overcome these constraints, it is recommended that future studies undertake extensive surveys, involving healthcare personnel and telecom providers, to gather firsthand information and get a more comprehensive knowledge of the practical consequences of implementing 5G technology in healthcare.

REFERENCES

Ahad, A., Tahir, M., & Yau, K. L. A. (2019). 5G-based smart healthcare network: Architecture, taxonomy, challenges and future research directions. *IEEE Access : Practical Innovations, Open Solutions, 7*, 100747–100762. DOI: 10.1109/ACCESS.2019.2930628

Ahad, A., Tahir, M., & Yau, K.-L. A. (2019). 5G-based smart healthcare network: Architecture, taxonomy, challenges and future research directions. *IEEE Access : Practical Innovations, Open Solutions, 7*, 100747–100762. DOI: 10.1109/ACCESS.2019.2930628

Alibakhshi-Kenari, M., Naser-Moghadasi, M., Sadeghzadeh, R. A., Virdee, B. S., & Limiti, E. (2016). Periodic array of complementary artificial magnetic conductor metamaterials-based multiband antennas for broadband wireless transceivers. *IET Microwaves, Antennas & Propagation*, *10*(15), 1682–1691. DOI: 10.1049/iet-map.2016.0069

Anand, A., ... (2023). Mitigating cyber-security risks using cyber-analytics. In *2023 7th International Conference on Trends in Electronics and Informatics (ICOEI)* (pp. 630–635). IEEE. DOI: 10.1109/ICOEI56765.2023.10126001

Castillejo, P., Martinez, J. F., Rodriguez-Molina, J., & Cuerva, A. (2013). Integration of wearable devices in a wireless sensor network for an e-health application. *IEEE Wireless Communications*, *20*(4), 38–49. DOI: 10.1109/MWC.2013.6590049

Chung, W. Y., Lee, Y. D., & Jung, S. J. (2008, August 20–25). *A wireless sensor network compatible wearable u-healthcare monitoring system using integrated ECG, accelerometer and SpO2*. In 2008 30th Annual International Conference of the IEEE Engineering in Medicine and Biology Society (pp. 1529–1532). IEEE. DOI: 10.1109/IEMBS.2008.4649424

De Brouwer, M., Ongenae, F., Bonte, P., & De Turck, F. (2018). Towards a cascading reasoning framework to support responsive ambient-intelligent healthcare interventions. *Sensors (Basel)*, *18*(10), 3514. DOI: 10.3390/s18103514 PMID: 30340363

Deloitte. (2015). *Connected health: How digital technology is transforming health and social care*. Deloitte.

Eid, M., Cha, J., & El Saddik, A. (2010). Admux: An adaptive multiplexer for haptic-audio-visual data communication. *IEEE Transactions on Instrumentation and Measurement*, *60*(1), 21–31. DOI: 10.1109/TIM.2010.2065530

Espinoza, A. V., Van Hooff, R. J., De Smedt, A., Moens, M., Yperzeele, L., Nieboer, K., Hubloue, I., De Keyser, J., Convents, A., & Tellez, H. F.. (2016). Development and pilot testing of 24/7 in-ambulance telemedicine for acute stroke: Prehospital stroke study at the Universitair Ziekenhuis Brussel-project. *Cerebrovascular Diseases (Basel, Switzerland)*, *42*(1–2), 15–22. DOI: 10.1159/000444175 PMID: 26950076

3GPP. (2017). *Study on scenarios and requirements for next generation access technologies* (3GPP TR 38.913 V14.2.0). https://www.3gpp.org/DynaReport/38913.htm

Gupta, P., & Ghosh, M. (2019). Revolutionizing healthcare with 5G. *Telecom Business Review*, *12*, 41.

Hamm, S., Schleser, A. C., Hartig, J., Thomas, P., Zoesch, S., & Bulitta, C. (2020). 5G as enabler for digital healthcare. *Current Directions in Biomedical Engineering*, *6*(1), 1–4. DOI: 10.1515/cdbme-2020-3001

Hartmann, M., Hashmi, U. S., & Imran, A. (2019). Edge computing in smart healthcare systems: Review, challenges, and research directions. *Transactions on Emerging Telecommunications Technologies*, *3710*. Advance online publication. DOI: 10.1002/ett.3710

Istepanian, R. S., Hu, S., Philip, N. Y., & Sungoor, A. (2011, August 30–September 3). *The potential of Internet of m-health Things "m-IoT" for non-invasive glucose level sensing*. In 2011 Annual International Conference of the IEEE Engineering in Medicine and Biology Society (pp. 5264–5266). IEEE. DOI: 10.1109/IEMBS.2011.6091282

Kamal, M. D., Tahir, A., Kamal, M. B., & Naeem, M. A. (2020). Future location prediction for emergency vehicles using big data: A case study of healthcare engineering. *Journal of Healthcare Engineering*, *6641571*, 1–11. Advance online publication. DOI: 10.1155/2020/6641571 PMID: 33354308

Kim, H., Kim, S. W., Park, E., Kim, J. H., & Chang, H. (2020). The role of fifth-generation mobile technology in prehospital emergency care: An opportunity to support paramedics. *Health Policy and Technology*, *9*(1), 109–114. DOI: 10.1016/j.hlpt.2020.01.002

Krasniqi, F., Gavrilovska, L., & Maraj, A. (2019). The analysis of key performance indicators (KPI) in 4G/LTE networks. In Poulkov, V. (Ed.), *Future access enablers for ubiquitous and intelligent infrastructures* (pp. 285–296). Springer. DOI: 10.1007/978-3-030-23976-3_25

Li, D. (2019). 5G and intelligence medicine—How the next generation of wireless technology will reconstruct healthcare? *Precision Clinical Medicine*, *2*(3), 205–208. DOI: 10.1093/pcmedi/pbz020 PMID: 31886033

Marshall, A., Yap, K. M., & Yu, W. (2008). Providing QoS for networked peers in distributed haptic virtual environments. *Advances in Multimedia*, *841590*(1), 841590. Advance online publication. DOI: 10.1155/2008/841590

Mutlag, A. A., Abd Ghani, M. K., Arunkumar, N. A., Mohammed, M. A., & Mohd, O. (2019). Enabling technologies for fog computing in healthcare IoT systems. *Future Generation Computer Systems*, *90*, 62–78. DOI: 10.1016/j.future.2018.07.049

National Science Foundation. (2016). *NSF follow-on workshop on ultra-low latency wireless networks*. NSF.

Ojaroudi Parchin, N., Jahanbakhsh Basherlou, H., Al-Yasir, Y. I., Abd-Alhameed, R. A., Abdulkhaleq, A. M., & Noras, J. M. (2019). Recent developments of reconfigurable antennas for current and future wireless communication systems. *Electronics (Basel)*, *8*(2), 128. DOI: 10.3390/electronics8020128

Ojaroudiparchin, N., Shen, M., & Pedersen, G. F. (2016, May 9–11). *Wide-scan phased array antenna fed by coax-to-microstriplines for 5G cell phones*. In 2016 21st International Conference on Microwave, Radar and Wireless Communications (MIKON) (pp. 1–4). IEEE. DOI: 10.1109/MIKON.2016.7492064

Padmashree, T., & Nayak, S. S. (2020, October 7–9). *5G technology for e-health.* In 2020 Fourth International Conference on I-SMAC (IoT in Social, Mobile, Analytics and Cloud) (I-SMAC) (pp. 211–216). IEEE. https://doi.org/DOI: 10.1109/I-SMAC49090.2020.9243366

Patil, A., ... (2024). Cyber resilience: Safeguarding India's markets in the post-pandemic cyber landscape. In *2024 4th International Conference on Innovative Practices in Technology and Management (ICIPTM)* (pp. 1–5). IEEE. DOI: 10.1109/ICIPTM59628.2024.10563229

Qi, J., Yang, P., Min, G., Amft, O., Dong, F., & Xu, L. (2017). Advanced internet of things for personalised healthcare systems: A survey. *Pervasive and Mobile Computing*, *41*, 132–149. DOI: 10.1016/j.pmcj.2017.06.018

Qureshi, H. N., Manalastas, M., Zaidi, S. M. A., Imran, A., & Al Kalaa, M. O. (2020). Service level agreements for 5G and beyond: Overview, challenges and enablers of 5G-healthcare systems. *IEEE Access : Practical Innovations, Open Solutions*, *9*, 1044–1061. DOI: 10.1109/ACCESS.2020.3046927 PMID: 35211361

Rasid, M. F., Musa, W. M., Kadir, N. A., Noor, A. M., Touati, F., Mehmood, W., Khriji, L., Al-Busaidi, A., & Mnaouer, A. B. (2014, May 28–30). *Embedded gateway services for Internet of Things applications in ubiquitous healthcare*. In 2014 2nd International Conference on Information and Communication Technology (ICoICT) (pp. 145–148). IEEE. DOI: 10.1109/ICoICT.2014.6914055

Ravindranathan, P.. (2024). Illuminating the dark: Gaining insights and managing risks with dark analytics. In *2024 International Conference on Intelligent and Innovative Technologies in Computing, Electrical and Electronics (IITCEE)* (pp. 1–6). IEEE. DOI: 10.1109/IITCEE59897.2024.10467380

Rohokale, V. M., Prasad, N. R., & Prasad, R. (2011, February 28–March 3). *A cooperative Internet of Things (IoT) for rural healthcare monitoring and control.* In 2011 2nd International Conference on Wireless Communication, Vehicular Technology, Information Theory and Aerospace & Electronic Systems Technology (Wireless VITAE) (pp. 1–6). IEEE. DOI: 10.1109/WIRELESSVITAE.2011.5940920

Saxena, Y.. (2024). Cloud renaissance: Thriving in the post-pandemic digital landscape. In *2024 Fourth International Conference on Advances in Electrical, Computing, Communication and Sustainable Technologies (ICAECT)* (pp. 1–6). IEEE. DOI: 10.1109/ICAECT60202.2024.10469149

Schaeffer, C., Haque, A., Booton, L., Halleck, J., & Coustasse, A. (2016). Big data management in United States hospitals: Benefits and barriers.

Schaich, F., Hamon, M. H., Hunukumbure, M., Lorca, J., Pedersen, K., Schubert, M., Kosmatos, E., Wunder, G., & Reaz, K. (2018, June 3–6). *The ONE5G approach towards the challenges of multi-service operation in 5G systems.* In 2018 IEEE 87th Vehicular Technology Conference (VTC Spring) (pp. 1–6). IEEE. https://doi.org/DOI: 10.1109/VTCSpring.2018.8417832

Sisodiya, M., ... (2024). The transformative power of robotic process automation: Redefining business in Industry 4.0. In *2024 14th International Conference on Cloud Computing, Data Science & Engineering (Confluence)* (pp. 498–503). IEEE. DOI: 10.1109/Confluence60223.2024.10463415

Terkelsen, C., Nørgaard, B., Lassen, J., Gerdes, J., Ankersen, J., Rømer, F., Nielsen, T., & Andersen, H. (2002). Telemedicine used for remote prehospital diagnosing in patients suspected of acute myocardial infarction. *Journal of Internal Medicine*, *252*(5), 412–420. DOI: 10.1046/j.1365-2796.2002.01051.x PMID: 12528759

Thuemmler, C., & Bai, C. (2017). *Health 4.0: How virtualization and big data are revolutionizing healthcare*. Springer. DOI: 10.1007/978-3-319-47617-9

Vankadara, Y.. (2024). 6G revolution: Redefining communication systems. In *2024 International Conference on Smart Systems for Applications in Electrical Sciences (ICSSES)* (pp. 1–6). IEEE. DOI: 10.1109/ICSSES62373.2024.10561292

Yang, G., Urke, A. R., & Øvsthus, K. (2018, March 22–23). *Mobility support of IoT solution in home care wireless sensor network*. In 2018 Ubiquitous Positioning, Indoor Navigation and Location-Based Services (UPINLBS) (pp. 475–480). IEEE. https://doi.org/DOI: 10.1109/UPINLBS.2018.8559724

Chapter 16
Ethical Considerations in Automated Healthcare

Wasswa Shafik
https://orcid.org/0000-0002-9320-3186
Dig Connectivity Research Laboratory (DCRLab), Uganda & School of Digital Science, Universiti Brunei Darussalam, Brunei

ABSTRACT

Automated healthcare systems, powered by artificial intelligence are revolutionizing medical diagnosis, treatment, and patient care by offering enhanced precision, efficiency, and scalability. However, their deployment raises critical ethical considerations. Issues such as patient privacy, data security, and informed consent are paramount, given the sensitive nature of healthcare data. Bias in algorithms can lead to unequal treatment and exacerbate healthcare disparities, while the lack of transparency and explainability in AI decision-making challenges trust and accountability. Furthermore, determining liability in cases of errors or harm caused by autonomous systems complicates legal and ethical responsibility. The balance between AI autonomy and human oversight is crucial to ensure safety and fairness. As automated healthcare continues to evolve, fostering ethical frameworks that prioritize equity, inclusivity, and patient rights is essential for building systems that enhance health outcomes while maintaining public trust and adherence to societal values.

1. INTRODUCTION

Automated healthcare, a class of automation, is defined by the processes within which we can refer to as medical and healthcare applications supporting patient's medical emotions. Healthcare, in itself, is an act of maintaining and restoring human health through services offered by healthcare professionals (Wasswa, 2025). Although the ultimate goal of a healthcare system is to automate, it excludes those activities regarding clinical and non-clinical roles and services (Prorok & Takacs, 2023). Automation is an action. Automated healthcare includes designing the diagnosing machine, monitoring the patient by machine, and telemedicine. Automation within the healthcare sector in a variety of sectors is being included in the sections below, but for this topic, this text targets mainly the automation of diagnostics and monitoring of patients (S. Kalaivani et al., 2023). Automated healthcare, a multipurpose system, is used in different applications all over the globe. Automated healthcare systems are those systems that

DOI: 10.4018/979-8-3373-1022-0.ch016

are capable of making any clinical or non-clinical medical decision without intervention from human professionals. The increasing change of thought with artificial intelligence and improved technologies has made the systems more efficient and further developed the system now (Göllner & Tropmann-Frick, 2023a).

The main advantages of the techniques are the saving of time and more accurate diagnosis. Automated systems are designed using the following techniques: remote monitoring, alerting systems, automatic diagnosis of diseases, etc. Automated healthcare is the practice of applying computational approaches and tools to support the delivery of medical care, the undertaking of biomedical research, and a range of other applications (Ramanathan et al., 2023). Automated healthcare is increasingly being used across health and care systems. Advanced computer systems now have the capabilities to produce diagnostic decisions and advise on the course of treatment as well as the monitoring of treatment response for a range of disorders and illnesses. In many instances, these systems are now providing an acceptable level of performance (Shafik, 2024g). The style and configuration in the approach to automated healthcare systems implementations have many advantages and positive outcomes for delivering large-scale analysis and highly consistent viewpoints. However, the technology also has several underlying issues or limitations as well as ethical considerations that cause resistance and hesitancies by both professionals and end-users (Babu et al., 2023).

Recent years have seen the expansion of what is often referred to as 'automated healthcare.' While there exists neither a unique nor a clear definition of this widespread phenomenon, we will here refer to healthcare automation as the use of technological resources with autonomous developing capabilities and some sense-making abilities in order to make complex tasks in healthcare easier (Monlezun, 2023a). Robotic surgery, artificially intelligent diagnosis algorithms, or machine learning-based personalized therapy regimens are all examples of healthcare automation (Nneka et al., 2024). Often, automated healthcare does not fully replace human work when making decisions regarding healthcare but rather becomes a part of healthcare systems, enabling clinicians to assess a certain health concern more reliably or introducing administrative tools to facilitate more effective patient management, using enabling technologies as sampled in Figure 1 (Shafik, 2024i, 2024m).

Figure 1. Healthcare enabling technologies

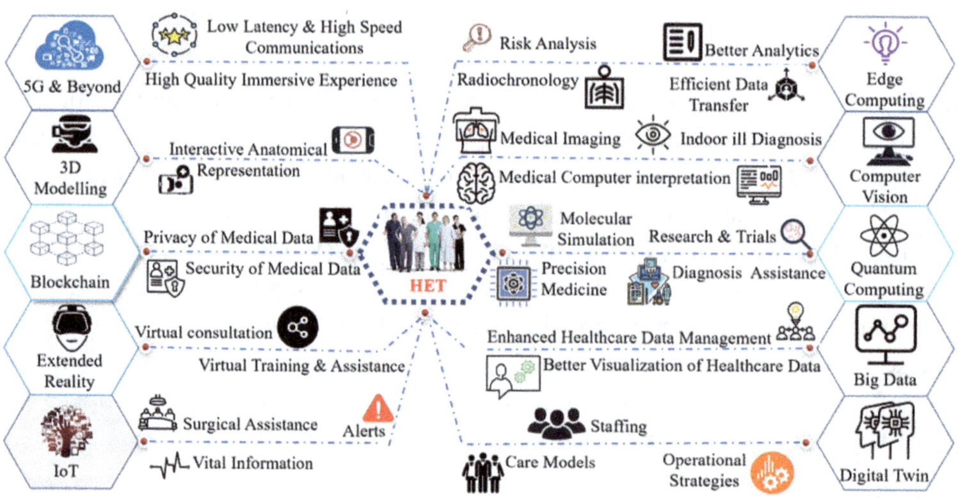

We distinguish two main automatons in healthcare. Caring automatons, such as assisted or rehabilitative robots or conversational agents like chatbots, all directly inscribe in or supplement the process of patient care. The second group comprises administrative automatons, which are healthcare algorithms or rules managing patient data or patient flow in the hospital, earmarking or automatic scheduling of specific diagnostic or therapeutic procedures for individuals, managing health savings accounts, or in silico predictive scoring systems, optimizing operations and patient flow within a healthcare enterprise (Di Nuovo, 2024). Throughout this chapter, we use automated healthcare or healthcare automation to refer to both automatic developments in patient care and administrative automation. The introduction of automated healthcare, either in patient care or at a more administrative level, impacts the healthcare enterprise as a whole, as reliance on algorithms influences the behavior of the professionals in this enterprise and, more importantly, impacts the patient-care relationship (Petersson et al., 2023). This view extends beyond well-established technological considerations of automated healthcare and allows us to begin to delineate a set of ethical challenges that may accompany fully realizing the potential of these technologies as they continue to develop (Monlezun, 2023b).

Automated healthcare offers several strengths over traditional care. One significant advantage is improving the quality of healthcare. Existing work shows that an AI model can achieve over 90% accuracy for diagnostic problems like breast cancer. In healthcare, even if human experts diagnose less accurately than the AI model, its supplementary diagnostic process can enhance diagnosis (Shafik, 2025k, 2025i; Shafik & Kalinaki, 2024; Su et al., 2024). Monitoring patients using AI can be much more real-time, predict further complications, and increase the probability of disease control, limiting adverse results (Stylianides et al., 2023). Additionally, AI can provide factual and data-driven information that is difficult to quantify, such as emotional instability. Generally, AI promises to provide high quality and accuracy in therapeutic and healthcare delivery. Another advantage of automated healthcare is that it is built on the promotion of effectiveness. Automated healthcare can increase the productivity of medical checkups and earlier detection, further boosting healthcare's effectiveness. Reducing the diagnostic process and administration investment can increase the number of patients receiving a medical diagnosis earlier before complications arise (Bellucci & Michele, 2023). Last but not least, the outcome of automating service and care in healthcare nurtures a more innovative care delivery structure, aiding in health-related challenges at home. Balancing the advantages, there are also some challenges in automated healthcare technology. One of the limitations is the lack of transparency; unreliable AI can produce damaging effects. There is a prospect for health inequality, given that the cost of implementing AI can vary significantly between high-end hospitals (Mooghali et al., 2023). The AI strategy can be readily dispensable and reused in underprivileged societies, and the technique needs to have a human-centric method that thoroughly considers the outcomes. Negative effects of improper implementation of AI in healthcare include autonomation, reduction of efficient care at scale for chronic diseases, and an outlier response with a proportion of the population not impacted. Automated healthcare can also induce ethical concerns regarding patient autonomy, as patient data is made available and integrated through health systems, potentially reducing the privacy of patients (Morpurgo & Occhipinti, 2023). In addition, the automated system is expected to cause liability problems, as developers may not be held accountable if their product does not work as planned. The efficiency of the fulfillment, psychological status of the above problems, responsibility, and regulations must be considered. In light of the advantages above and disadvantages, implementing automated healthcare systems should be done carefully, with compliance to ethical frameworks, because the possible dangers are significant when integrating responsibility for health (Fukizi, 2023).

2. BENEFITS AND CHALLENGES OF AUTOMATION IN HEALTHCARE

Automated healthcare promises substantial efficiency gains for highly labor-intensive processes. Reductions in clinical workloads and potential bureaucratic overhead could save professionals valuable time while also potentially reducing the costs of delivering healthcare services (Qin et al., 2024; Wang et al., 2024). In addition, automation could assist in reducing human error and administrative overhead. Automated records could be available for quick consultation, which would be particularly beneficial in emergency care situations (Meszaros et al., 2022; Shafik, 2023). Improved tracking and automation could also improve the efficiency of resource allocation across healthcare systems, using predictive models and machine learning to reduce queuing and waiting times for care. For patients with chronic diseases requiring ongoing medication, diagnostics, and healthcare interventions, automation could assist in improving long-term patient outcomes and reduce the overhead in following up with long-term patients (Aranovich & Matulionyte, 2023; Shafik, 2024p). The proliferation of automation also has a number of potential pitfalls and challenges. The most prominent is the displacement of jobs within the healthcare system, potentially leading to increases in unemployment and the devaluation of traditional healthcare curriculums. This would require non-trivial retraining or upskilling of a significant proportion of the healthcare workforce to adapt to the changing nature of healthcare predicated on automation rather than intervention-based care (Polevikov, 2023; Solanki et al., 2023). Ultimately, technological advancements regularly confront society with ethical dilemmas. In the healthcare system, it draws the line for how much human involvement to include in the build-out of AI in the service of caring for another human (Shafik, 2025e). The nature of this problem is that we seek both a highly innovative, technologically savvy healthcare system that could improve patient well-being by creating a frictionless health service experience and simultaneously is human-centered (Iniesta, 2023; Shafik, Kalinaki, et al., 2024). Automation in the healthcare space presents both opportunities and challenges specific to healthcare delivery.

2.1. Improved Efficiency and Accuracy

Automation has resulted in more efficient healthcare for professionals and patients. Certain technologies allow medical professionals to spend less time on administrative duties and more time interacting directly with their patients. Accessible and easy-to-use scheduling software can streamline the process of booking appointments, allowing the front desk to focus on other pressing tasks (Pourzolfaghar et al., 2023; Shafik, 2024c). Automated check-in kiosks also have the potential to save time and resources. Online, phone and text-based booking has become particularly popular during the pandemic as health providers maximize social distancing measures. Automated transcription tools are another valuable resource that saves time for medical professionals. Not only do they streamline the documentation process, but they are significantly more affordable than traditional human transcription services (Shafik, 2024d; Subasi et al., 2023). Once a patient has been seen, automated prescription systems ensure their medications can be filled without delay. At the diagnostic and treatment level, precision is key. Automated systems interpret statistical data more accurately and are more accurate at diagnosing cancer than their human counterparts. Automated systems also enable physicians to more easily access patient records, pull up images, and more easily access relevant information. This kind of computing power can help healthcare providers make better decisions, enhancing their effectiveness (Monlezun, 2023d; Shafik, 2024o). Statistical data also supports the claim that automated healthcare systems provide better patient outcomes using the current health innovation entities and stakeholders, as illustrated in Figure 2.

Figure 2. Health innovation Entities and Stakeholders

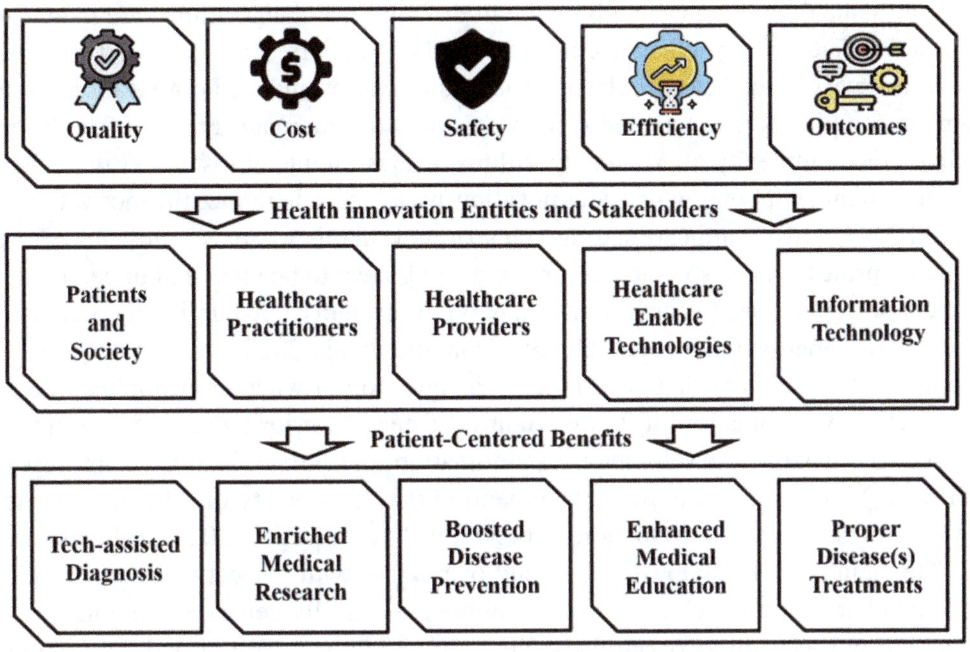

Time savings also provide less tangible benefits, such as less stress on staff. Individuals who do not have to concentrate on individual clerical tasks can engage more with their patients (Shafik, 2024q). The automation of certain healthcare tasks also leads to a safer healthcare environment by reducing human error. Automating predictive systems, checks and balances, and procedures ensures that certain treatment plans do not proceed if established fail-safes are not in place (Monlezun, 2023c; Shafik, Tufail, et al., 2024). If a patient is on a treatment plan that affects their kidneys, an automated system may prevent further treatment if their kidney function has decreased outside of an established safe zone. Evidence suggests that treating patients outside of these standards leads to poor outcomes. Ultimately, automation in healthcare improves efficiency within a system that has historically seen medical professionals overworked (Di Nuovo, 2024; Petersson et al., 2023). As systems are able to process more effective treatments, providing better outcomes for patients, demand for medical professionals may increase in kind. It is worth noting, for ethical considerations, that the biases held by human developers and overseers in the AI process can be perpetuated in any automated system. An ongoing relationship and ongoing human oversight on the part of the physicians is critical in ensuring the accuracy and fairness of automated healthcare processes (Prorok & Takacs, 2023).

2.2. Potential Risks and Ethical Concerns

Robots are used either to assist human professionals or to reduce the burden they carry, which is certainly beneficial. However, what would happen if the system controlling this robot fails during the intervention of a patient? The outcomes might be dramatic and will cost a lot in terms of patient care. In order to avoid such risks, the development of an ethical argument on the implementation of automated healthcare services is necessary (S. Kalaivani et al., 2023). Such an innovation will bring a wide range of ethical issues; moreover, these also include privacy, bias and fairness, transparency, and accountability. In healthcare, the same dilemma may apply to the use of automated algorithms: are patients willing to trade a human-led understanding of their needs for faster, data-supported diagnosis and decision-making? At the heart of the query is the heavily related issue of automation-induced obfuscation, or the practice of concealing the complexity in automated systems (Göllner & Tropmann-Frick, 2023a; Ramanathan et al., 2023). Given the complexity of AI and algorithms, values might get lost under the opaque layer of predictions and recommendations, which does not allow us, as users, to retrace the motivations for certain outputs (Shafik, 2024f). In a healthcare setting, transparency, in this sense, is a must-have for the trust in human healthcare professionals, so practices and reasoning have to be clear and understood. There is a risk that medical personnel may become over-reliant on the systems, outsourcing their decision-making capacities to their automation (Babu et al., 2023; Stylianides et al., 2023).

The ethical line drawing here should be around the question of whether or not health outcomes are negatively impacted by automation. It is important to foster and prioritize human judgment and care (Shafik, 2025f). The balanced development of automation and human healthcare professionals' care is the middle way. Moreover, it is important to mention that the opacity of AI can also impact equity in treatment decisions with the introduction of bias in the data (Treacy, 2023). Ethical concerns with automation. The main concern that arises over and over again with respect to automation is related to the so-called 'data barrier' in which a significant number of serially generated patient records convert the care instead of a direct link between the patient and the human care provider, into an exercise to extract similar information so that other data can be compared and aggregated (Sakhare et al., 2023). From a different angle, unlike the numerous potential practical applications for AI in healthcare, there is also a significant threat of wide-scale, catastrophic data breaches. Concerns have also been raised about the significant amount of data that is collected, how it is used, and the security of these systems from internal subversion and external hacking (Alexandropoulou et al., 2023). A major criticism of the relentless drive to create an autonomous and data-driven framework model for healthcare is that not all valuable patient care outcomes can be measured and understood only through the clinical domain of personalized medicine, nor should they be automated so they can be rendered obsolete in the face of such heights and mergers (Monlezun, 2023a). In a 'treating like' environment, the full diversity and potential offered by humanity and innovation will be lost, and the argument that personalized data-driven care and recommendation systems rely on the average can be but a step away. Wariness is therefore required, especially on our part as experts in the field, with individual responsibility embraced in the way they use these emerging technologies (Göllner & Tropmann-Frick, 2023b).

3. KEY ETHICAL PRINCIPLES IN HEALTHCARE AUTOMATION

Beneficence and non-maleficence represent the commitment of healthcare providers and researchers to benefit patients and avoid harm. Whether physical, psychological, or social, technologies from a variety of domains designed for use in healthcare contexts should add value to or not negatively impact these domains. In automated decision-making, potential harms must be properly managed, particularly if patients are expected to commit to automated decisions (Monlezun, 2023d). The principle of autonomy emphasizes the importance of patient's informed consent and the right to respect their choices. Automation has the potential to herald qualitative changes in patient autonomy, which may be seen as either enhancing or impeding. The membership principle of beneficence and non-maleficence may place a prima facie obligation to value equity independent of patient choice (Walsh et al., 2023). Nonetheless, such respect can be limited if machines are expected to encourage public health behavior and thus may have a duty to be effective rather than fair in design and application. The requirement to respect autonomy would still have to be upheld, as people must not be forced into making lifestyle changes. According to the law, healthcare providers, researchers, and developers should respect patient decisions to refuse necessary care. For example, devices that enable home hemodialysis can be used without supervision by healthcare professionals (Morpurgo & Occhipinti, 2023). These patients are trusting the technology, as well as themselves, with life and death decisions. By understanding the ethics of automation in healthcare, it becomes possible better to appreciate the relationship between ethical issues and accountability, although further research is needed to identify the nuances of design, development, and policy responses. Case studies are useful tools as they provide real-world examples that can enhance understanding by translating ethical concepts into practice (Monlezun, 2023c).

3.1. Beneficence and non-maleficence

Beneficence, the moral imperative to promote others' well-being, plays directly into the ethical justification of implementing new technologies in healthcare, especially if they involve some form of intervention (Shafik, 2024h). As an example, in the realm of automated interventions to arrive at a personalized chronic disease management plan, if a patient is successfully treated and progresses satisfactorily, it could be claimed that the automated care process may bring about good health outcomes in alignment with the principle of beneficence (Karpova, 2023). In the automated healthcare process example given, it can be assumed that the primary aim of this technological advancement is to ultimately benefit the patient, i.e., make them better, which makes this principle quite relevant. Non-maleficence, or the obligation to not inflict harm, is a significant requirement in the biomedical field (Shafik, 2025c). This is particularly true when a novel technology or process is being brought into operative scenarios. The ethical consideration comes in when one is confronted with the possible negative side effects of the technology or intervention (Fukizi, 2023). In automated healthcare, non-maleficence is raised as a potential loss of patient autonomy by an over-reliance on or overconfidence in the advice of an automated system. It also has to do with the integration of the technology within existing healthcare systems and mechanisms. This receptivity of the technology and its potential effect on patients can be evaluated in a live healthcare environment. These principles have been chosen to frame the ethical discourse for automating healthcare, as they epitomize the ethical concerns typically raised by the introduction of any innovation (Mooghali et al., 2023). They also provide an interpretation point for ethical analysis of healthcare practice.

3.2. Autonomy and Informed Consent

Autonomy is a fundamental principle in healthcare ethics and is usually expressed through the need for informed consent. The principle of autonomy reflects the right of patients to have information about their health, options for treatment, and the ability to make decisions based on that information. In the world of automated healthcare, the concept of informed consent continues to exist. However, the process of obtaining this can change with automation (Subasi et al., 2023). The process of sharing information remains the same in written consent processes, but there typically is no in-person conversation about the options and no possibility for the patient to ask questions to clarify information. A general requirement for consent is that individuals understand the information being presented. Informed consent relies on this notion. However, in practice, comprehending complex algorithms is difficult for patients (Tidjon & Khomh, 2023). In healthcare, the difficulty becomes exacerbated because comprehension becomes synonymous with understanding why the algorithm was used, as patients like to understand why decisions are being made. It is, therefore, extremely important that healthcare providers communicate clearly that not only is an automated tool being used but that the patient has the right to either consent to its use or not (Alahmed et al., 2023). The concept of informed consent is particularly important in healthcare because clinicians are entrusted with power, and patients may not challenge that power by asking questions. This is why healthcare professionals need to explain the tool and its capabilities, but very importantly also its limitations, to prevent any confusion regarding trust. Typically, healthcare professionals trust these tools and their results more than a standard patient would, forcing biases in interpretation. Overall, upholding patient autonomy in healthcare processes is an ethical requirement (Petersson et al., 2023). Additionally, when collecting consent in research, this should be done in such a way that all patients can understand and make their own decisions irrespective of intelligence level, background, or other inherent characteristics (Shafik, 2025l). The principle of autonomy is further entrenched in the recommendation that patients should remain informed and make the decision on consent continuously rather than simply at the initiation of the automation process and sustainable practices, as illustrated in Figure 3 (Aranovich & Matulionyte, 2023).

Figure 3. Sustainable practices

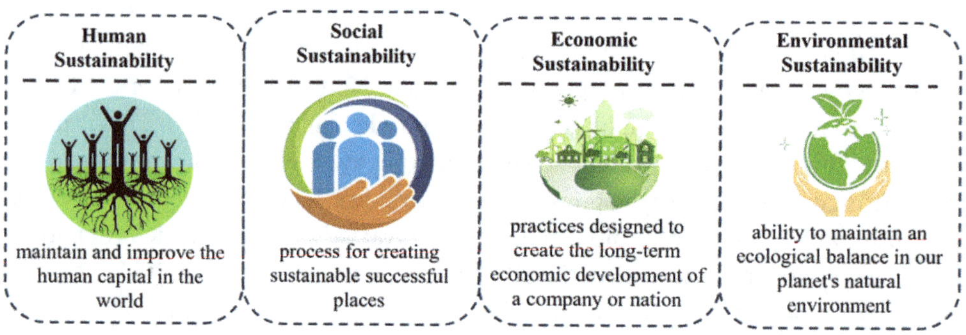
Human Sustainability
maintain and improve the human capital in the world
Social Sustainability
process for creating sustainable successful places
Economic Sustainability
practices designed to create the long-term economic development of a company or nation
Environmental Sustainability
ability to maintain an ecological balance in our planet's natural environment

4. ETHICAL FRAMEWORKS IN HEALTHCARE

Ethical Crosswalks in Automated Healthcare. Considering the ethical frameworks relevant to automated healthcare practice is crucial for identifying potential dilemmas or objections to such systems. These approaches to making ethical decisions add subtle dimensions to institutions' and practitioners' decisions regarding their compliance with current healthcare standards. The most commonly cited approach to ethical decision-making is called principlism, rooted in four major ethical considerations (Khan & Alamäki, 2023). These are reverence for autonomy (agreeing that with full understanding, competent adults are best equipped to make their own health decisions), beneficence (obligation to promote maximal possible benefit), non-maleficence (obligation to avoid any element of harm), and justice (often interpreted as impartiality) (Ramanayake et al., 2023). Alternatively, a system called utilitarianism operates where the acceptable answer to any ethical dilemma is the one that increases the overall happiness of the population. The major problem experienced when applying utilitarian ethical rules to healthcare decision-making is the suppression of individual patients' rights to a favorable outcome (Shafik, 2024l). Finally, virtue ethics proposes that, in making an ethical decision, the most important thing to do is to act like a good person. These ethos-compliant decisions are reflective of the decision-makers image of moral intelligence and wholism (Polevikov, 2023). The ethical frameworks presented offer differing perspectives on the complexities of ethical conduct. The most comprehensive of these, in this particular instance, is the use of principlism, which will form the foundation for our further discussion (Monlezun, 2023b). The strengths and weaknesses of these ethical frameworks show that principlism does not provide any true advantages or profundity associated with its theorization used within medical ethics. Virtue ethics, on the other hand, focuses on the person commissioning the act and stresses the responsibilities involved with an agent or character. This addresses what kind of person should execute medical procedures and their moral attributes (Iniesta, 2023).

4.1. Principlism

The principlist approach consists of using the four fundamental principles as a guide for decision-making around healthcare. It is the most widely recognized ethical framework in healthcare. The four foundational principles are autonomy, beneficence, non-maleficence, and justice. Autonomy refers to respecting the individual patient's right to self-determination, including giving or withholding informed consent (Meszaros et al., 2022). According to the literal interpretation of the principle of autonomy, informed consent by autonomous patients is required, and automated care should be part of the informed consent obtained from the patient. Beneficence obliges practitioners to do good for patients, while non-maleficence obliges practitioners not to inflict any harm. In automated care, one must strive for technological solutions that are good for the patient and do no harm; hence, they should not only avoid negative effects but actually have positive effects (Sharma et al., 2023; L. Singh, 2022). Justice is, in the first instance, about equitable distribution of accountability. Automated care should, in an equitable way, inform all involved about the possibilities of care automation, the decisions being made by the software, and the persons and organizations that are accountable. Furthermore, justice also implies that everyone should have access to the benefits of automated healthcare and that the burdens of the possible negative side effects are divided fairly (Nasir et al., 2024). In addition to autonomy, non-maleficence, and beneficence also lead to ethical constraints, obligations, and responsibilities for technological solutions. Indeed, in light of these principles, it is clear that technology should offer an appropriate level of care quality and not harm or exploit the patient. By analyzing the tenability of the use of the four principles and the universal norms, it is clear what principles and norms guide responsible practices in care and preferably also in the implementation of care by technology (Plummer, 2024). In the above section, we argued that autonomy stands in a significant relationship to automation. Up to today, care needs a fundamental degree of human involvement both on the part of the patient and on the part of the healthcare provider (Shafik, 2025m). However, new technologies in e-health care are a challenge to these well-known principles in bioethical as well as medical debates. When we follow a micro-ethical approach, i.e., the interrelations between the doctor and the patient, we can ask several questions on the basis of the principle of non-maleficence (Khalifa & Albadawy, 2024).

4.2. Utilitarianism

There are various normative ethical theories, each prescribing its criteria on how a moral decision should be made. Therefore, these ethical theories imply different considerations in terms of achieving the greatest good for people or the promotion of an individual's interest. The first moral theory is utilitarianism, which adopts the principle of 'the greatest good for the greatest number.' In following this act consequentialist paradigm, the central focus in deciding what is right is grounded in considerations of aggregated outcomes or harms (Alahmed et al., 2023; Tidjon & Khomh, 2023). Utilitarianism can guide decisions in a variety of ways, depending on the nature of the ethical question being asked and the framework applied. In terms of automated healthcare, it is a normative theory that can guide the decision-making of automated interventions in collective outcomes and growing concern with fairness (Shafik, 2025g). It is placed at the endpoints of justice and beneficence, whereby the outcomes of automated interventions perpetrate justice through efficiency and distress in the population (Petersson et al., 2023). Therefore, the main consideration of the utilitarianism framework is the utilitarian mandate, which emphasizes the assessment of benefits and harms in deciding the right implicit or explicit actions through three main factors: namely, who is affected, what types of benefits, and the general effects of benefits and harms. In this context, utilitarianism orients the technology away from thinking about individual considerations and duties toward a larger public good perspective (Aranovich & Matulionyte, 2023). In addition, utilitarianism normatively legitimizes automated interventions by suggesting that algorithmic decisions must promote the greatest benefits in light of the greatest contributors of pain: the benefit of the many in light of the cost to the few. In other words, it places lesser importance upon the harmful results to a few individuals under a promise of the greatest good that every individual may operate or benefit from streamlined care processes, removing subjectivity and maximizing the fairness of considering outcomes. Otherwise, how could one balance the potential public health benefits that could flow from workforce regulations concerning health professionals and longer working hours with such potential restrictions on their rights to work and make a living (Bellucci & Michele, 2023; Khan & Alamäki, 2023)?

4.3. Virtue Ethics

An ethical theory that focuses on the character traits of individuals. As a profession, healthcare is characterized by certain virtues, such as compassion, which are necessary to maintain an ethical attitude when performing care work. Individuals who possess the virtues fitting for their profession enable the realization of good care for their patients (S. Kalaivani et al., 2023). In healthcare, integrity, accountability, beneficence, compassion, empathy, and professional and personal responsibility are emphasized as the moral virtues required for the professional practice of care ethics. Automated healthcare should aim to enhance the development and exercise of these virtues by healthcare professionals and not allow these challenging and humane virtues to deteriorate (Ramanathan et al., 2023). Human judgment is necessary for a healthcare process in which the virtues of caregivers may shed light on and reinforce each other. It is uncertain how the implementation or use of automated healthcare processes may contribute to these virtues. Automated systems may relieve healthcare professionals of tiresome tasks so that they have more time for genuine human contact with the patient (R. Singh et al., 2024). Automated healthcare could enhance professionalism by supporting healthcare professionals in making the best decisions with respect to each individual patient, as the system is based on more detailed and complex information than those professionals have (S. Kalaivani et al., 2023).

On the other hand, the use of technology in healthcare poses challenges to the virtues. First, the call for efficiency could overshadow the virtue of compassion and empathy, as efficiency does not allow for the moral sentiment of resentment. The healthcare professional has the choice to be resentful about the inefficiency of the healthcare process, but automation may cause resentment to become a moral default. Other professionals may think highly of professionals who take over these tiresome responsibilities from other professionals, while it is supposed to belong to the job of every professional (Babu et al., 2023). Third, a technology that restrains empathy hampers the self-realization and well-being of the professional. If professionals can do hardly anything but keep the patient going and sometimes cause suffering due to the maze of technology that most of the time they do not understand, they might suffer in their professional integrity (Shafik, 2024b). Automated healthcare should aim for a more humane and safer healthcare by enhancing virtues, also when reasonable human resistance against standardization is taken into account (Alexandropoulou et al., 2023; Sakhare et al., 2023). Requiring certain humane virtues from healthcare professionals and processes that enable these virtues fosters an atmosphere of trust, respect, and appreciation. Because virtue ethics is a process-oriented ethics, it might help in guiding the conduct of healthcare professionals with regard to the use of automated technology such that it prevents dehumanizing victimization of patients and the gradual loss of humane advantages that are important in good care. Similar to the sections mentioned above, virtue ethics raises the question of the humanization of care. How can we ensure that automated healthcare yields the best possible (Fukizi, 2023)? In other words, how should we act virtuously as developers or users of automated technology in healthcare?

5. ETHICAL ISSUES IN AUTOMATED HEALTHCARE

The introduction of automated healthcare solutions raises various challenges from an ethics perspective. Here, we discuss the main ethical issues in the field and propose how they can be addressed. The key issue of data privacy and security is complemented by problems related to bias and informed consent (Shafik, 2024k). The discussion of the ethics of data privacy and security highlights the potential negative consequences for trust in an automated healthcare system, raising the need for a clear and widely accepted security strategy (Meszaros et al., 2022). Data in automated healthcare contain information on the history, current condition, and clinical outcomes of patients, but also about the limitations and operational requirements of the equipment used for generating the data. This concerns digital data as well as imaging data from modalities such as magnetic resonance imaging, X-ray computed tomography, and ultrasound. Instead of a system security perspective, one can approach the challenge from a patient data angle, which includes data protection and data security (Arbelaez Ossa et al., 2024; Nasir et al., 2024). Harm can occur—not only the misuse of patient data, but also if the data are accurate, the system providing automated healthcare allows, does not allow, or overrules providing care in the physical care context. Furthermore, to allow decisions that concern therapeutic measures, the patient offer, seeking informed consent from patients to use automated healthcare is necessary (Shafik, 2025h). Currently, it may be idiosyncratic and unethical to decide on automated healthcare measures for patients without their consent (Fukizi, 2023). Patients need to be informed on limitations of decision-making and the advantages and disadvantages of the system they agree to when seeking care. Patients need sufficient understanding and teach-back to staff tutors or explain the system content in their own words. If every form of patient understanding of the system content is insufficient, then it should be remediated before consent is sought. Staff needs to use their clinical expertise to determine whether the overall understanding is sufficient (Babu et al., 2023; Stylianides et al., 2023).

5.1. Data Privacy and Security

With the substantial technological advancements in medicine, the healthcare industry has seen a significant increase in the automation of various tasks. Examples of automated healthcare systems include the presence of virtual doctors, which use expert systems to provide patient-specific medical advice and treatment, smart health and fitness tracking applications, and machine learning-based diagnosis and predictions (Prorok & Takacs, 2023). For automated healthcare systems to be deployed and used effectively, several ethical considerations of these systems must be explored and addressed. One of these ethical considerations is the impact that these automated healthcare systems have on patients' privacy and data security. In this section, we discuss and consider this topic in detail as ealier detailed in (Shafik, 2025j). Data privacy and security are critical areas of ethical concern with healthcare systems and institutions (Göllner & Tropmann-Frick, 2023a). Healthcare data, in electronic form, is not only very sensitive in nature, as it contains patients' identification and treatment data that, if leaked, could lead to embarrassment, discrimination, and social taboos, which can be a threat to society as a whole. Additionally, because of the importance of healthcare services, it can lead to bodily harm, mental suffering, loss of reputation, loss of jobs, and even financial damages (Sakhare et al., 2023; Treacy, 2023; Göllner & Tropmann-Frick, 2023b; Monlezun, 2023a).

5.2. Algorithmic Bias

For all the potential that automated healthcare holds, critics have raised concerns about different ethical problems, including algorithmic bias. If machines learn from biased data, the decisions they make can perpetuate or even exacerbate existing disparities. This has wide-reaching ethical implications. Moreover, it highlights the need for healthcare providers to be transparent about their use of automated decision-making systems (Walsh et al., 2023). Engineers may not be aware of sources of bias in their systems or may be uncertain about what to do about it. Time pressures and strict guidelines around the sharing of personal and sensitive data could prevent thorough evaluation of these systems by those with the power to change them. Even if all the data that a decision-making system uses is complete and reliable, algorithms can be biased when they are trained on data that is already skewed (Karpova, 2023; Monlezun, 2023c). This can happen when decisions discriminate against individuals who were already systematically overlooked or mistreated in data about a certain area. It is the developers' responsibility to try to make the decision-making process as fair as possible (Shafik, 2025d). Both of these notorious examples show how using biased data can lead to flawed decisions. Policymakers introduced the moderated allocation algorithm without paying attention to its underlying data. No examination of biased data was performed when employers used the algorithm (Mooghali et al., 2023; Subasi et al., 2023). Knowing these two case studies, catching hidden biases in hiring or policing algorithms seems more plausible. Machine learning algorithms, including the use of AI in healthcare, are subject to the principle of 'Garbage in, garbage out.' It is notable that a judgment has taken this principle into consideration. It is impossible to examine all cases where errors in the algorithm do not lead to unjust results. Healthcare providers have the responsibility to be transparent about their use of automated systems, explaining the elements of patient care to which the systems can be applied (Tidjon & Khomh, 2023). Continuous monitoring and evaluation of algorithms are necessary.

5.3. Informed Consent

In healthcare, the ethical principles of autonomy, doing no harm, and justice are chiefly manifested in the requirement for informed consent. One major question in the application of these principles and the duty to obtain informed consent is whether patients understand the implications of having part of their care automated and whether they adhere to the designed pathways and implications (Prorok & Takacs, 2023). Furthermore, the design of such give and take of informed consent may be compromised too, for instance, if systems lack the data to accurately predict outcomes or when there is mutual uncertainty in decision-making. Consequently, the informed consent processes, regulatory and guidance systems should clearly explain all of the above issues in an open and transparent dialogue between provider and patient (Ramanathan et al., 2023). This raises important issues around the complexity, which could limit the standardized understanding by various affected or involved parties from industry to clinical users. Starting points and ideologies of complexity have significant gaps; for example, a complex system constructed upon algorithms yields results, but dealing with stakeholders requires human judgment and a degree of enlightening communication. A further issue is the variability of the technology and clinical area, which puts a barrier in a blanket approach to best practice guidelines (Babu et al., 2023; Stylianides et al., 2023). Initial evidence may show how autonomic systems still mostly perform in non-decision support for downstream processes of clinical intervention. However, this technology will continually evolve in breadth of service and more integrative intertwines with model development for acute clinical care (Shafik, 2024e). Additionally, as autonomous technology closes the gaps of uncertainty, the consenting process may become more formalized due to transparency being more assured. On the contrary, under this logical pursuit, the empirical evidence which may show that autonomous technology can handle classical cases may therefore inhibit the chase to address the challenges (Monlezun, 2023a). The discussion above is a snapshot of the hurdles for ethically managing informed consent and consenting processes. Not implementing processes that can adequately handle the ethical concerns of designing autonomous or automated systems may lead to these machines being perceived as upholding negligent practices. As such, it is important to keep patient autonomy at the heart of the operations, keep the dialogue open and honest, and retain trust in autonomy, thereby reinforcing the pledge on duty of care and clinical responsibility (Göllner & Tropmann-Frick, 2023a; Prorok & Takacs, 2023).

5.4. Transparency and Accountability in Automated Healthcare Systems

In discussions of machine learning and AI in medicine, transparency in automated systems is often portrayed as vital for building trust: patients and healthcare providers need to understand and accept the judgments made by the decision-support systems they use (Wasswa Shafik, 2024). In a clinical setting, a certain level of understanding of the functioning of an algorithm needs to exist if there is to be a constructive assessment of its outcomes. An essential part of understanding is the why behind a decision and its consequences for treatment (Babu et al., 2023). Providing an ethical hypercare approach to build a technical fix for ethical rules like non-maleficence after the fact is morally unsound engineering practice (Petersson et al., 2023). Recommendations and guidelines for the introduction and deployment of AI in healthcare underline the need for accountability mechanisms that secure just and responsible outcomes and address the potential needs of stakeholders (Subasi et al., 2023). Technically, many algorithms are difficult to decipher—no input/output functionality description is easily available (Alexandropoulou et al., 2023). Being able to open the so-called "black box" could present an opportunity for technicians and the lay public alike to detect significant ethical shortcomings at an early stage. It is thus important to disclose decision architecture and tools to open black boxes when possible. Transparency fosters discussion and debate and increases both patient and clinician engagement (Göllner & Tropmann-Frick, 2023b). A culture of openness around the development and deployment of algorithms is clearly an important build on standardized, ethically endowed processes. In fact, transparency as the first cornerstone of corporate responsibility refers to a fundamental ethical standard in business ethics, encompassing honesty in sales and overall transparency to improve efficiency and effectiveness in decision-making processes in the context of administrations and HR departments. Transparent algorithms build trust, foster ethical integration, and promote shared values in the use of AI in medicine (Morpurgo & Occhipinti, 2023).

5.5. Bias and Fairness in Automated Healthcare

Bias in algorithms used by automated healthcare systems can reflect or even exacerbate existing inequalities in healthcare, such as when minorities or marginalized patient populations receive lower quality care than wealthier patients. A diagnostic tool that disproportionately fails to diagnose minority patients as needing care could result in those individuals or populations failing to receive the same care as majorities in the population (Fukizi, 2023; Walsh et al., 2023). Automated healthcare may have the potential to reduce the time to treatment, costs, and the variability in human operator outcomes. However, the design of algorithms must carefully consider and correct for underlying biases in healthcare and other systems that the algorithm analyzes. In cases in which algorithms are intended to make treatment recommendations or provide diagnoses, it is paramount that the algorithm's recommendations, regardless of accuracy, are fair and equitable (Prorok & Takacs, 2023).

Fairness, as a value in the allocation of healthcare resources, is generally defined as providing equitable treatment or just outcomes to diverse populations. Automated healthcare systems that are designed to fail more or less often or provide more or less aggressive treatment recommendations when treating persons of differing demographic characteristics may be vulnerable to claims of unfairness (Shafik, 2024j). If a computer algorithm fails to detect a particular form of a disease in older patients at the same rate it fails to detect the disease in younger patients, the result may be that fewer older patients receive treatment, which could bias the older patients' mortality rates compared to what could be expected for younger populations (Babu et al., 2023). Besides being unfair to older patients who are affected by the systemic change, the poor detection rate of older patients leads to kappa paradoxes in those populations. By only collecting data on patients receiving treatment, methodologies that are biased against vulnerable or older populations cannot improve healthcare outcomes or patient experiences. One proxy by which unbiased and fair data can be collected is to over-sample potentially vulnerable health condition states (Sakhare et al., 2023). Algorithmic bias that is unfair and systematically affects the outcomes of health condition states is statistically repairable, and initiatives to promote fairness should also focus on improving health outcomes for those problem conditions. Systematically testing and evaluating algorithms on which populations are adversely affected is a necessary step towards ensuring fair treatment of those patients (Shafik, 2024n, 2024a).

5.6. Data Privacy and Security in Automated Healthcare

Data collected by such systems is highly sensitive, and its unauthorized access can be harmful to patients. It is critical for safety, patient acceptance, and the success of automated healthcare that data privacy and security measures are robust and function effectively (Shafik, 2025b). At a minimum, data must be stored and processed in a way that prevents unauthorized people from accessing it. Since patient data has the highest legal protection, with the expectation of electronic forms requiring it, it is best to proceed under the assumption that no personally identifiable information or protected health information will be collected (S. Kalaivani et al., 2023). The primary goal of health data protection policy is to prevent the disclosure of patient data to third parties who are not authorized to access it. This restrains the data that can be collected in an automated health system to only that which is needed to support the designated functions (Alahmed et al., 2023). In order to ensure that the data is secure and being processed only as intended, all information systems must follow data protection mechanisms and policies that are informed by a basic knowledge of the applicable regulations and their implications. This act exists to ensure that an individual's confidentiality preferences regarding their Electronic Protected Health Information are honored. Automated healthcare systems must adhere to principles of privacy and protection mechanisms in order to engender patient trust and confidence (Göllner & Tropmann-Frick, 2023a).

The potential of any device, including a medical device, to expose patient data to breaches and/or to be accidentally destroyed is driven by several factors. These include, for instance, the feasibility of exploitation by an attacker, the trustworthiness of system components, the security of the software system, sensible defaults for operation, and having system owners follow security practices, such as changing default passwords (Shafik, 2025a). The misuse of patient data by exploited software or hardware is an ethical issue that would be mitigated by accurately assessing the potential vulnerability of the data to loss. It is worth reiterating that remaining ethical with data depends on accurate risk assessment and management, as this is what informs all decisions in the data collection process from the outset (Ramanathan et al., 2023). Nowadays, advanced health systems are designed to help patients have greater control over their own health data. In addition, they can allow patients to monitor their data and make their processor instructions as transparent as possible in order to ensure that they are not misused (Monlezun, 2023b; Polevikov, 2023). In this way, patients will gain trust. Awareness of the need to protect data should result in robust hardware assets with considerable simplicity, making them relatively immune to unforeseen problems. If these issues are comprehensively addressed in system architecture, it is anticipated that a reduction in system complexity will lead to increased system performance and durability (Stylianides et al., 2023). With such considerations in place, healthcare practitioners will be able to ensure that the data they collect is robustly protected, provided that these same considerations are also extended to the software aspects of systems and the broader work that is done by programmers. However, hardware protection is only as good as the protection measures that are implemented to mitigate hacker activity; the two must work in concert in order to maximize healthcare data and therefore patient safety (Sakhare et al., 2023).

6. CONCLUSION

Automated healthcare is increasingly important in modern medical practice. Advances in sensor technology, automation, and machine learning enable the development of specialized and context-aware healthcare devices that have the potential to orchestrate medical intervention for individual patients or entire healthcare systems efficiently. Automation in healthcare holds the promise to optimize the patient's care pathway using granular data and efficient allocation of resources and treatments. Automated healthcare is a fast-changing field, with sensors and medical devices gaining the active capacity to sense various aspects of the human body accurately and over prolonged periods. Some of these devices go beyond sensing to diagnosing disease, characterizing illness, and proposing treatments. Doctors, then, are poised to increasingly delegate to these devices the responsibility for initiating appropriate therapy to optimize patient outcomes. Understanding the ethical implications of this trend is important. Subsequently, what is automation? In modern terms, automation can be defined as the use of control systems and information technologies to both reduce human intervention in technical systems and replace human involvement in systems with the potential to facilitate efficient use of resources and enhanced decision-making. Technological improvements have fostered the emergence of many highly automated devices and information systems. Though the notion of automated systems is over 420 years old, the use of automation has become important only in the past few decades, with the aim of enhancing the reliability of mechanical processes, reducing human workload, and improving system efficiency and safety. In healthcare, automation would enable such mechanical decision pathways and processes, which can currently be loop or open-loop decision making. Automated systems are considered to be an evolution of mechanization.

REFERENCES

Alahmed, Y., Abadla, R., Ameen, N., & Shteiwi, A. (2023). Bridging the Gap Between Ethical AI Implementations. *International Journal of Membrane Science and Technology*, *10*(3), 3034–3046. Advance online publication. DOI: 10.15379/ijmst.v10i3.2953

Alexandropoulou, C. A., Panagiotopoulos, I., Kleanthous, S., Dimitrakopoulos, G., Constantinou, I., Politi, E., Ntalaperas, D., Papageorgiou, X., Stylianides, C., Ioannides, N., Palazis, L., Pattichis, C. S., & Panayides, A. S. (2023). AI-Enabled Solutions, Explainability and Ethical Concerns for Predicting Sepsis in ICUs: A Systematic Review. *Proceedings 2023 IEEE 19th International Conference on E-Science, e-Science 2023*. DOI: 10.1109/e-Science58273.2023.10254863

Aranovich, T. de C., & Matulionyte, R. (2023). Ensuring AI explainability in healthcare: Problems and possible policy solutions. *Information & Communications Technology Law*, *32*(2), 259–275. Advance online publication. DOI: 10.1080/13600834.2022.2146395

Arbelaez Ossa, L., Lorenzini, G., Milford, S. R., Shaw, D., Elger, B. S., & Rost, M. (2024). Integrating ethics in AI development: A qualitative study. *BMC Medical Ethics*, *25*(1), 10. Advance online publication. DOI: 10.1186/s12910-023-01000-0 PMID: 38262986

Babu, C. V. S., Akshayah, N. S., & Vinola, P. M. (2023). Artificial intelligence in healthcare: Assessing impacts, challenges, and recommendations for achieving healthcare independence. In *Perspectives on Artificial Intelligence in Times of Turbulence*. Theoretical Background to Applications., DOI: 10.4018/978-1-6684-9814-9.ch005

Bellucci, B., & Michele, E. (2023). Focusing on the integration of AI in healthcare sector of USA: Focusing on the roles of AI adoption and innovative capabilities. *Journal of Commercial Biotechnology*, *28*(5). Advance online publication. DOI: 10.5912/jcb2142

Di Nuovo, A. (2024). Letter to the Editor: "How Can Biomedical Engineers Help Empower Individuals With Intellectual Disabilities? The Potential Benefits and Challenges of AI Technologies to Support Inclusivity and Transform Lives." In *IEEE Journal of Translational Engineering in Health and Medicine* (Vol. 12). DOI: 10.1109/JTEHM.2023.3331977

Fukizi, K. Y. (2023). Collaborative Decision-Making Assistant for Healthcare Professionals: A Human-Centered AI Prototype Powered by Azure Open AI. *COMPASS 2023 - Proceedings of the ACM SIGCAS/SIGCHI Conference on Computing and Sustainable Societies*. DOI: 10.1145/3588001.3609370

Göllner, S., & Tropmann-Frick, M. (2023a). Bridging the Gap between Theory and Practice: Towards Responsible AI Evaluation. *CEUR Workshop Proceedings*, **•••**, 3580.

Göllner, S., & Tropmann-Frick, M. (2023b). VERIFAI - A Step Towards Evaluating the Responsibility of AI-Systems. *Lecture Notes in Informatics (LNI), Proceedings - Series of the Gesellschaft Fur Informatik (GI), P-331*. DOI: 10.18420/BTW2023-63

Iniesta, R. (2023). The human role to guarantee an ethical AI in healthcare: A five-facts approach. *AI and Ethics*. Advance online publication. DOI: 10.1007/s43681-023-00353-x

Kalaivani, S., Nasreen Banu, D., Parvin Begum, I., & Sivasamy, J. (2023). Cognitive Robotics: Integrating Artificial Intelligence and Embodied Intelligence for Advanced Problem Solving. *Journal of Artificial Intelligence and Capsule Networks*, *5*(4). Advance online publication. DOI: 10.36548/jaicn.2023.4.002

Karpova, E. A. (2023). AI in Health Ethical Review: A Value Design Methodology. *Chelovek*, *34*(3), 129. Advance online publication. DOI: 10.31857/S023620070026109-6

Khalifa, M., & Albadawy, M. (2024). Artificial Intelligence for Clinical Prediction: Exploring Key Domains and Essential Functions. In *Computer Methods and Programs in Biomedicine Update* (Vol. 5). DOI: 10.1016/j.cmpbup.2024.100148

Khan, U. A., & Alamäki, A. (2023). Designing an Ethical and Secure Pain Estimation System Using AI Sandbox for Contactless Healthcare. *International Journal of Online and Biomedical Engineering*, *19*(15), 166–201. Advance online publication. DOI: 10.3991/ijoe.v19i15.43663

Meszaros, J., Minari, J., & Huys, I. (2022). The future regulation of artificial intelligence systems in healthcare services and medical research in the European Union. *Frontiers in Genetics*, *13*, 927721. Advance online publication. DOI: 10.3389/fgene.2022.927721 PMID: 36267404

Monlezun, D. J. (2023a). Chapter 4 - AI+public health: effective and fair collaboration. In *The Thinking Healthcare System.*

Monlezun, D. J. (2023b). Chapter 8 - AI+health ethics: moral interoperability and pluralism. In *The Thinking Healthcare System.*

Monlezun, D. J. (2023c). Chapter 9 - The future's (AI) thinking healthcare system: blueprint, roadmap, and DNA. In *The Thinking Healthcare System.*

Monlezun, D. J. (2023d). The future's (AI) thinking healthcare system. In *The Thinking Healthcare System*. DOI: 10.1016/B978-0-443-18906-7.00008-8

Mooghali, M., Stroud, A. M., Yoo, D. W., & Barry, B. A. & ... (2023). Barriers and Facilitators to Trustworthy and Ethical AI-enabled Medical Care From Patient and Healthcare Provider Perspectives: A Literature Review. *MedRxiv*.

Morpurgo, F., & Occhipinti, C. (2023). Let the AI assisted medicine remain human Developing a care centered model of ethical decision making in AI based healthcare. *CEUR Workshop Proceedings*, •••, 3486.

Nasir, S., Khan, R. A., & Bai, S. (2024). Ethical Framework for Harnessing the Power of AI in Healthcare and Beyond. *IEEE Access : Practical Innovations, Open Solutions*, *12*, 31014–31035. Advance online publication. DOI: 10.1109/ACCESS.2024.3369912

Nneka, O. O., Okafor, K. C., Nwabueze, C. A., Mbachu, C. B., Iloh, J. P., Chinebu, T. I., Adebisi, B., & Chukwunenye Anthony, O. (2024). A computational fractional order model for optimal control of wearable healthcare monitoring devices for maternal health. *Healthcare Analytics*, *5*, 100308. Advance online publication. DOI: 10.1016/j.health.2024.100308

Petersson, L., Vincent, K., Svedberg, P., Nygren, J. M., & Larsson, I. (2023). Ethical Perspectives on Implementing AI to Predict Mortality Risk in Emergency Department Patients: A Qualitative Study. *Studies in Health Technology and Informatics*, *302*. Advance online publication. DOI: 10.3233/SHTI230234 PMID: 37203776

Plummer, D. (2024). Ethical AI and the Future of Healthcare: Combining Academic Theory and Industry Practice to Ensure Patient-Centered Care. *European Journal of Technology*, *8*(1), 1–13. Advance online publication. DOI: 10.47672/ejt.1727

Polevikov, S. (2023). Advancing AI in healthcare: A comprehensive review of best practices. In *Clinica Chimica Acta* (Vol. 548). DOI: 10.1016/j.cca.2023.117519

Pourzolfaghar, Z., Alfano, M., & Helfert, M. (2023). Application of ethical AI requirements to an AI solution use-case in healthcare domain. *American Journal of Business*, *38*(3), 112–128. Advance online publication. DOI: 10.1108/AJB-12-2022-0201

Prorok, M., & Takacs, I. (2023). Legal and Moral Issues Related to Artificial Intelligence Technology in Business. *SISY 2023 - IEEE 21st International Symposium on Intelligent Systems and Informatics, Proceedings*. DOI: 10.1109/SISY60376.2023.10417881

Qin, W. F., Xue, Y., Peng, H., Li, G., Chen, W., Zhao, X., Pang, J., & Zhou, B. (2024). Wearable real-time multi-health parameter monitoring system. *International Journal of Clothing Science and Technology*, *36*(1), 17–33. Advance online publication. DOI: 10.1108/IJCST-04-2023-0054

Ramanathan, A., Vijaya Rani, K. R., Bhupathyraaj, M., Chacko, L., & Alharbi, H. F. (2023). An Ethical Outlook on the Applications of Artificial Intelligence in Medicine and Pharmacy. In *Artificial Intelligence in Pharmaceutical Sciences*. DOI: 10.1201/9781003343981-10

Ramanayake, R., Wicke, P., & Nallur, V. (2023). Immune moral models? Pro-social rule breaking as a moral enhancement approach for ethical AI. *AI & Society*, *38*(2), 801–813. Advance online publication. DOI: 10.1007/s00146-022-01478-z PMID: 35645466

Sakhare, N. N., Limkar, S., Mahadik, R. V., Phursule, R., Godbole, A., Shirkande, S. T., & Patange, A. (2023). Ethical considerations of AI applications in medicine: A policy framework for responsible deployment. In *Journal of Krishna Institute of Medical Sciences University* (Vol. 12, Issue 4).

Shafik, W. (2023). Wearable Medical Electronics in Artificial Intelligence of Medical Things. In *Handbook of Security and Privacy of AI-Enabled Healthcare Systems and Internet of Medical Things*. https://doi.org/DOI: 10.1201/9781003370321-2

Shafik, W. (2024a). 2 Deep Field of Learning Artificial Impacts Intelligence in the. *Deep Learning Concepts in Operations Research*, 9.

Shafik, W. (2024b). Artificial Intelligence and the Medical Tourism. In *Examining Tourist Behaviors and Community Involvement in Destination Rejuvenation* (pp. 207–233). IGI Global. DOI: 10.4018/979-8-3693-6819-0.ch016

Shafik, W. (2024c). Artificial Intelligence-Enabled Internet of Medical Things (AIoMT) in Modern Healthcare Practices. In *Clinical Practice and Unmet Challenges in AI-Enhanced Healthcare Systems* (pp. 42–69). IGI Global. DOI: 10.4018/979-8-3693-2703-6.ch003

Shafik, W. (2024d). Artificial Intelligence-Enabled Internet of Medical Things for Enhanced Healthcare Systems. In *Smart Healthcare Systems* (pp. 119–134). CRC Press., DOI: 10.1201/9781032698519-9

Shafik, W. (2024e). Blockchain's impetus for secure IoT-enabled applications in smart city. In *Big Data and Blockchain Technology for Secure IoT Applications* (pp. 48–71). CRC Press., DOI: 10.1201/9781032663005-4

Shafik, W. (2024f). Community and Artificial Intelligence-Enabled Disaster Management and Preparedness. In *Navigating Natural Hazards in Mountainous Topographies: Exploring the Challenges and Opportunities of Living* (pp. 243–266). Springer. DOI: 10.1007/978-3-031-65862-4_13

Shafik, W. (2024g). Connected healthcare—the impact of Internet of Things on medical services. In *Artificial Intelligence and Internet of Things based Augmented Trends for Data Driven Systems* (pp. 181–217). CRC Press., DOI: 10.1201/9781003497318-10

Shafik, W. (2024h). Consumer. *Advances in Marketing, Customer Relationship Management, and E-Services*, •••, 75–108. DOI: 10.4018/979-8-3693-9122-8.ch004

Shafik, W. (2024i). Digital healthcare systems in a federated learning perspective. In *Federated Learning for Digital Healthcare Systems* (pp. 1–35). Elsevier., DOI: 10.1016/B978-0-443-13897-3.00001-1

Shafik, W. (2024j). Digital healthcare systems in a federated learning perspective. In *Federated Learning for Digital Healthcare Systems* (pp. 1–35). Elsevier. DOI: 10.1016/B978-0-443-13897-3.00001-1

Shafik, W. (2024k). Generative AI for Social Good and Sustainable Development. In *Generative AI: Current Trends and Applications* (pp. 185–217). Springer. DOI: 10.1007/978-981-97-8460-8_10

Shafik, W. (2024l). IoMT Future Trends and Challenges: Emerging Technologies, Policy Implications, and Research Questions. *Lightweight Digital Trust Architectures in the Internet of Medical Things (IoMT)*, 348–370.

Shafik, W. (2024m). IoT-Enabled Secure and Intelligent Smart Healthcare. In *Secure and Intelligent IoT-Enabled Smart Cities* (pp. 308–333). IGI Global., DOI: 10.4018/979-8-3693-2373-1.ch015

Shafik, W. (2024n). Science of Emotional Intelligence. In *Enhancing and Predicting Digital Consumer Behavior with AI* (pp. 284–310). IGI Global. DOI: 10.4018/979-8-3693-4453-8.ch015

Shafik, W. (2024o). Smart Health Revolution: Exploring Artificial Intelligence of Internet of Medical Things. In *Healthcare Industry Assessment: Analyzing Risks, Security, and Reliability* (pp. 201–229). Springer. DOI: 10.1007/978-3-031-65434-3_9

Shafik, W. (2024p). The Future of Healthcare: AIoMT—Redefining Healthcare with Advanced Artificial Intelligence and Machine Learning Techniques. In *Artificial Intelligence and Machine Learning in Drug Design and Development* (pp. 605–634). Wiley., DOI: 10.1002/9781394234196.ch19

Shafik, W. (2024q). Toward a More Ethical Future of Artificial Intelligence and Data Science. In *The Ethical Frontier of AI and Data Analysis* (pp. 362–388). IGI Global., DOI: 10.4018/979-8-3693-2964-1.ch022

Shafik, W. (2025a). Artificial Intelligence Assisted Internet of Medical Things (AIoMTs) in Sustainable Healthcare Ecosystem. *Wellness Management Powered by AI Technologies*, 75–101.

Shafik, W. (2025b). Artificial Intelligence-Enabled Cybersecurity and Internet of Things Applications in Smart Cities. In *Building Tomorrow's Smart Cities With 6G Infrastructure Technology* (pp. 301–334). IGI Global Scientific Publishing.

Shafik, W. (2025c). Digital twins tools and technologies. In *Digital Twins for Smart Cities and Villages* (pp. 55–80). Elsevier., https://doi.org/https://doi.org/10.1016/B978-0-443-28884-5.00003-8 DOI: 10.1016/B978-0-443-28884-5.00003-8

Shafik, W. (2025d). Generative Adversarial Networks: Security, Privacy, and Ethical Considerations. In *Generative Artificial Intelligence (AI) Approaches for Industrial Applications* (pp. 93–117). Springer.

Shafik, W. (2025e). Human-Artificial Intelligence Collaborations in Polycystic Ovary Syndrome (PCOS) Clinical Trials and Research. In *AI-Based Nutritional Intervention in Polycystic Ovary Syndrome (PCOS)* (pp. 307–330). Springer Nature Singapore. DOI: 10.1007/978-981-96-2120-0_13

Shafik, W. (2025f). Introduction to Machine Learning and Its Applications to Neuroscience. In *Machine Learning for Neurodegenerative Disorders* (pp. 1–32). CRC Press., DOI: 10.1201/9781032661025-1

Shafik, W. (2025g). Investigating Generative Artificial Intelligence Readiness in the Internet of Medical Things: Are We Progressing Technologically? In *Convergence of Internet of Medical Things (IoMT) and Generative AI* (pp. 31–58). IGI Global Scientific Publishing.

Shafik, W. (2025h). Quantum Computing and Generative Adversarial Networks (GANs): Ethics, Privacy, and Security. In *Quantum AI and its Applications in Blockchain Technology* (pp. 111–156). IGI Global Scientific Publishing.

Shafik, W. (2025i). Revolutionizing Skin Cancer Diagnosis With Artificial Intelligence: Insights Into Machine Learning Techniques. In *Impact of Digital Solutions for Improved Healthcare Delivery* (pp. 167–194). IGI Global.

Shafik, W. (2025j). Revolutionizing Skin Cancer Diagnosis With Artificial Intelligence: Insights Into Machine Learning Techniques. In *Impact of Digital Solutions for Improved Healthcare Delivery* (pp. 167–194). IGI Global.

Shafik, W. (2025k). Smart biomedical devices for smart healthcare. In *Machine Learning Models and Architectures for Biomedical Signal Processing* (pp. 421–448). Elsevier. DOI: 10.1016/B978-0-443-22158-3.00017-X

Shafik, W. (2025l). Sustainable Agriculture and Diet for Urban Development. In *Sustainable Smart Cities and the Future of Urban Development* (pp. 165–192). IGI Global Scientific Publishing.

Shafik, W. (2025m). Sustainable Agriculture and Diet in the Metaverse Era: Sustainable Farming and Nutritious Eating in the Metaverse. In *Food in the Metaverse and Web 3.0 Era: Intersecting Food, Technology, and Culture* (pp. 159–184). IGI Global Scientific Publishing.

Shafik, W., & Kalinaki, K. (2024). Societal and Ethical Implications of Technology-Enhanced Agriculture and Healthcare: An African Context. *2024 IST-Africa Conference (IST-Africa)*, 1–11. DOI: 10.23919/IST-Africa63983.2024.10569306

Shafik, W., Kalinaki, K., Fahim, K. E., & Adam, M. (2024). Safeguarding Data Privacy and Security in Federated Learning Systems. In *Federated Deep Learning for Healthcare* (pp. 170–190). CRC Press., DOI: 10.1201/9781032694870-13

Shafik, W., Tufail, A., Liyanage, C. D. S., & Apong, R. A. A. H. M. (2024). Medical Robotics and AI-Assisted Diagnostics Challenges for Smart Sustainable Healthcare. In *AI-Driven Innovations in Digital Healthcare: Emerging Trends, Challenges, and Applications* (pp. 304–323). IGI Global. DOI: 10.4018/979-8-3693-3218-4.ch016

Sharma, V., Mishra, N., Kukreja, V., Alkhayyat, A., & Elngar, A. A. (2023). Framework for Evaluating Ethics in AI. *International Conference on Innovative Data Communication Technologies and Application, ICIDCA 2023 - Proceedings*. DOI: 10.1109/ICIDCA56705.2023.10099747

Singh, L. (2022). Automated Kantian Ethics: A Faithful Implementation. *Lecture Notes in Computer Science (Including Subseries Lecture Notes in Artificial Intelligence and Lecture Notes in Bioinformatics), 13404 LNAI*. DOI: 10.1007/978-3-031-15791-2_16

Singh, R., Shafik, W., Crowther, D., & Kumar, V. (Eds.). (2024). *Transforming Healthcare Sector Through Artificial Intelligence and Environmental Sustainability* (1st ed., Vol. 1). Springer Nature Singapore., DOI: 10.1007/978-981-97-9555-0

Solanki, P., Grundy, J., & Hussain, W. (2023). Operationalising ethics in artificial intelligence for healthcare: A framework for AI developers. *AI and Ethics*, *3*(1), 223–240. Advance online publication. DOI: 10.1007/s43681-022-00195-z

Stylianides, C., Alexandropoulou, C. A., Sulaiman, W., Panagiotopoulos, I., Kleanthous, S., Dimitrakopoulos, G., Constantinou, I., Vassiliou, S., Garcia, F., Politi, E., Ntalaperas, D., Papageorgiou, X., Ioannides, N., Palazis, L., Pattichis, C. S., & Panayides, A. S. (2023). AI-based solutions for predicting sepsis in ICUs. *2023 IEEE EMBS Special Topic Conference on Data Science and Engineering in Healthcare, Medicine and Biology, IEEECONF 2023*. DOI: 10.1109/IEEECONF58974.2023.10404309

Su, B., Wang, B., Cao, Y., Dou, H., Zhang, T., & He, X. (2024). A multi-functional flexible piezoresistive sensor based on sericin-functionalized CNTs decorated carbon foams for wearable thermal-therapy devices. *Ceramics International*, *50*(7), 10305–10313. Advance online publication. DOI: 10.1016/j.ceramint.2023.12.342

Subasi, A., Ozaltin, O., Mitra, A., Subasi, M. E., & Sarirete, A. (2023). Trustworthy artificial intelligence in healthcare. In *Accelerating Strategic Changes for Digital Transformation in the Healthcare Industry: Volume 2* (Vol. 2). DOI: 10.1016/B978-0-443-15299-3.00015-4

Tidjon, L. N., & Khomh, F. (2023). The Different Faces of AI Ethics Across the World: A Principle-to-Practice Gap Analysis. *IEEE Transactions on Artificial Intelligence*, *4*(4), 820–839. Advance online publication. DOI: 10.1109/TAI.2022.3225132

Treacy, S. (2023). Mechanisms and Constraints Underpinning Ethically Aligned Artificial Intelligence Systems: An Exploration of Key Performance Areas. *Human-Centric Intelligent Systems*, *3*(3), 189–196. Advance online publication. DOI: 10.1007/s44230-023-00036-0

Walsh, G., Stogiannos, N., van de Venter, R., Rainey, C., Tam, W., McFadden, S., McNulty, J. P., Mekis, N., Lewis, S., O'Regan, T., Kumar, A., Huisman, M., Bisdas, S., Kotter, E., Pinto dos Santos, D., Sá dos Reis, C., van Ooijen, P., Brady, A. P., & Malamateniou, C. (2023). Responsible AI practice and AI education are central to AI implementation: a rapid review for all medical imaging professionals in Europe. *BJR|Open, 5*(1). DOI: 10.1259/bjro.20230033

Wang, C., Wang, Z., Guan, W., Wang, W., Xu, L., Li, L., Huang, S., & Wang, W. (2024). Trustworthy Health Monitoring Based on Distributed Wearable Electronics With Edge Intelligence. *IEEE Transactions on Consumer Electronics*, *70*(1), 2333–2341. Advance online publication. DOI: 10.1109/TCE.2024.3358803

Wasswa, S. (2025). The Role of Emotional Intelligence in Career Development and Career Success. In K. D. Pushan, G. Sachin, K. Shafali, G. Anita, Rita Karmakar, & Pronaya Bhattacharya (Eds.), *Emotional Intelligence in the Digital Era: Concepts, Frameworks, and Applications* (1st ed., Vol. 1, pp. 108–128). Taylor & Francis Group. DOI: 10.1201/9781032715377-7

Wasswa Shafik. (2024). Challenges and Future Prospectives of Ultrasound-Assisted Extraction. In Bancha Yingngam, M. S. A. (Ed.), *Ultrasound Assisted Extraction: Methods and Applications* (1st ed., Vol. 1). Nova, Science and Technology.

Compilation of References

3GPP. (2017). *Study on scenarios and requirements for next generation access technologies* (3GPP TR 38.913 V14.2.0). https://www.3gpp.org/DynaReport/38913.htm

Abatal, A., Mzili, M., Mzili, T., Cherrat, K., Yassine, A., & Abualigah, L. (2024). Intelligent Interconnected Healthcare System: Integrating IoT and Big Data for Personalized Patient Care. *International Journal of Online & Biomedical Engineering*, *20*(11), 46–65. DOI: 10.3991/ijoe.v20i11.49893

Abbasi, N., Nizamullah, F. N. U., & Zeb, S. (2023). AI in healthcare: Integrating advanced technologies with traditional practices for enhanced patient care. *BULLET: Jurnal Multidisiplin Ilmu*, *2*(3), 546–556.

Abbas, S. R., Abbas, Z., Zahir, A., & Lee, S. W. (2024). Federated Learning in Smart Healthcare: A Comprehensive Review on Privacy, Security, and Predictive Analytics with IoT Integration. *Health Care*, *12*(24), 2587. PMID: 39766014

Abdellatif, A. A., Samara, L., Mohamed, A., Erbad, A., Chiasserini, C. F., Guizani, M., O'Connor, M. D., & Laughton, J. (2021). MEdge-Chain: Leveraging Edge Computing and Blockchain for Efficient Medical Data Exchange. *IEEE Internet of Things Journal*, *8*(21), 15762–15775. DOI: 10.1109/JIOT.2021.3052910

Abdulmalek, S., Nasir, A., Jabbar, W. A., Almuhaya, M. A. M., Bairagi, A. K., Md, A. M. K., & Kee, S. H. (2022). IoT-Based Healthcare-Monitoring System towards Improving Quality of Life: A Review. *Healthcare (Basel)*, *10*(10), 1993. Advance online publication. DOI: 10.3390/healthcare10101993 PMID: 36292441

Abràmoff, M. D., Tarver, M. E., Loyo-Berrios, N., Trujillo, S., Char, D., Obermeyer, Z., Eydelman, M. B., & Maisel, W. H. (2023). Considerations for addressing bias in artificial intelligence for health equity. npj. *Digital Medicine*, *6*(1), 170. DOI: 10.1038/s41746-023-00913-9 PMID: 37700029

Adenekan, T. K. (2024). *AI-Driven Diagnostic Models for Cardiovascular Health: Exploring Security and Business Analytics in Aortic Stenosis Detection*. ResearchGate.

Adeniyi, A. E., Awokola, J. A., Alam, S., Bharany, S., Agboola, P., Shuaib, M., & Ahmed, R. (2023). A Hybrid Framework of Blockchain and IoT Technology in the Pharmaceutical Industry: A Comprehensive Study. In *Mobile Information Systems* (Vol. 2023). DOI: 10.1155/2023/3265310

Agali, K., Masrom, M., Abdul Rahim, F., & Yahya, Y. (2024). IoT-based remote monitoring system: A new era for patient engagement. *Healthcare Technology Letters*, *11*(6), 437–446. DOI: 10.1049/htl2.12089 PMID: 39720747

Agrawal, R., & Poovaiah, R. (2021). CoSpeak: Peer Feedback on Voice Stories to Inform Learning Spoken English. *Companion Publication of the 2021 Conference on Computer Supported Cooperative Work and Social Computing*, 1–4. DOI: 10.1145/3462204.3481750

Ahad, A., Tahir, M., & Yau, K. L. A. (2019). 5G-based smart healthcare network: Architecture, taxonomy, challenges and future research directions. *IEEE Access : Practical Innovations, Open Solutions*, *7*, 100747–100762. DOI: 10.1109/ACCESS.2019.2930628

Ahmed, M., Hassan, H., Eldeeb, A., & Khattab, T. (2023). Towards Contactless Remote Health Monitoring using Ambient RF Sensing. *2023 21st Mediterranean Communication and Computer Networking Conference (MedComNet)*, 135–142.

Ahmed, S. S. T., Thanuja, K., Guptha, N. S., & Narasimha, S. (2016, January). Telemedicine approach for remote patient monitoring system using smart phones with an economical hardware kit. In 2016 international conference on computing technologies and intelligent data engineering (ICCTIDE'16) (pp. 1-4). IEEE.

Ahmed, M. U., Begum, S., & Funk, P. (2016). Artificial intelligence in health and medicine: Where do we stand? *International Journal of Medical Informatics*, *84*(1), 74–86.

Ahmed, S., & Cho, S. H. (2023). Machine learning for healthcare radars: Recent progresses in human vital sign measurement and activity recognition. *IEEE Communications Surveys and Tutorials*, *26*(1), 461–495. DOI: 10.1109/COMST.2023.3334269

Aileni, R. M., Suciu, G., Valderrama Sukuyama, C. A., & Pasca, S. (2020). Internet of Things and communication technology synergy for remote services in healthcare. *IoT and ICT for Healthcare Applications*, 59–82.

Ajazmoharkan, Z., Choudhury, T., Gupta, S. C., & Raj, G. 2017. "Internet of Things and Its Applications in E-Learning." *3rd IEEE International Conference On* 10(1):447–52. DOI: 10.1109/CIACT.2017.7977333

Akhter, N. (2023).. . *Harnessing IOT and Artificial Intelligence for Sustainable Healthcare.*, (March). Advance online publication. DOI: 10.25215/138757678X.35

Al Kuwaiti, A., Nazer, K., Al-Reedy, A., Al-Shehri, S., Al-Muhanna, A., Subbarayalu, A. V., Al Muhanna, D., & Al-Muhanna, F. A. (2023). A Review of the Role of Artificial Intelligence in Healthcare. *Journal of Personalized Medicine*, *13*(6), 1–22. DOI: 10.3390/jpm13060951 PMID: 37373940

Alahi, E. E., Sukkuea, A., Tina, F. W., Nag, A., Kurdthongmee, W., Suwannarat, K., & Mukhopadhyay, S. C. 2023. "Integration of IoT-Enabled Technologies and Artificial Advancements and Future Trends." *Sensors (Switzerland)* 23(5206).

Alahmed, Y., Abadla, R., Ameen, N., & Shteiwi, A. (2023). Bridging the Gap Between Ethical AI Implementations. *International Journal of Membrane Science and Technology*, *10*(3), 3034–3046. Advance online publication. DOI: 10.15379/ijmst.v10i3.2953

Alam, S. (2023, February). Security concerns in smart agriculture and blockchain-based solution. In 2022 OPJU international technology conference on emerging technologies for sustainable development (OTCON) (pp. 1-6). IEEE.

Alam, S., Shuaib, M., Ahmad, S., Jayakody, D. N. K., Muthanna, A. S., Bharany, S., & Elgendy, I. A. (2022). Blockchain-Based Solutions Supporting Reliable Healthcare for Fog Computing and Internet of Medical Things (IoMT) Integration. In *Sustainability (Switzerland)* (Vol. 14, Issue 22). DOI: 10.3390/su142215312

Alam, S. (2023). Security concerns in smart agriculture and blockchain-based solution. *2022 OPJU International Technology Conference on Emerging Technologies for Sustainable Development (OTCON)*, 1–6. DOI: 10.1109/OTCON56053.2023.10113953

Alam, S. (2023b). The current state of blockchain consensus mechanism: Issues and future works. *International Journal of Advanced Computer Science and Applications*, *14*(8). Advance online publication. DOI: 10.14569/IJACSA.2023.0140810

Alam, S., Bhatia, S., Shuaib, M., Khubrani, M. M., Alfayez, F., Malibari, A. A., & Ahmad, S. (2023). An overview of blockchain and IoT integration for secure and reliable health records monitoring. *Sustainability (Basel)*, *15*(7), 5660. DOI: 10.3390/su15075660

Alam, S., Jasim Mohammad, O. K., Alfurhood, B. S., Saxena, K. K., Anand, M., Mahaveerakannan, R., & Savitha, V. (2023). Effective sound detection system in commercial car vehicles using Msp430 launchpad development. *Multimedia Tools and Applications*. Advance online publication. DOI: 10.1007/s11042-023-15373-2

Al-Anazi, S., Al-Omari, A., Alanazi, S., Marar, A., Asad, M., Alawaji, F., & Alwateid, S. (2024). Artificial intelligence in respiratory care: Current scenario and future perspective. *Annals of Thoracic Medicine*, *19*(2), 117–130.

Albahri, O. S., Zaidan, A. A., Zaidan, B. B., Hashim, M., Albahri, A. S., & Alsalem, M. A. (2018). Real-time remote health-monitoring Systems in a Medical Centre: A review of the provision of healthcare services-based body sensor information, open challenges and methodological aspects. *Journal of Medical Systems*, *42*(9), 1–47. DOI: 10.1007/s10916-018-1006-6 PMID: 30043085

Aldahiri, A., Alrashed, B., & Hussain, W. (2021). Trends in Using IoT with Machine Learning in Health Prediction System. *Forecasting*, *3*(1), 181–206. DOI: 10.3390/forecast3010012

Al-Dmour, R., Al-Dmour, H., Basheer Amin, E., & Al-Dmour, A. (2025). Impact of AI and big data analytics on healthcare outcomes: An empirical study in Jordanian healthcare institutions. *Digital Health*, *11*, 20552076241311052. DOI: 10.1177/20552076241311051 PMID: 39777060

Alexandropoulou, C. A., Panagiotopoulos, I., Kleanthous, S., Dimitrakopoulos, G., Constantinou, I., Politi, E., Ntalaperas, D., Papageorgiou, X., Stylianides, C., Ioannides, N., Palazis, L., Pattichis, C. S., & Panayides, A. S. (2023). AI-Enabled Solutions, Explainability and Ethical Concerns for Predicting Sepsis in ICUs: A Systematic Review. *Proceedings 2023 IEEE 19th International Conference on E-Science, e-Science 2023*. DOI: 10.1109/e-Science58273.2023.10254863

Alharthi, H. (2018). Healthcare predictive analytics: An overview with a focus on Saudi Arabia. *Journal of Infection and Public Health*, *11*(6), 749–756. DOI: 10.1016/j.jiph.2018.02.005 PMID: 29526444

Alibakhshi-Kenari, M., Naser-Moghadasi, M., Sadeghzadeh, R. A., Virdee, B. S., & Limiti, E. (2016). Periodic array of complementary artificial magnetic conductor metamaterials-based multiband antennas for broadband wireless transceivers. *IET Microwaves, Antennas & Propagation*, *10*(15), 1682–1691. DOI: 10.1049/iet-map.2016.0069

Al-kahtani, M. S., Khan, F., & Taekeun, W. (2022). Application of Internet of Things and Sensors in Healthcare. *Sensors (Basel)*, *22*(15), 5738. Advance online publication. DOI: 10.3390/s22155738 PMID: 35957294

Al-Marridi, A. Z., Mohamed, A., & Erbad, A. 2018. "Convolutional Autoencoder Approach for EEG Compression and Reconstruction in M-Health Systems." *2018 14th International Wireless Communications and Mobile Computing Conference, IWCMC 2018* 370–75. DOI: 10.1109/IWCMC.2018.8450511

Al-Nbhany, W. A. N. A., Zahary, A. T., & Al-Shargabi, A. A. (2024). Blockchain-IoT healthcare applications and trends: A review. *IEEE Access : Practical Innovations, Open Solutions*, *12*, 4178–4212. DOI: 10.1109/ACCESS.2023.3349187

Alowais, S. A., Alghamdi, S. S., Alsuhebany, N., Alqahtani, T., Alshaya, A. I., Almohareb, S. N., Aldairem, A., Alrashed, M., Bin Saleh, K., Badreldin, H. A., Al Yami, M. S., Al Harbi, S., & Albekairy, A. M. (2023). Revolutionizing healthcare: The role of artificial intelligence in clinical practice. *BMC Medical Education*, *23*(1), 689. DOI: 10.1186/s12909-023-04698-z PMID: 37740191

Alqahtani, N., Alam, S., Aqeel, I., Shuaib, M., Mohsen Khormi, I., Khan, S. B., & Malibari, A. A. (2023). Deep belief networks (DBN) with IoT-based Alzheimer's disease detection and classification. *Applied Sciences (Basel, Switzerland)*, *13*(13), 7833. DOI: 10.3390/app13137833

Alshamrani, M. (2022). IoT and artificial intelligence implementations for remote healthcare monitoring systems: A survey. *Journal of King Saud University. Computer and Information Sciences*, *34*(8), 4687–4701. DOI: 10.1016/j.jksuci.2021.06.005

Alsharif, A., & Nabil, M. (2020). A Blockchain-based Medical Data Marketplace with Trustless Fair Exchange and Access Control. *GLOBECOM 2020 - 2020 IEEE Global Communications Conference*, 1–6. DOI: 10.1109/GLOBECOM42002.2020.9348192

Alshehri, F., & Muhammad, G. (2021). A Comprehensive Survey of the Internet of Things (IoT) and AI-Based Smart Healthcare. *IEEE Access : Practical Innovations, Open Solutions*, *9*, 3660–3678. DOI: 10.1109/ACCESS.2020.3047960

Al-Talafheh, K., Aplop, F., Al-Yousef, A., Obiedat, M., & Khazaaleh, M. (2024). Predictive Big Data Analytics Capability Model to Enhancing Healthcare Organization Performance. *International Journal of Advances in Soft Computing & Its Applications*, *16*(3), 149–165. DOI: 10.15849/IJASCA.241130.09

Amann, J., Blasimme, A., Vayena, E., Frey, D., & Madai, V. I. (2020). Explainability for artificial intelligence in healthcare: A multidisciplinary perspective. *BMC Medical Informatics and Decision Making*, *20*(1), 310. DOI: 10.1186/s12911-020-01332-6 PMID: 33256715

Amin, S. U., & Shamim Hossain, M. (2021). Edge Intelligence and Internet of Things in Healthcare: A Survey. *IEEE Access : Practical Innovations, Open Solutions*, *9*, 45–59. DOI: 10.1109/ACCESS.2020.3045115

Amos, J. D., Zhang, Z., Tian, Y., Lowry, G. V., Wiesner, M. R., & Hendren, C. O. (2024). Knowledge and Instance Mapping: Architecture for premeditated interoperability of disparate data for materials. *Scientific Data, 11*(1), 173. DOI: 10.1038/s41597-024-03006-8 PMID: 38321063

Anand, A., ... (2023). Mitigating cyber-security risks using cyber-analytics. In *2023 7th International Conference on Trends in Electronics and Informatics (ICOEI)* (pp. 630–635). IEEE. DOI: 10.1109/ICOEI56765.2023.10126001

Ango, R., Masih, R. K., Reddy, C. K. K., Shuaib, M., Singh, M., & Alam, S. (2024). Fraud Detection in Banking using the Kaggle Credit Card Dataset and XGBoost Model. *2024 International Conference on IoT Based Control Networks and Intelligent Systems (ICICNIS)*, 968–973. DOI: 10.1109/ICICNIS64247.2024.10823227

Antevski, K., Girletti, L., Bernardos, C. J., de la Oliva, A., Baranda, J., & Mangues-Bafalluy, J. (2021). A 5G-based eHealth monitoring and emergency response system: Experience and lessons learned. *IEEE Access : Practical Innovations, Open Solutions, 9*, 131420–131429. DOI: 10.1109/ACCESS.2021.3114593

Aqeel, I., Khormi, I. M., Khan, S. B., Shuaib, M., Almusharraf, A., Alam, S., & Alkhaldi, N. A. (2023). Load Balancing Using Artificial Intelligence for Cloud-Enabled Internet of Everything in Healthcare Domain. In *Sensors* (Vol. 23, Issue 11). DOI: 10.3390/s23115349

Ara, A., & Mifa, A. F. (2024). Integrating artificial intelligence and big data in mobile health: A systematic review of innovations and challenges in healthcare systems. *Global Mainstream Journal of Business, Economics. Development & Project Management, 3*(01), 1–16.

Arabahmadi, M., & Farahbakhsh, R. (2022). Deep Learning for Smart Healthcare: A Survey on Brain Tumor. *Sensors (Basel), 22*, 1–27. DOI: 10.3390/s22051960 PMID: 35271115

Arachchige, G., Kithmini, P. B., & But, J. (2023). Evaluation of Blockchain Networks' Scalability Limitations in Low-Powered Internet of Things (IoT) Sensor Networks. *Future Internet, 15*(9), 317. Advance online publication. DOI: 10.3390/fi15090317

Aranovich, T. de C., & Matulionyte, R. (2023). Ensuring AI explainability in healthcare: Problems and possible policy solutions. *Information & Communications Technology Law, 32*(2), 259–275. Advance online publication. DOI: 10.1080/13600834.2022.2146395

Arbelaez Ossa, L., Lorenzini, G., Milford, S. R., Shaw, D., Elger, B. S., & Rost, M. (2024). Integrating ethics in AI development: A qualitative study. *BMC Medical Ethics, 25*(1), 10. Advance online publication. DOI: 10.1186/s12910-023-01000-0 PMID: 38262986

Arif, M., Adak, M., Ahmad, A. A., Nayak, C., Aqeel, I., Alam, S., & Siddiqua, A. (2024). Energy optimization approach based machine learning on linear reflector systems. *Journal of Theoretical and Applied Information Technology, 102*(6).

Arora, A., Ranjan, P., & Srivastava, R. K. (2023). Application of machine learning in medical diagnostics: A systematic review. *Journal of Medical Systems, 47*(3), 17–29.

Aruna, E., & Sahayadhas, A. (2024). Blockchain-Inspired Lightweight Dynamic Encryption Schemes for a Secure Health Care Information Exchange System. *Engineering, Technology & Applied Science Research, 14*(4 SE-), 15050–15055. DOI: 10.48084/etasr.7390

Ashfaq, Z., Mumtaz, R., Rafay, A., Mohammad, S., Zaidi, H., Saleem, H., Mumtaz, S., Shahid, A., De Poorter, E., & Moerman, I. (2022). Applied Sciences Embedded AI-Based Digi-Healthcare. *Applied Sciences (Basel, Switzerland), 12*(519), 1–17.

Atreja, A., Francis, S., Kurra, S., & Kabra, R. (2019). Digital medicine and evolution of remote patient monitoring in cardiac electrophysiology: A state-of-the-art perspective. *Current Treatment Options in Cardiovascular Medicine, 21*(12), 1–10. DOI: 10.1007/s11936-019-0787-3 PMID: 31832887

Awasthy, R., Malhotra, M., Seavers, M. L., & Newman, M. (2024). Admission prioritization of heart failure patients with multiple comorbidities. *Frontiers in Digital Health, 6*, 1379336. DOI: 10.3389/fdgth.2024.1379336 PMID: 39015480

Babu, C. V. S., Akshayah, N. S., & Vinola, P. M. (2023). Artificial intelligence in healthcare: Assessing impacts, challenges, and recommendations for achieving healthcare independence. In *Perspectives on Artificial Intelligence in Times of Turbulence*. Theoretical Background to Applications., DOI: 10.4018/978-1-6684-9814-9.ch005

Badawy, M., Ramadan, N., & Hefny, H. A. (2023). Healthcare Predictive Analytics Using Machine Learning and Deep Learning Techniques: A Survey. *Journal of Electrical Systems and Information Technology, 10*(1), 40. Advance online publication. DOI: 10.1186/s43067-023-00108-y

Badiganti, P. K., Peddirsi, S., Alla, T. J. R., & Tripathi, S. L. (2022). Design and Implementation of Smart Healthcare Monitoring System Using FPGA. *Lecture Notes in Networks and Systems, 329*, 205–213. DOI: 10.1007/978-981-16-6246-1_18

Baig, M. M., & Gholamhosseini, H. (2013). Smart health monitoring systems: An overview of design and modeling. *Journal of Medical Systems, 37*(2), 1–14. DOI: 10.1007/s10916-012-9898-z PMID: 23321968

Bajpai, A., Srivastava, V., Shuaib, M., Jaiswal, A., Bharany, S., Alam, S., & Ahmad, S. (2024). An Efficient Hybrid Model to Summarize the Text Using Transfer Learning. In *Lecture Notes in Electrical Engineering* (Vol. 1146). LNEE., DOI: 10.1007/978-981-97-0037-0_5

Baker, S., & Xiang, W. (2023). Artificial Intelligence of Things for Smarter Healthcare: A Survey of Advancements, Challenges, and Opportunities. *IEEE Communications Surveys and Tutorials, 25*(2), 1261–1293. DOI: 10.1109/COMST.2023.3256323

Banbury, A., Roots, A., & Nancarrow, S. (2014). Rapid review of applications of e-health and remote monitoring for rural residents. *The Australian Journal of Rural Health, 22*(5), 211–222. DOI: 10.1111/ajr.12127 PMID: 25303412

Bansal, A., Kumar, S., Bajpai, A., Tiwari, V. N., Nayak, M., Venkatesan, S., & Narayanan, R. (2015). Remote health monitoring system for detecting cardiac disorders. *IET Systems Biology, 9*(6), 309–314. DOI: 10.1049/iet-syb.2015.0012 PMID: 26577166

Bauder, C. J., Moadi, A.-K., Theilmann, P. T., & Fathy, A. E. (2023). Development of a multi-functional remote health monitoring system. *2023 International Microwave and Antenna Symposium (IMAS)*, 103–106. DOI: 10.1109/IMAS55807.2023.10066893

Bauer, C. R., Reddy, K. A., & Singh, M. (2022). Deep learning in medical imaging: Emerging applications and challenges. *Computer Methods and Programs in Biomedicine*, *227*, 107–122.

Bellino, F., Turvani, G., Garlando, U., & Riente, F. (2022). An integrated multi-sensor system for remote bee health monitoring. *2022 IEEE Workshop on Metrology for Agriculture and Forestry (MetroAgriFor)*, 334–338. DOI: 10.1109/MetroAgriFor55389.2022.9965130

Bellucci, B., & Michele, E. (2023). Focusing on the integration of AI in healthcare sector of USA: Focusing on the roles of AI adoption and innovative capabilities. *Journal of Commercial Biotechnology*, *28*(5). Advance online publication. DOI: 10.5912/jcb2142

Benhaddou, D., Balakrishnan, M., & Yuan, X. (2008, April). Remote healthcare monitoring system architecture using sensor networks. In 2008 IEEE Region 5 Conference (pp. 1-6). IEEE.

Ben-Israel, D., Jacobs, W. B., Casha, S., Lang, E., & Clarke, D. B. (2021). The impact of machine learning on patient care: A systematic review. *Neurosurgery*, *87*(1), 14–24.

Bhan, R., Pamula, R., Faruki, P., & Gajrani, J. (2023). Blockchain-enabled secure and efficient data sharing scheme for trust management in healthcare smartphone network. *The Journal of Supercomputing*, *79*(14), 16233–16274. DOI: 10.1007/s11227-023-05272-6 PMID: 37359328

Bharany, S., Alam, S., Shuaib, M., & Talwar, B. (2023). *Sentiment Analysis of Twitter Data for COVID-19 Posts BT - Data Intelligence and Cognitive Informatics* (I. J. Jacob, S. Kolandapalayam Shanmugam, & I. Izonin, Eds.; pp. 457–466). Springer Nature Singapore.

Bi, H., Liu, J., & Kato, N. (2021). Deep learning-based privacy preservation and data analytics for IoT enabled healthcare. *IEEE Transactions on Industrial Informatics*, *18*(7), 4798–4807. DOI: 10.1109/TII.2021.3117285

Bossenko, I., Randmaa, R., Piho, G., & Ross, P. (2024). Interoperability of health data using FHIR Mapping Language: transforming HL7 CDA to FHIR with reusable visual components. *Frontiers in Digital Health, Volume 6-*. https://www.frontiersin.org/journals/digital-health/articles/10.3389/fdgth.2024.1480600

Bulla, C., Parushetti, C., Teli, A., Aski, S., & Koppad, S. (2020). A Review of AI Based Medical Assistant Chatbot. *HBRP Publication*, *3*(2), 1–14. DOI: 10.5281/zenodo.3902215

Burrell, D. N., Burton, S. L., Nobles, C., Springs, D., Huff, A. J., Brown-Jackson, K. L., Richardson, K., Wright, J. B., Muller, S. R., & Jones, A. J. (2023). The Managerial Ethical and Operational Challenges of Hospital Cybersecurity. In Burrell, D. (Ed.), *Transformational Interventions for Business, Technology, and Healthcare* (pp. 444–458). IGI Global Scientific Publishing., DOI: 10.4018/979-8-3693-1634-4.ch026

Butt, U. M., Letchmunan, S., Ali, M., Hassan, F. H., Baqir, A., & Sherazi, H. H. R. (2021). Machine learning based diabetes classification and prediction for healthcare applications. *Journal of Healthcare Engineering*, *2021*(1), 9930985. DOI: 10.1155/2021/9930985 PMID: 34631003

Cano-Marin, E., Mora-Cantallops, M., & Sanchez-Alonso, S. (2023). The power of big data analytics over fake news: A scientometric review of Twitter as a predictive system in healthcare. *Technological Forecasting and Social Change*, *190*, 122386. DOI: 10.1016/j.techfore.2023.122386

Carter, D., Kolencik, J., & Cug, J. (2021). Smart internet of things-enabled mobile-based health monitoring systems and medical big data in COVID-19 telemedicine. *American Journal of Medical Research (New York, N.Y.)*, *8*(1), 20–29. DOI: 10.22381/ajmr8120212

Castillejo, P., Martinez, J. F., Rodriguez-Molina, J., & Cuerva, A. (2013). Integration of wearable devices in a wireless sensor network for an E-health application. *IEEE Wireless Communications*, *20*(4), 38–49. DOI: 10.1109/MWC.2013.6590049

Chanda, B., Mallick, P. K., & Chae, G.-S. (2021). An analytical study of the role of m-iot in healthcare domain. *Hybrid Artificial Intelligence and IoT in Healthcare*, 75–96.

Char, D. S., Abràmoff, M. D., & Feudtner, C. (2020). Identifying ethical considerations for machine learning healthcare applications. *The American Journal of Bioethics*, *20*(11), 7–17. DOI: 10.1080/15265161.2020.1819469 PMID: 33103967

Chataut, R., Phoummalayvane, A., & Akl, R. (2023). Unleashing the Power of IoT: A Comprehensive Review of IoT Applications and Future Prospects in Healthcare, Agriculture, Smart Homes, Smart Cities, and Industry 4.0. *Sensors (Basel)*, *23*(16), 7194. Advance online publication. DOI: 10.3390/s23167194 PMID: 37631731

Chavali, D., Dhiman, V. K., & Katari, S. C. (2024). AI-Powered Virtual Health Assistants. *Transforming Patient Engagement Through Virtual Nursing.*, *2*(2), 613–624. DOI: 10.5281/zenodo.10691495

Chen, J., Shi, Y., Yi, C., Du, H., Kang, J., & Niyato, D. (2024). Generative AI-driven human digital twin in IoT-healthcare: A comprehensive survey. *IEEE Internet of Things Journal*, *11*(21), 34749–34773. DOI: 10.1109/JIOT.2024.3421918

Chen, Z., Cruciani, L., Fan, K., Fontana, M., Lievore, E., De Cobelli, O., Musi, G., Ferrigno, G., & De Momi, E. (2024). Towards Safer Robot-Assisted Surgery: A Markerless Augmented Reality Framework. *Neural Networks*, *178*(March), 106469. DOI: 10.1016/j.neunet.2024.106469 PMID: 38925030

Chinthala, K. K. R., Thakur, M. S., Shuaib, M., & Alam, S. (2022). Prospects of Computational Intelligence in Society: Human-Centric Solutions, Challenges, and Research Areas. *Journal of Computational and Cognitive Engineering*.

Chiranjeevi, P., & Rajaram, A. (2024). A smart recommender model based on learning method for sentiment classification. *Multimedia Tools and Applications*, •••, 1–21. DOI: 10.1007/s11042-024-20347-z

Chiuchisan, I., Costin, H. N., & Geman, O. 2014. "Adopting the Internet of Things Technologies in Health Care Systems." *EPE 2014 - Proceedings of the 2014 International Conference and Exposition on Electrical and Power Engineering* (Epe 2014):532–35. DOI: 10.1109/ICEPE.2014.6969965

Choudhury, T., & Dhar, P. (2023). AI in healthcare: Ethical dilemmas and regulatory challenges. *Ethics, Medicine, and Public Health*, *24*, 100–118.

Chronaki, C. E., & Vardas, P. (2013). Remote monitoring costs, benefits, and reimbursement: A European perspective. *Europace : European Pacing, Arrhythmias, and Cardiac Electrophysiology : Journal of the Working Groups on Cardiac Pacing, Arrhythmias, and Cardiac Cellular Electrophysiology of the European Society of Cardiology*, *15*(suppl_1), i59–i64. DOI: 10.1093/europace/eut110 PMID: 23737233

Chua, M., Kim, D., Choi, J., Lee, N. G., Deshpande, V., Schwab, J., Lev, M. H., Gonzalez, R. G., Gee, M. S., & Do, S. (2023). Tackling prediction uncertainty in machine learning for healthcare. *Nature Biomedical Engineering*, *7*(6), 711–718. DOI: 10.1038/s41551-022-00988-x PMID: 36581695

Chui, K. T., Alhalabi, W., Sally, S. H. P., Ordóñez de Pablos, P., Liu, R. W., & Zhao, M. (2017). Disease Diagnosis in Smart Healthcare: Innovation, Technologies and Applications. *Sustainability (Basel)*, *9*(12), 1–23. DOI: 10.3390/su9122309

Chung, W. Y., Lee, Y. D., & Jung, S. J. (2008, August 20–25). *A wireless sensor network compatible wearable u-healthcare monitoring system using integrated ECG, accelerometer and SpO2*. In 2008 30th Annual International Conference of the IEEE Engineering in Medicine and Biology Society (pp. 1529–1532). IEEE. DOI: 10.1109/IEMBS.2008.4649424

Cogin, J. A., Ng, J. L., & Lee, I. (2016). Controlling healthcare professionals: How human resource management influences job attitudes and operational efficiency. *Human Resources for Health*, *14*(1), 55. DOI: 10.1186/s12960-016-0149-0 PMID: 27649794

Colace, F., De Santo, M., Marongiu, F., Santaniello, D., & Troiano, A. (2022). In Gupta, B. B., & Mourelle, L. M. (Eds.), *Secure Medical Data Sharing Through Blockchain and Decentralized Models BT - Robotics and AI for Cybersecurity and Critical Infrastructure in Smart Cities (N. Nedjah, A. A. Abd El-Latif* (pp. 249–262). Springer International Publishing., DOI: 10.1007/978-3-030-96737-6_13

Coman, L.-I., Ianculescu, M., Paraschiv, E.-A., Alexandru, A., & Bădărău, I.-A. (2024). Smart solutions for diet-related disease management: Connected care, remote health monitoring systems, and integrated insights for advanced evaluation. *Applied Sciences (Basel, Switzerland)*, *14*(6), 2351. DOI: 10.3390/app14062351

Comito, C., Falcone, D., & Forestiero, A. (2022). AI-Driven Clinical Decision Support: Enhancing Disease Diagnosis Exploiting Patients Similarity. *IEEE Access : Practical Innovations, Open Solutions*, *10*, 6878–6888. DOI: 10.1109/ACCESS.2022.3142100

Coronato, A., Naeem, M., De Pietro, G., & Paragliola, G. (2020). Reinforcement Learning for Intelligent Healthcare Applications: A Survey. *Artificial Intelligence in Medicine*, *109*, 101964. DOI: 10.1016/j.artmed.2020.101964 PMID: 34756216

Corthis, P. B., Ramesh, G. P., García-Torres, M., & Ruíz, R. (2024). Effective Identification and Authentication of Healthcare IoT Using Fog Computing with Hybrid Cryptographic Algorithm. *Symmetry*, *16*(6), 726. DOI: 10.3390/sym16060726

Costa, T., Borges-Tiago, T., Martins, F., & Tiago, F. (2024). System interoperability and data linkage in the era of health information management: A bibliometric analysis. *The HIM Journal*, *18333583241277950*, 18333583241277952. Advance online publication. DOI: 10.1177/18333583241277952 PMID: 39282893

Dalloul, A. H., Miramirkhani, F., & Kouhalvandi, L. (2023). A review of recent innovations in remote health monitoring. *Micromachines, 14*(12), 2157. DOI: 10.3390/mi14122157 PMID: 38138326

De Brouwer, M., Ongenae, F., Bonte, P., & De Turck, F. (2018). Towards a cascading reasoning framework to support responsive ambient-intelligent healthcare interventions. *Sensors (Basel), 18*(10), 3514. DOI: 10.3390/s18103514 PMID: 30340363

Deepa, P., Badrinath, P., Mohanaprasanth, N., Pranesh, S., & Sriram, E. (2024). AI-Powered Doctolib: Revolutionizing Healthcare Appointment Management. *Asian Journal of Basic Science & Research, 6*(4), 90–102. DOI: 10.38177/AJBSR.2024.6407

Deloitte. (2015). *Connected health: How digital technology is transforming health and social care.* Deloitte.

Deo, R. C. (2015). Machine learning in medicine. *Circulation, 132*(20), 1920–1930. DOI: 10.1161/CIRCULATIONAHA.115.001593 PMID: 26572668

Dhatterwal, J. S., Kaswan, K. S., & Kumar, N. (2023). Robotic Process Automation in Healthcare. In Bhattacharyya, S., Banerjee, J. S., & De, D. (Eds.), *Confluence of Artificial Intelligence and Robotic Process Automation. Smart Innovation, Systems and Technologies* (Vol. 335). Springer., DOI: 10.1007/978-981-19-8296-5_7

Di Nuovo, A. (2024). Letter to the Editor: "How Can Biomedical Engineers Help Empower Individuals With Intellectual Disabilities? The Potential Benefits and Challenges of AI Technologies to Support Inclusivity and Transform Lives." In *IEEE Journal of Translational Engineering in Health and Medicine* (Vol. 12). DOI: 10.1109/JTEHM.2023.3331977

Dilsizian, S. E., & Siegel, E. L. (2014). Artificial intelligence in medicine and cardiac imaging. *Cardiology Clinics, 32*(2), 225–234. PMID: 24793799

Din, U., Ikram, A. A., Guizani, M., & Zuair, M. (2019). A Decade of Internet of Things: Analysis in the Light of Healthcare Applications. *IEEE Access : Practical Innovations, Open Solutions, 7*, 89967–89979. DOI: 10.1109/ACCESS.2019.2927082

Dubey, A. (2024). *C Kishor Kumar Reddy, Srinath Doss and Marlia Mohd Hanafiah, "Exploring the Advancements and Future Directions of Digital Twins in Healthcare 6.0.* IGI Global.

Du, L., & Xie, T. (2024). Towards Secure Internet of Things-Enabled Healthcare: Integrating Elliptic Curve Digital Signatures and Rivest Cipher Encryption. *International Journal of Advanced Computer Science and Applications, 15*(8). Advance online publication. DOI: 10.14569/IJACSA.2024.0150858

Edoh, N. L., Chigboh, V. M., Zouo, S. J., & Olamijuwon, J. (2024). *Improving healthcare decision-making with predictive analytics: A conceptual approach to patient risk assessment and care optimization.*

Eid, M., Cha, J., & El Saddik, A. (2010). Admux: An adaptive multiplexer for haptic-audio-visual data communication. *IEEE Transactions on Instrumentation and Measurement, 60*(1), 21–31. DOI: 10.1109/TIM.2010.2065530

Erlinawati, N. D., Anurogo, D., Hasyim, D. M., & Ardi, A. (2024). Application of the Internet of Things (IoT) in Health: The Future of Personal Care. *Journal of World Future Medicine. Health and Nursing, 2*(1), 79–92. PMID: 38291421

Escorcia-Gutierrez, J., Mansour, R. F., Leal, E., Villanueva, J., Jimenez-Cabas, J., Soto, C., & Soto-Díaz, R. (2024). Privacy preserving blockchain with energy aware clustering scheme for IoT healthcare systems. *Mobile Networks and Applications*, *29*(1), 1–12. DOI: 10.1007/s11036-023-02115-9

Espinoza, A. V., Van Hooff, R. J., De Smedt, A., Moens, M., Yperzeele, L., Nieboer, K., Hubloue, I., De Keyser, J., Convents, A., & Tellez, H. F.. (2016). Development and pilot testing of 24/7 in-ambulance telemedicine for acute stroke: Prehospital stroke study at the Universitair Ziekenhuis Brussel-project. *Cerebrovascular Diseases (Basel, Switzerland)*, *42*(1–2), 15–22. DOI: 10.1159/000444175 PMID: 26950076

Esteva, A., Kuprel, B., Novoa, R. A., Ko, J., Swetter, S. M., Blau, H. M., & Thrun, S. (2017). Dermatologist-level classification of skin cancer with deep neural networks. *Nature*, *542*(7639), 115–118. DOI: 10.1038/nature21056 PMID: 28117445

Eswaran, U., Eswaran, V., Murali, K., & Eswaran, V. (2024). Elevating healthcare: the synergy of ai and biosensors in disease management. i-Manager's Journal on Artificial Intelligence & Machine Learning (JAIM), 2(1).

Eswaran, U., Eswaran, V., Murali, K., & Eswaran, V. (2024). Predictive Healthcare Analytics. In Exploring the Advancements and Future Directions of Digital Twins in Healthcare 6.0 (pp. 171-199). IGI Global.

Eswaran, V., Eswaran, U., Eswaran, V., & Murali, K. (2024b). Revolutionizing healthcare: The application of image processing techniques. In *Medical Robotics and AI-Assisted Diagnostics for a High-Tech Healthcare Industry* (p. 16). IGI Global., DOI: 10.4018/979-8-3693-2105-8.ch019

Etli, D., Djurovic, A., & Lark, J. (2024). The Future of Personalized Healthcare: AI-Driven Wearables For Real-Time Health Monitoring And Predictive Analytics. *Current Research in Health Sciences*, *2*(2), 10–14.

Farias, F. A. C. D., Dagostini, C. M., Bicca, Y. D. A., Falavigna, V. F., & Falavigna, A. (2020). Remote patient monitoring: A systematic review. *Telemedicine Journal and e-Health*, *26*(5), 576–583. DOI: 10.1089/tmj.2019.0066 PMID: 31314689

Fayaz, M., Amin, M., & Iqbal, M. (2024). Artificial intelligence in decision-making: A descriptive analysis of its impact on strategic planning. *Journal of Business and Management Research*, *3*(2), 222–235. http://jbmr.com.pk/index.php/Journal/article/view/228

Fotouhi, H., Causevic, A., Lundqvist, K., & Björkman, M. (2016, June). Communication and Security in Health Monitoring Systems--A Review. In 2016 IEEE 40th annual computer software and applications conference (COMPSAC) (Vol. 1, pp. 545-554). IEEE.

Friedman, J. H. (1991). Multivariate adaptive regression splines. *Annals of Statistics*, *19*(1), 1–67.

Fukizi, K. Y. (2023). Collaborative Decision-Making Assistant for Healthcare Professionals: A Human-Centered AI Prototype Powered by Azure Open AI. *COMPASS 2023 - Proceedings of the ACM SIGCAS/SIGCHI Conference on Computing and Sustainable Societies*. DOI: 10.1145/3588001.3609370

Ganiya, R. K., Veeraiah, D., Thatha, V. N., Rao, K. S., Rao, J. N., Manjith, R., & Rajaram, A. (2024). Revolutionizing vascular health through the temporal convolutional transformer for drug screening and model evolution. *Biomedical Signal Processing and Control*, *95*, 106390. DOI: 10.1016/j.bspc.2024.106390

Gao, J., Yang, Y., Lin, P., & Park, D. S. (2018). Editorial: Computer Vision in Healthcare Applications. *Journal of Healthcare Engineering*, *2018*, 1–4. Advance online publication. DOI: 10.1155/2018/5157020 PMID: 29686826

Gates, J. D., Yulianti, Y., & Pangilinan, G. A. (2024). Big data analytics for predictive insights in healthcare. *International Transactions on Artificial Intelligence*, *3*(1), 54–63. DOI: 10.33050/italic.v3i1.622

Gatsios, D., Rigas, G., & Konitsiotis, S. (2021). Design of a clinical decision support system powered by mhealth for the management of Parkinson's disease. *2021 6th South-East Europe Design Automation, Computer Engineering,Computer Networks and Social Media Conference (SEEDA-CECNSM)*, 1–4.

Gaudet-Blavignac, C., Raisaro, J. L., Touré, V., Österle, S., Crameri, K., & Lovis, C. (2021). A National, Semantic-Driven, Three-Pillar Strategy to Enable Health Data Secondary Usage Interoperability for Research Within the Swiss Personalized Health Network: Methodological Study. *JMIR Medical Informatics*, *9*(6), e27591. DOI: 10.2196/27591 PMID: 34185008

Ghadi, Y. Y., Mazhar, T., & Shahzad, T. Muhammad Amir khan, Alaa Abd-Alrazaq, Arfan Ahmed, and Habib Hamam. 2024. *The Role of Blockchain to Secure Internet of Medical Things*. Vol. 14. Nature Publishing Group UK.

Ghaffar, A., Arshad, A., Siddqiue, M. U., & Nasir, A. (2024). AI Strategy in Healthcare CHRM: Analyzing the Influence Organization Effective Performance Evidence from the Private Hospitals of Lahore Pakistan. *Journal of Health and Rehabilitation Research*, *4*(1), 639–645. DOI: 10.61919/jhrr.v4i1.339

Ghosh, A. M., Halder, D., & Hossain, S. A. (2016, May). Remote health monitoring system through IoT. In 2016 5th International Conference on Informatics, Electronics and Vision (ICIEV) (pp. 921-926). IEEE.

Goffman, R. M., Harris, S. L., May, J. H., Milicevic, A. S., Monte, R. J., Myaskovsky, L., Rodriguez, K. L., Tjader, Y. C., & Vargas, D. L. (2017). Modeling patient no-show history and predicting future outpatient appointment behavior in the Veterans Health Administration. *Military Medicine*, *182*(5-6), e1708–e1714. DOI: 10.7205/MILMED-D-16-00345 PMID: 29087915

Göllner, S., & Tropmann-Frick, M. (2023a). Bridging the Gap between Theory and Practice: Towards Responsible AI Evaluation. *CEUR Workshop Proceedings*, ●●●, 3580.

Göllner, S., & Tropmann-Frick, M. (2023b). VERIFAI - A Step Towards Evaluating the Responsibility of AI-Systems. *Lecture Notes in Informatics (LNI), Proceedings - Series of the Gesellschaft Fur Informatik (GI), P-331*. DOI: 10.18420/BTW2023-63

Gong, C., & Wu, J. (2022). Federated learning in healthcare: A review and future directions. *Journal of Biomedical Informatics*, *128*, 104026.

Gosh, P. (2018). *AI Early Diagnosis Could Save Heart and Cancer Patients*. BBC.

Greco, L., Percannella, G., Ritrovato, P., Tortorella, F., & Vento, M. (2020). Trends in IoT Based Solutions for Health Care: Moving AI to the Edge. *Pattern Recognition Letters*, *135*, 346–353. DOI: 10.1016/j.patrec.2020.05.016 PMID: 32406416

Guido, R., Ferrisi, S., Lofaro, D., & Conforti, D. (2024). An overview on the advancements of support vector machine models in healthcare applications: A review. *Information (Basel)*, *15*(4), 235. DOI: 10.3390/info15040235

Guntur, S. R., Gorrepati, R. R., & Dirisala, V. R. (2018). Internet of Medical things: Remote healthcare and health monitoring perspective. In *Medical big data and internet of medical things* (pp. 271–297). CRC Press. DOI: 10.1201/9781351030380-11

Gupta, P., & Ghosh, M. (2019). Revolutionizing healthcare with 5G. *Telecom Business Review*, *12*, 41.

Gurusamy, A., & Mohamed, I. A. (2021). The role of AI and machine learning in full stack development for healthcare applications. *Journal of Knowledge Learning and Science Technology ISSN: 2959-6386 (Online)*, *1*(1), 116–123.

Habibur, M., Hasan, M. H., Sadik, M. S., Estehad, M., Rahatul, M., Kumar, P., & Rahman, A. (2024). Impact of Internet of Things (IoT) on healthcare in transforming patient care and overcoming operational challenges. *Journal of Angiotherapy*, *8*(11), 1–8. DOI: 10.25163/angiotherapy.81110041

Hakim, T., Ahmi, A., & Alam, S. (2024). A Decade in Blockchain: A Bibliometric Reflection on the Growth and Interdisciplinary Reach of a Disruptive Technology. *Journal of Information and Communication Technology*, *23*(4), 627–665. DOI: 10.32890/jict2024.23.4.3

Haleem, A., Javaid, M., Singh, R. P., Suman, R., & Rab, S. (2021). Blockchain Technology Applications in Healthcare: An Overview. *International Journal of Intelligent Networks*, *2*(May), 130–139. DOI: 10.1016/j.ijin.2021.09.005

Hamm, S., Schleser, A. C., Hartig, J., Thomas, P., Zoesch, S., & Bulitta, C. (2020). 5G as enabler for digital healthcare. *Current Directions in Biomedical Engineering*, *6*(1), 1–4. DOI: 10.1515/cdbme-2020-3001

Haq, A. U., Jian, P. L., Ahmad, S., Khan, S., Alshara, M. A., & Alotaibi, R. M. (2021). Diagnostic Approach for Accurate Diagnosis of COVID-19 Employing Deep Learning and Transfer Learning Techniques through Chest X-Ray Images Clinical Data in E-Healthcare. *Sensors (Basel)*, *21*(24), 8219. DOI: 10.3390/s21248219 PMID: 34960313

Haque, A., Guo, M., & Albayda, J. (2022). Emerging applications of reinforcement learning in personalized medicine. *Nature Machine Intelligence*, *4*(5), 371–382.

Haque, M. A., Ahmad, S., Sonal, D., Haque, S., Kumar, K., & Rahman, M. (2023). Analytical Studies on the Effectiveness of IoMT for Healthcare Systems. *Iraqi Journal of Science*, •••, 4719–4728. DOI: 10.24996/ijs.2023.64.9.34

Harris, S. L., May, J. H., & Vargas, L. G. (2016). Predictive analytics model for healthcare planning and scheduling. *European Journal of Operational Research*, *253*(1), 121–131. DOI: 10.1016/j.ejor.2016.02.017

Hartmann, M., Hashmi, U. S., & Imran, A. (2019). Edge computing in smart healthcare systems: Review, challenges, and research directions. *Transactions on Emerging Telecommunications Technologies, 3710*. Advance online publication. DOI: 10.1002/ett.3710

Hasan, A., Badhautiya, A., & Pandey, A. (2024). HealthNet: IoT-based healthcare monitoring and management system. *International Journal for Research in Applied Science and Engineering Technology, 12*(3), 473–481. DOI: 10.22214/ijraset.2024.58851

Heart, T., Ben-Assuli, O., & Shabtai, I. (2017). A review of PHR, EMR and EHR integration: A more personalized healthcare and public health policy. *Health Policy and Technology, 6*(1), 20–25. DOI: 10.1016/j.hlpt.2016.08.002

Heba, M. (2022). Healthcare Workers' Resilience Toolkit for Disaster Management and Climate Change Adaptation. *International Journal of Environmental Research and Public Health, 19*(19), 12440–12440. DOI: 10.3390/ijerph191912440 PMID: 36231739

Hegde, M. G., Shenoy, P. D., & Venugopal, K. R. (2023). A Comparative Study of Neural Network and Machine Learning on Privacy Preserving Federated Learning for Healthcare Applications. *2023 IEEE Technology & Engineering Management Conference-Asia Pacific (TEMSCON-ASPAC)*, 1–6.

Hendawi, R., & Li, J. (2024). Comprehensive Personal Health Knowledge Graph for Effective Management and Utilization of Personal Health Data. *2024 IEEE First International Conference on Artificial Intelligence for Medicine, Health and Care (AIMHC)*, 92–100. DOI: 10.1109/AIMHC59811.2024.00026

Herrera Perez, J. L., Fajes Alfonso, A., & Alvarez, D. (1989). Retinopatia Diabetica E Hiperlipoproteinemia. *Revista Cubana de Medicina, 28*(4), 333–340.

Herzog, N. J. (n.d.). *Dilek Celik &. Rejwan Bin Sulaiman*. Artificial Intelligence in Healthcare and Medical Records Security.

Hoang, H. D., Duy, P. T., Tien, N. T., Hien, D. T. T., & Pham, V.-H. (2022). A Blockchain-based approach and Attribute-based Encryption for Healthcare Record Data Exchange. *2022 RIVF International Conference on Computing and Communication Technologies (RIVF)*, 65–70. DOI: 10.1109/RIVF55975.2022.10013886

Hossain, S., Ahmed, A., Khadka, U., Sarkar, S., & Khan, N. (2024). AI-driven Predictive Analytics, Healthcare Outcomes, Cost Reduction, Machine Learning, Patient Monitoring. *AIJMR-Advanced International Journal of Multidisciplinary Research, 2*(5).

Huang, Z., Lu, X., & Duan, H. (2018). Health information sharing in IoT healthcare: Machine learning techniques and privacy concerns. *Computers in Biology and Medicine, 96*, 90–101.

Huifeng, W., Kadry, S. N., & Raj, E. D. (2020). Continuous Health Monitoring of Sportsperson Using IoT Devices Based Wearable Technology. *Computer Communications, 160*, 588–595. DOI: 10.1016/j.comcom.2020.04.025

Ianculescu, M., Coardo , D., Bica, O., & Vevera, V. (2020, October). Security and privacy risks for remote healthcare monitoring systems. In 2020 International Conference on e-Health and Bioengineering (EHB) (pp. 1-4). IEEE. DOI: 10.1109/EHB50910.2020.9280103

Ibeh, C. V., Elufioye, O. A., Olorunsogo, T., Asuzu, O. F., Nduubuisi, N. L., & Daraojimba, A. I. (2024). Data analytics in healthcare: A review of patient-centric approaches and healthcare delivery. *World Journal of Advanced Research and Reviews*, *21*(02), 1750–1760. DOI: 10.30574/wjarr.2024.21.2.0246

Ibikunle, O. E., Usuemerai, P. A., Abass, L. A., Alemede, V., Nwankwo, E. I., & Mbata, A. O. (2024). Artificial intelligence in healthcare forecasting: Enhancing market strategy with predictive analytics. *International Journal of Applied Research in Social Sciences*, *6*(10).

Iliashenko, O., Bikkulova, Z., & Dubgorn, A. (2019). Opportunities and challenges of artificial intelligence in healthcare. *E3S Web of Conferences, 110*, 2028.

Indrakumari, R., Poongodi, T., Suresh, P., & Balamurugan, B. (2019). *The Growing Role of Internet of Things in Healthcare Wearables*. Elsevier Inc.

Iniesta, R. (2023). The human role to guarantee an ethical AI in healthcare: A five-facts approach. *AI and Ethics*. Advance online publication. DOI: 10.1007/s43681-023-00353-x

Iqbal, M. S., Abd-Alrazaq, A., & Househ, M. (2022). Artificial Intelligence Solutions to Detect Fraud in Healthcare Settings: A Scoping Review. *Studies in Health Technology and Informatics*, *295*(July), 20–23. DOI: 10.3233/SHTI220649 PMID: 35773795

Irshad, R. R., Alattab, A. A., Omar, A. S. A., Sohail, S. S., Aziz, A., Madsen, D. Ø., & Alalayah, K. M. (2023). An Optimization-Linked Intelligent Security Algorithm for Smart Healthcare Organizations. *Healthcare (Basel)*, *11*(4), 580. Advance online publication. DOI: 10.3390/healthcare11040580 PMID: 36833114

Islam, M., Usman, M., Mahmood, A., Abbasi, A. A., & Song, O.-Y. (2020). Predictive analytics framework for accurate estimation of child mortality rates for Internet of Things enabled smart healthcare systems. *International Journal of Distributed Sensor Networks*, *16*(5), 1550147720928897. DOI: 10.1177/1550147720928897

Ismail, W. N., Hassan, M. M., Alsalamah, H. A., & Fortino, G. (2020). CNN-Based Health Model for Regular Health Factors Analysis in Internet-of-Medical Things Environment. *IEEE Access : Practical Innovations, Open Solutions*, *8*, 52541–52549. DOI: 10.1109/ACCESS.2020.2980938

Istepanian, R. S., Hu, S., Philip, N. Y., & Sungoor, A. (2011, August 30–September 3). *The potential of Internet of m-health Things "m-IoT" for non-invasive glucose level sensing*. In 2011 Annual International Conference of the IEEE Engineering in Medicine and Biology Society (pp. 5264–5266). IEEE. DOI: 10.1109/IEMBS.2011.6091282

Janowski, A. (2023). Natural Language Processing Techniques for Clinical Text Analysis in Healthcare. *Journal of Advanced Analytics in Healthcare Management*, *7*(1), 51–76. https://research.tensorgate.org/index.php/JAAHM/article/view/37

Javed, H., Abaid, Z., Akbar, S., Ullah, K., Ahmad, A., Saeed, A., Ali, H., Ghadi, Y. Y., Alahmadi, T. J., Alkahtani, H. K., & Raza, A. (2023). Blockchain-based logging to defeat malicious insiders: The case of remote health monitoring systems. *IEEE Access : Practical Innovations, Open Solutions*, *12*, 12062–12079. DOI: 10.1109/ACCESS.2023.3346432

Javed, H., Muqeet, H. A., Javed, T., Rehman, A. U., & Sadiq, R. (2023). Ethical frameworks for machine learning in sensitive healthcare applications. *IEEE Access : Practical Innovations, Open Solutions*, *12*, 16233–16254. DOI: 10.1109/ACCESS.2023.3340884

Jiang, F., Jiang, Y., Zhi, H., Dong, Y., Li, H., Ma, S., Wang, Y., Dong, Q., Shen, H., & Wang, Y. (2017). Artificial Intelligence in Healthcare: Past, Present, and Future. *Stroke and Vascular Neurology*, *2*(4), 230–243. DOI: 10.1136/svn-2017-000101 PMID: 29507784

Johnson, A. E. W., Pollard, T. J., & Mark, R. G. (2016). Reproducibility in critical care: A vision for improving healthcare. *Critical Care Medicine*, *44*(1), e102–e109.

Joshi, H., Kumar Reddy, C. K., Ouaissa, M., Mohd Hanafiah, M., & Doss, S. (2024). Intelligent systems and IoT applications in clinical health. In IGI Global. https://doi.org/DOI: 10.4018/979-8-3693-8990-4

Kalaivani, K., Kshirsagarr, P. R., Sirisha Devi, J., Bandela, S. R., Colak, I., Nageswara Rao, J., & Rajaram, A. (2023). Prediction of biomedical signals using deep learning techniques. *Journal of Intelligent & Fuzzy Systems*, *44*(6), 9769–9782. DOI: 10.3233/JIFS-230399

Kalaivani, S., Nasreen Banu, D., Parvin Begum, I., & Sivasamy, J. (2023). Cognitive Robotics: Integrating Artificial Intelligence and Embodied Intelligence for Advanced Problem Solving. *Journal of Artificial Intelligence and Capsule Networks*, *5*(4). Advance online publication. DOI: 10.36548/jaicn.2023.4.002

Kalamkar, S., & Mary, G. A. 2020. "Clinical Data Fusion and Machine Learning Techniques for Smart Healthcare." *2020 International Conference on Industry 4.0 Technology, I4Tech 2020* 211–16. DOI: 10.1109/I4Tech48345.2020.9102706

Kalaria, C., Singh, S., & Prajapati, B. G. (2023). Intelligent Healthcare Supply Chain. Human-Machine Interface: Making Healthcare Digital, 449-481.

Kamal, M. D., Tahir, A., Kamal, M. B., & Naeem, M. A. (2020). Future location prediction for emergency vehicles using big data: A case study of healthcare engineering. *Journal of Healthcare Engineering*, *6641571*, 1–11. Advance online publication. DOI: 10.1155/2020/6641571 PMID: 33354308

Kang, H., & Park, Y. (2021). Predictive analytics for chronic disease management using AI. *Healthcare Analytics*, *3*(2), 53–65.

Kanksha, A. B., Pande, S., Malik, R., & Khamparia, A. (2021). An Intelligent Unsupervised Technique for Fraud Detection in Health Care Systems. *Intelligent Decision Technologies*, *15*(1), 127–139. DOI: 10.3233/IDT-200052

Karmakar, K., Saif, S., Das, P., Neogy, S., & Biswas, S. (2022). FDRF: Fault detection and recovery framework for seamless data transmission in remote health monitoring using WBAN. *Wireless Personal Communications*, *123*(1), 325–356. DOI: 10.1007/s11277-021-09134-3

Karpova, E. A. (2023). AI in Health Ethical Review: A Value Design Methodology. *Chelovek*, *34*(3), 129. Advance online publication. DOI: 10.31857/S023620070026109-6

Karthik, A., Aalam, S. S., Sivakumar, M., Sundari, M. V. R., Rose, J. D., Elangovan, M., & Rajaram, A. (2024). Improving brain tumor treatment with better imaging and real-time therapy using quantum dots. *Biomedical Signal Processing and Control*, *95*, 106286. DOI: 10.1016/j.bspc.2024.106286

Karthik, A., Hamatta, H. S. A., Patthi, S., Krubakaran, C., Pradhan, A. K., Rachapudi, V., Shuaib, M., & Rajaram, A. (2024). Ensemble-based multimodal medical imaging fusion for tumor segmentation. *Biomedical Signal Processing and Control*, *96*, 106550. DOI: 10.1016/j.bspc.2024.106550

Karthik, A., Sahoo, S. K., Kumar, A., Patel, N., Chinnaraj, P., Maguluri, L. P., & Rajaram, A. (2025). Unified approach for accurate brain tumor Multi-Classification and segmentation through fusion of advanced methodologies. *Biomedical Signal Processing and Control*, *100*, 106872. DOI: 10.1016/j.bspc.2024.106872

Kaza, V. S., Alamer, A., Alam, S., Shuaib, M., Basudan, S., & Sheneamer, A. (2024). Detecting and forecasting cryptojacking attack trends in Internet of Things and wireless sensor networks devices. *PeerJ. Computer Science*, *10*, e2491. DOI: 10.7717/peerj-cs.2491 PMID: 39650421

Kelly, C. J., Karthikesalingam, A., Suleyman, M., Corrado, G., & King, D. (2019). Key challenges for delivering clinical impact with artificial intelligence. *BMC Medicine*, *17*(1), 195. DOI: 10.1186/s12916-019-1426-2 PMID: 31665002

Khalifa, M., & Albadawy, M. (2024). Artificial Intelligence for Clinical Prediction: Exploring Key Domains and Essential Functions. In *Computer Methods and Programs in Biomedicine Update* (Vol. 5). DOI: 10.1016/j.cmpbup.2024.100148

Khan, J., Li, J., Haq, A. U., Parveen, S., Khan, G. A., Shahid, M., Monday, H. N., Ullah, S., & Sun, R. 2019. "Medical Image Encryption into Smart Healthcare IOT System." *2019 16th International Computer Conference on Wavelet Active Media Technology and Information Processing, ICCWAMTIP 2019* 378–82. DOI: 10.1109/ICCWAMTIP47768.2019.9067592

Khan, A., Zubair, S., Shuaib, M., Sheneamer, A., Alam, S., & Assiri, B. (2024). Development of a robust parallel and multi-composite machine learning model for improved diagnosis of Alzheimer's disease: Correlation with dementia-associated drug usage and AT (N) protein biomarkers. *Frontiers in Neuroscience*, *18*, 1391465. DOI: 10.3389/fnins.2024.1391465 PMID: 39308946

Khan, H. A., Abdulla, R., Selvaperumal, S. K., & Bathich, A. (2021). IoT Based on Secure Personal Healthcare Using RFID Technology and Steganography. *International Journal of Electrical and Computer Engineering*, *11*(4), 3300–3309. DOI: 10.11591/ijece.v11i4.pp3300-3309

Khan, J., Khan, G. A., Jian, P. L., Alajmi, M. F., Haq, A. U., Khan, S., Ahmad, N., Parveen, S., Shahid, M., Ahmad, S., Raji, M., Ahamad, B., Alghamdi, A. A., & Ali, A. (2022). Secure Smart Healthcare Monitoring in Industrial Internet of Things (IIoT) Ecosystem with Cosine Function Hybrid Chaotic Map Encryption. *Scientific Programming*, *2022*, 1–22. Advance online publication. DOI: 10.1155/2022/8853448

Khan, M. M., & Alkhathami, M. (2024). Anomaly detection in IoT-based healthcare: Machine learning for enhanced security. *Scientific Reports*, *14*(1), 5872. DOI: 10.1038/s41598-024-56126-x PMID: 38467709

Khan, U. A., & Alamäki, A. (2023). Designing an Ethical and Secure Pain Estimation System Using AI Sandbox for Contactless Healthcare. *International Journal of Online and Biomedical Engineering*, *19*(15), 166–201. Advance online publication. DOI: 10.3991/ijoe.v19i15.43663

Khoi, N. M., Saguna, S., Mitra, K., & Åhlund, C. (2015, October). IReHMo: An efficient IoT-based remote health monitoring system for smart regions. In 2015 17th international conference on e-health networking, application & services (HealthCom) (pp. 563-568). IEEE.

Khubrani, M. M., & Alam, S. (2021). A detailed review of blockchain-based applications for protection against pandemic like COVID-19. *Telkomnika, 19*(4), 1185–1196. DOI: 10.12928/telkomnika.v19i4.18465

Khubrani, M., & Alam, S. (2023). Blockchain-Based Microgrid for Safe and Reliable Power Generation and Distribution: A Case Study of Saudi Arabia. *Energies, 16*(16), 5963. DOI: 10.3390/en16165963

Kim, H., Kim, S. W., Park, E., Kim, J. H., & Chang, H. (2020). The role of fifth-generation mobile technology in prehospital emergency care: An opportunity to support paramedics. *Health Policy and Technology, 9*(1), 109–114. DOI: 10.1016/j.hlpt.2020.01.002

Kishor Kumar Reddy, C., Daduvy, A., Madana Mohana, R., Assiri, B., Shuaib, M., Alam, S., & Abdullah Sheneamer, M. (2024). Enhancing Precision Agriculture and Land Cover Classification: A Self –Attention 3D Convolutional Neural Network Approach for Hyperspectral Image Analysis. *IEEE Access : Practical Innovations, Open Solutions, 12*, 125592–125608. Advance online publication. DOI: 10.1109/ACCESS.2024.3420089

Kishor Kumar Reddy, C., Kaza, V. S., Madana Mohana, R., Alhameed, M., Jeribi, F., Alam, S., & Shuaib, M. (2025). Detecting anomalies in smart wearables for hypertension: A deep learning mechanism. *Frontiers in Public Health, 12*, 1426168. DOI: 10.3389/fpubh.2024.1426168 PMID: 39850864

Knight, D. R. T., Aakre, C. A., Anstine, C. V., Munipalli, B., Biazar, P., Mitri, G., Valery, J. R., Brigham, T., Niazi, S. K., Perlman, A. I., Halamka, J. D., & Abu Dabrh, A. M. (2023). Artificial intelligence for patient scheduling in the real-world health care setting: A metanarrative review. *Health Policy and Technology, 12*(4), 100824. DOI: 10.1016/j.hlpt.2023.100824

Knudsen, J. E., Ghaffar, U., Ma, R., & Hung, A. J. (2024). Clinical Applications of Artificial Intelligence in Robotic Surgery. *Journal of Robotic Surgery, 18*(1), 1–10. DOI: 10.1007/s11701-024-01867-0 PMID: 38427094

Ko, D.-G., Mai, F., Shan, Z., & Zhang, D. (2019). Operational efficiency and patient-centered health care: A view from online physician reviews. *Journal of Operations Management, 65*(4), 353–379. DOI: 10.1002/joom.1028

Krapivin, V., & Shutko, A. M. (2012). *Information technologies for remote monitoring of the environment*. Springer Science & Business Media. DOI: 10.1007/978-3-642-20567-5

Krasniqi, F., Gavrilovska, L., & Maraj, A. (2019). The analysis of key performance indicators (KPI) in 4G/LTE networks. In Poulkov, V. (Ed.), *Future access enablers for ubiquitous and intelligent infrastructures* (pp. 285–296). Springer. DOI: 10.1007/978-3-030-23976-3_25

Kumar, V., Ali, A. A., Mittal, P., Aqeel, I., Shuaib, M., Alam, S., & Aalsalem, M. Y. (2024). E2SVM: Electricity-Efficient SLA-aware Virtual Machine Consolidation approach in cloud data centers. *PLoS ONE, 19*(6 June). DOI: 10.1371/journal.pone.0303313

Kumar, D., & Suthar, N. (2024). Predictive analytics and early intervention in healthcare social work: A scoping review. *Social Work in Health Care, 63*(4–5), 208–229. DOI: 10.1080/00981389.2024.2316700 PMID: 38349783

Kumar, M., Kumar, A., Verma, S., Bhattacharya, P., Ghimire, D., Kim, S., & Hosen, A. S. M. S. (2023). Healthcare Internet of Things (H-IoT): Current trends, future prospects, applications, challenges, and security issues. *Electronics (Basel), 12*(9), 2050. DOI: 10.3390/electronics12092050

Kumar, M., Verma, S., Kumar, A., Ijaz, M. F., & Rawat, D. B. (2022). ANAF-IoMT: A novel architectural framework for IoMT-enabled smart healthcare system by enhancing security based on RECC-VC. *IEEE Transactions on Industrial Informatics, 18*(12), 8936–8943. DOI: 10.1109/TII.2022.3181614

Kumar, R., & Sharma, R. (2022). Leveraging Blockchain for Ensuring Trust in IoT: A Survey. *Journal of King Saud University. Computer and Information Sciences, 34*(10), 8599–8622. DOI: 10.1016/j.jksuci.2021.09.004

Kumar, S., & Sharma, A. (2023). Machine learning algorithms for drug discovery and development. *Journal of Cheminformatics, 15*(4), 41–55.

Kunbi, A., Silver Cross, D. P., & Oladele, S. (2024). Increased Patient Engagement with Wireless Monitoring Systems.

Kwon, A., Lee, H.-Y., Shin, S.-Y., Yang, K., Sung, Y., Lee, K., Byeon, N.-S., Lim, T.-H., & Lee, J.-H. (2024). Current Health Data Standardization Project and Future Directions to Ensure Interoperability in Korea. *Healthcare Informatics Research, 30*(2), 93–102. DOI: 10.4258/hir.2024.30.2.93 PMID: 38755100

Landolina, M., Perego, G. B., Lunati, M., Curnis, A., Guenzati, G., Vicentini, A., Parati, G., Borghi, G., Zanaboni, P., Valsecchi, S., & Marzegalli, M. (2012). Remote monitoring reduces healthcare use and improves quality of care in heart failure patients with implantable defibrillators: The evolution of management strategies of heart failure patients with implantable defibrillators (EVOLVO) study. *Circulation, 125*(24), 2985–2992. DOI: 10.1161/CIRCULATIONAHA.111.088971 PMID: 22626743

Lazuardi, L., Sanjaya, G. Y., Ali, P. B., Siahaan, R. G. M., Achmad, L., & Wulandari, H. (2021). Interoperability of Health Digitalization: Case Study on Use of Information Technology for Maternal and Child Health Services in Indonesia. *Business Information Systems, 1*(SE-Applications), 317–327. DOI: 10.52825/bis.v1i.53

LeBaron, V. (2022). Challenges and opportunities in designing and deploying remote health monitoring technology for older adults with cancer. *Innovation in Aging, 6*(6), igac057. DOI: 10.1093/geroni/igac057 PMID: 36452048

Lee, D., & Yoon, S. N. (2021). Application of Artificial Intelligence-Based Technologies in the Healthcare Industry: Opportunities and Challenges. *International Journal of Environmental Research and Public Health, 18*(1), 271. DOI: 10.3390/ijerph18010271 PMID: 33401373

Lee, J. H., & Jeong, K. (2021). AI-driven medical imaging: Trends and future outlook. *Medical Image Analysis, 75*, 102301.

Li, D. (2019). 5G and intelligence medicine—How the next generation of wireless technology will reconstruct healthcare? *Precision Clinical Medicine*, *2*(3), 205–208. DOI: 10.1093/pcmedi/pbz020 PMID: 31886033

Lightsey, H. M.IV, Yeung, C. M., Samartzis, D., & Makhni, M. C. (2021). The past, present, and future of remote patient monitoring in spine care: An overview. *European Spine Journal : Official Publication of the European Spine Society, the European Spinal Deformity Society, and the European Section of the Cervical Spine Research Society*, *30*(8), 2102–2108. DOI: 10.1007/s00586-021-06921-1 PMID: 34241698

Li, J., & Carayon, P. (2021). Health Care 4.0: A Vision for Smart and Connected Health Care. *IISE Transactions on Healthcare Systems Engineering*, *11*(3), 171–180. DOI: 10.1080/24725579.2021.1884627 PMID: 34497970

Liu, Y., Wei, S., & Zhang, X. (2020). Privacy-preserving healthcare using blockchain and AI. *Journal of Medical Systems*, *44*(5), 78–91.

Lopes, M. A., Almeida, Á. S., & Almada-Lobo, B. (2015). Handling healthcare workforce planning with care: Where do we stand? *Human Resources for Health*, *13*(1), 38. DOI: 10.1186/s12960-015-0028-0 PMID: 26003337

Loupian, E. A., Bourtsev, M. A., Proshin, A. A., & Kobets, D. A. (2018). Evolution of remote monitoring information systems development concepts. Sovremennye problemy distantsionnogo zondirovaniya Zemli iz kosmosa, 15(3), 53-66.

MacKey, T. K., & Liang, B. A. (2012). Combating Healthcare Corruption and Fraud with Improved Global Health Governance. *BMC International Health and Human Rights*, *12*(1), 23. Advance online publication. DOI: 10.1186/1472-698X-12-23 PMID: 23088820

Magrupov, T. M., Yuldashev, Z. M., & Abdihalikov, S. P. (2021). A Medical Hardware-Software System for Remote Monitoring of Heart Diseases., 24(2), 78-86.

Maguluri, L. P., Chouhan, K., Balamurali, R., Rani, R., Hashmi, A., Kiran, A., & Rajaram, A. (2024). Adversarial deep learning for improved abdominal organ segmentation in CT scans. *Multimedia Tools and Applications*, *83*(35), 82107–82129. DOI: 10.1007/s11042-024-18578-1

Mahmoudian, Y., Nemati, A., & Safaei, A. S. (2023). A forecasting approach for hospital bed capacity planning using machine learning and deep learning with application to public hospitals. *Healthcare Analytics*, *4*, 100245. DOI: 10.1016/j.health.2023.100245

Majumder, S., Mondal, T., & Deen, M. J. (2017). Wearable sensors for remote health monitoring. *Sensors (Basel)*, *17*(1), 130. DOI: 10.3390/s17010130 PMID: 28085085

Maleki Varnosfaderani, S., & Forouzanfar, M. (2024). The Role of AI in Hospitals and Clinics: Transforming Healthcare in the 21st Century. *Bioengineering (Basel, Switzerland)*, *11*(4), 337. DOI: 10.3390/bioengineering11040337 PMID: 38671759

Marshall, A., Yap, K. M., & Yu, W. (2008). Providing QoS for networked peers in distributed haptic virtual environments. *Advances in Multimedia*, *841590*(1), 841590. Advance online publication. DOI: 10.1155/2008/841590

Martínez-Caro, E., Cegarra-Navarro, J. G., García-Pérez, A., & Fait, M. (2017, July). 2018. "Healthcare Service Evolution towards the Internet of Things: An End-User Perspective.". *Technological Forecasting and Social Change*, *136*, 268–276. DOI: 10.1016/j.techfore.2018.03.025

Masih, R. K., Alam, S., Tabassum, S., Shuaib, M., & Ahmad, S. (2023). An Analysis of the Significant Role Played by Mobile Cloud Forensics and its Key Obstacles. In *2023 International Conference in Advances in Power, Signal, and Information Technology, APSIT 2023*. DOI: 10.1109/APSIT58554.2023.10201715

Mastour, H., Khoshgoftar, Z., Ahmady, S., & Sohrabi, S. (2025). Implementing an Internet of Things-based learning platform into medical education: Addressing educational challenges with innovative solutions. *Medical Teacher*, ●●●, 1–4. DOI: 10.1080/0142159X.2024.2445036 PMID: 39773016

Mathew, P. S., Pillai, A. S., & Palade, V. (2018). Applications of Iot in Healthcare. *Lecture Notes on Data Engineering and Communications Technologies*, *14*, 263–288. DOI: 10.1007/978-3-319-70688-7_11

Matthews, P., & Rhodes-Maquaire, C. (2024). Personalisation and Recommendation for Mental Health Apps: A Scoping Review. *Behaviour & Information Technology*, ●●●, 1–16. DOI: 10.1080/0144929X.2024.2356630

McKinney, S. M., Sieniek, M., Godbole, V., Godwin, J., Antropova, N., Ashrafian, H., Back, T., Chesus, M., Corrado, G. S., Darzi, A., Etemadi, M., Garcia-Vicente, F., Gilbert, F. J., Halling-Brown, M., Hassabis, D., Jansen, S., Karthikesalingam, A., Kelly, C. J., King, D., & Shetty, S. (2020). International evaluation of an AI system for breast cancer screening. *Nature*, *577*(7788), 89–94. DOI: 10.1038/s41586-019-1799-6 PMID: 31894144

Merhej, J., Harb, H., Abouaissa, A., & Idoumghar, L. (2024). Toward a New Era of Smart and Secure Healthcare Information Exchange Systems: Combining Blockchain and Artificial Intelligence. In *Applied Sciences* (Vol. 14, Issue 19). DOI: 10.3390/app14198808

Meszaros, J., Minari, J., & Huys, I. (2022). The future regulation of artificial intelligence systems in healthcare services and medical research in the European Union. *Frontiers in Genetics*, *13*, 927721. Advance online publication. DOI: 10.3389/fgene.2022.927721 PMID: 36267404

Minoi, J. L., & Yeo, A. W. (2014, December). Remote health monitoring system in a rural population: Challenges and opportunities. In *2014 IEEE Conference on Biomedical Engineering and Sciences (IECBES)* (pp. 895-900). IEEE. DOI: 10.1109/IECBES.2014.7047641

Minutolo, A., Esposito, M., & De Pietro, G. (2016, December). 2017. "Optimization of Rule-Based Systems in MHealth Applications.". *Engineering Applications of Artificial Intelligence*, *59*, 103–121. DOI: 10.1016/j.engappai.2016.12.007

Mirbabaie, M., Stieglitz, S., & Frick, N. R. J. (2021). *Artificial Intelligence in Disease Diagnostics: A Critical Review and Classification on the Current State of Research Guiding Future Direction* (Vol. 11). Springer Berlin Heidelberg.

Mirjalali, S., Peng, S., Fang, Z., Wang, C., & Wu, S. (2022). Wearable sensors for remote health monitoring: Potential applications for early diagnosis of Covid-19. *Advanced Materials Technologies*, *7*(1), 2100545. DOI: 10.1002/admt.202100545 PMID: 34901382

Mitchell, M. D., Williams, K., Brennan, P. J., & Umscheid, C. A. (2010). Integrating local data into hospital-based healthcare technology assessment: Two case studies. *International Journal of Technology Assessment in Health Care, 26*(3), 294–300. DOI: 10.1017/S0266462310000334 PMID: 20584358

Mohamad Jawad, H. H., Bin Hassan, Z., Zaidan, B. B., Mohammed Jawad, F. H., Mohamed Jawad, D. H., & Alredany, W. H. D. (2022). A systematic literature review of enabling IoT in healthcare: Motivations, challenges, and recommendations. *Electronics (Basel), 11*(19), 3223. DOI: 10.3390/electronics11193223

Mohammed, K. I., Zaidan, A. A., Zaidan, B. B., Albahri, O. S., Alsalem, M. A., Albahri, A. S., Hadi, A., & Hashim, M. (2019). Real-time remote-health monitoring systems: A review on patients prioritisation for multiple-chronic diseases, taxonomy analysis, concerns and solution procedure. *Journal of Medical Systems, 43*(7), 1–21. DOI: 10.1007/s10916-019-1362-x PMID: 31187288

Mohanarangan, V. Devarajan., Rajya, Lakshmi, Gudivaka., Basava, Ramanjaneyulu, Gudivaka., Raj, Kumar, Gudivaka., T., Ganesan., Priyan, Malarvizhi, Kumar. (2024). Computer Vision-Based Radial Basis Function Networks in Healthcare Applications. DOI: 10.2139/ssrn.4809360

Monika Singh, T., Kishor Kumar Reddy, C., Ramana Murthy, B. V., Nag, A., & Doss, S. (2025). AI and Education: Bridging the Gap to Personalized, Efficient, and Accessible Learning. In M. Ouaissa, M. Ouaissa, H. Lamaazi, M. El Hamlaoui, & K. Reddy C. (Eds.), Internet of Behavior-Based Computational Intelligence for Smart Education Systems (pp. 131-160). IGI Global. DOI: 10.4018/979-8-3693-8151-9.ch005

Monlezun, D. J. (2023a). Chapter 4 - AI+public health: effective and fair collaboration. In *The Thinking Healthcare System.*

Monlezun, D. J. (2023b). Chapter 8 - AI+health ethics: moral interoperability and pluralism. In *The Thinking Healthcare System.*

Monlezun, D. J. (2023c). Chapter 9 - The future's (AI) thinking healthcare system: blueprint, roadmap, and DNA. In *The Thinking Healthcare System.*

Monlezun, D. J. (2023d). The future's (AI) thinking healthcare system. In *The Thinking Healthcare System.* DOI: 10.1016/B978-0-443-18906-7.00008-8

Mooghali, M., Stroud, A. M., Yoo, D. W., & Barry, B. A. & ... (2023). Barriers and Facilitators to Trustworthy and Ethical AI-enabled Medical Care From Patient and Healthcare Provider Perspectives: A Literature Review. *MedRxiv.*

Morpurgo, F., & Occhipinti, C. (2023). Let the AI assisted medicine remain human Developing a care centered model of ethical decision making in AI based healthcare. *CEUR Workshop Proceedings, •••*, 3486.

Munavalli, J. R., Boersma, H. J., Rao, S. V., & van Merode, G. G. (2021). Real-time capacity management and patient flow optimization in hospitals using AI methods. In Masmoudi, M., Jarboui, B., & Siarry, P. (Eds.), *Artificial intelligence and data mining in healthcare.* Springer., DOI: 10.1007/978-3-030-45240-7_3

Mutlag, A. A., Abd Ghani, M. K., Arunkumar, N. A., Mohammed, M. A., & Mohd, O. (2019). Enabling technologies for fog computing in healthcare IoT systems. *Future Generation Computer Systems, 90*, 62–78. DOI: 10.1016/j.future.2018.07.049

Mykowiecka, A., Marciniak, M., & Kupść, A. (2009). Rule-Based Information Extraction from Patients' Clinical Data. *Journal of Biomedical Informatics, 42*(5), 923–936. DOI: 10.1016/j.jbi.2009.07.007 PMID: 19646551

Nadakuditi, S., Kumar, B., & Kumar, T. (2024). AI and Machine Learning in Healthcare-Applications, Challenges and Ethics. *International Journal of Health Sciences, 7*(4), 36–43. DOI: 10.47941/ijhs.1949

Naddeo, S., Verde, L., Forastiere, M., De Pietro, G., & Sannino, G. (2017, February). A real-time m-health monitoring system: An integrated solution combining the use of several wearable sensors and mobile devices. In Special Session on Smart Medical Devices-From Lab to Clinical Practice (Vol. 6, pp. 545-552). SciTePress.

Naik, N., & Acharya, U. R. (2022). Role of natural language processing in healthcare data analysis. *Computer Methods and Programs in Biomedicine, 227*, 106924.

Nasir, S., Khan, R. A., & Bai, S. (2024). Ethical Framework for Harnessing the Power of AI in Healthcare and Beyond. *IEEE Access : Practical Innovations, Open Solutions, 12*, 31014–31035. Advance online publication. DOI: 10.1109/ACCESS.2024.3369912

Nasrullah, A. (2024). Utilizing Machine Learning for Predictive Analytics. *Advances in Healthcare Technology., 1*(1), 57–67. DOI: 10.60087/japmi.vol01.issue01.p67

National Science Foundation. (2016). *NSF follow-on workshop on ultra-low latency wireless networks*. NSF.

Nedungadi, P., Jayakumar, A., & Raman, R. (2018). Personalized health monitoring system for managing well-being in rural areas. *Journal of Medical Systems, 42*(1), 1–11. DOI: 10.1007/s10916-017-0854-9 PMID: 29242996

Ng, M., Borst, E., Garrity, A., Hirschfeld, E., & Lee, J. (2020). Evolution of do-it-yourself remote monitoring technology for type 1 diabetes. *Journal of Diabetes Science and Technology, 14*(5), 854–859. DOI: 10.1177/1932296819895537 PMID: 31893941

Nianga, Z. W. (2024). Leveraging AI for Strategic Management in Healthcare: Enhancing Operational and Financial Performance. *Journal of Intelligence and Knowledge Engineering (ISSN: 2959-0620), 2*(3), 1.

Nicholson, L., Vakharia, A. J., & Erenguc, S. S. (2004). Outsourcing inventory management decisions in healthcare: Models and application. *European Journal of Operational Research, 154*(1), 271–290. DOI: 10.1016/S0377-2217(02)00700-2

Nithya, B., & Ilango, V. 2017. "Predictive Analytics in Health Care Using Machine Learning Tools and Techniques." *Proceedings of the 2017 International Conference on Intelligent Computing and Control Systems, ICICCS 2017* 2018-January:492–99. DOI: 10.1109/ICCONS.2017.8250771

Niu, B., Mukhtarova, N., Alagoz, O., & Hoppe, K. (2022). Cost-effectiveness of telehealth with remote patient monitoring for postpartum hypertension. *The Journal of Maternal-Fetal & Neonatal Medicine*, *35*(25), 7555–7561. DOI: 10.1080/14767058.2021.1956456 PMID: 34470135

Nneka, O. O., Okafor, K. C., Nwabueze, C. A., Mbachu, C. B., Iloh, J. P., Chinebu, T. I., Adebisi, B., & Chukwunenye Anthony, O. (2024). A computational fractional order model for optimal control of wearable healthcare monitoring devices for maternal health. *Healthcare Analytics*, *5*, 100308. Advance online publication. DOI: 10.1016/j.health.2024.100308

Núñez, J. C., Cabido, R., Pantrigo, J. J., Montemayor, A. S., & Vélez, J. F. (2018). Convolutional Neural Networks and Long Short-Term Memory for Skeleton-Based Human Activity and Hand Gesture Recognition. *Pattern Recognition*, *76*, 80–94. DOI: 10.1016/j.patcog.2017.10.033

Nurshod, A., Khujamatov, K., & Lazarev, A. (2021, November). Remote monitoring system architectures in healthcare. In 2021 International Conference on Information Science and Communications Technologies (ICISCT) (pp. 01-05). IEEE. DOI: 10.1109/ICISCT52966.2021.9670405

Obermeyer, Z., & Emanuel, E. J. (2016). Predicting the future—Big data, machine learning, and clinical medicine. *The New England Journal of Medicine*, *375*(13), 1216–1219. DOI: 10.1056/NEJMp1606181 PMID: 27682033

Obijuru, A., Arowoogun, J. O., Onwumere, C., Odilibe, I. P., Anyanwu, E. C., & Daraojimba, A. I. (2024). Big data analytics in healthcare: A review of recent advances and potential for personalized medicine. *International Medical Science Research Journal*, *4*(2), 170–182. DOI: 10.51594/imsrj.v4i2.810

Ojaroudi Parchin, N., Jahanbakhsh Basherlou, H., Al-Yasir, Y. I., Abd-Alhameed, R. A., Abdulkhaleq, A. M., & Noras, J. M. (2019). Recent developments of reconfigurable antennas for current and future wireless communication systems. *Electronics (Basel)*, *8*(2), 128. DOI: 10.3390/electronics8020128

Ojaroudiparchin, N., Shen, M., & Pedersen, G. F. (2016, May 9–11). *Wide-scan phased array antenna fed by coax-to-microstriplines for 5G cell phones*. In 2016 21st International Conference on Microwave, Radar and Wireless Communications (MIKON) (pp. 1–4). IEEE. DOI: 10.1109/MIKON.2016.7492064

Olawade, D. B., David-Olawade, A. C., Wada, O. Z., Asaolu, A. J., Adereni, T., & Ling, J. (2024). Artificial intelligence in healthcare delivery: Prospects and pitfalls. *Journal of Medicine, Surgery, and Public Health*, *3*, 100108. https://doi.org/https://doi.org/10.1016/j.glmedi.2024.100108. DOI: 10.1016/j.glmedi.2024.100108

Oniani, S., Marques, G., Barnovi, S., Pires, I. M., & Bhoi, A. K. (2020). Artificial intelligence for internet of things and enhanced medical systems. In *Bio-inspired neurocomputing* (pp. 43–59). Springer.

Ozturk, B. A., Tayyeh, H. K., Namiq, H. E., Mahajan, H. B., Junnarkar, A. A., Uke, N., Shamaileh, A. A., Deshpande, S. D., Futane, P. R., & Rane, M. (2024). The Blockchain for Healthcare 4.0 Apply in Standard Secure Medical Data Processing Architecture. *Internet Technology Letters, n/a*(n/a), e614. https://doi.org/https://doi.org/10.1002/itl2.614

Padmashree, T., & Nayak, S. S. (2020, October 7–9). *5G technology for e-health*. In 2020 Fourth International Conference on I-SMAC (IoT in Social, Mobile, Analytics and Cloud) (I-SMAC) (pp. 211–216). IEEE. https://doi.org/DOI: 10.1109/I-SMAC49090.2020.9243366

Panayides, A. S., Amini, A., Filipovic, N. D., Sharma, A., Tsaftaris, S. A., Young, A., Foran, D., Do, N., Golemati, S., Kurc, T., Huang, K., Nikita, K. S., Veasey, B. P., Zervakis, M., Saltz, J. H., & Pattichis, C. S. (2020). AI in Medical Imaging Informatics: Current Challenges and Future Directions. *IEEE Journal of Biomedical and Health Informatics*, *24*(7), 1837–1857. DOI: 10.1109/JBHI.2020.2991043 PMID: 32609615

Pandimurugan, V., & Sultan Ahmad, A. (2024). CNN-Based Deep Learning Model for Early Identification and Categorization of Melanoma Skin Cancer Using Medical Imaging. *SN Computer Science*, *5*(7), 1–20. DOI: 10.1007/s42979-024-03270-w

Parihar, Akshay, Jigna B. Prajapati, Bhupendra G. Prajapati, Binti Trambadiya, Arti Thakkar, and Pinalkumar Engineer. 2024. "Role of IOT in Healthcare: Applications, Security & Privacy Concerns." *Intelligent Pharmacy* (December 2023). .DOI: 10.1016/j.ipha.2024.01.003

Park, S. H., & Han, K. (2018). Methodologic guide for evaluating clinical performance and effect of AI in medical imaging. *Radiology*, *286*(3), 800–809. DOI: 10.1148/radiol.2017171920 PMID: 29309734

Patil, A., ... (2024). Cyber resilience: Safeguarding India's markets in the post-pandemic cyber landscape. In *2024 4th International Conference on Innovative Practices in Technology and Management (ICIPTM)* (pp. 1–5). IEEE. DOI: 10.1109/ICIPTM59628.2024.10563229

Patil, S., & Shankar, H. (2023). Transforming healthcare: Harnessing the power of AI in the modern era. *International Journal of Multidisciplinary Sciences and Arts*, *2*(2), 60–70. DOI: 10.47709/ijmdsa.v2i1.2513

Pendyala, S. K. (2024). Healthcare Data Analytics: Leveraging Predictive Analytics For Improved Patient Outcomes. *International Journal Of Computer Engineering And Technology (Ijcet)*, *15*(6), 548–565.

Petersson, L., Vincent, K., Svedberg, P., Nygren, J. M., & Larsson, I. (2023). Ethical Perspectives on Implementing AI to Predict Mortality Risk in Emergency Department Patients: A Qualitative Study. *Studies in Health Technology and Informatics*, *302*. Advance online publication. DOI: 10.3233/SHTI230234 PMID: 37203776

Peyroteo, M., Ferreira, I. A., Elvas, L. B., Ferreira, J. C., & Lapão, L. V. (2021). Remote monitoring systems for patients with chronic diseases in primary health care: Systematic review. *JMIR mHealth and uHealth*, *9*(12), e28285. DOI: 10.2196/28285 PMID: 34932000

Phuong, J., Hong, S., Palchuk, M. B., Espinoza, J., Meeker, D., Dorr, D. A., & Adams, W. G. (2022). Advancing interoperability of patient-level social determinants of health data to support COVID-19 research. *AMIA Joint Summits on Translational Science Proceedings AMIA Summit on Translational Science*, *2022*, 396.

Pierre, K., Haneberg, A. G., Kwak, S., Peters, K. R., Hochhegger, B., Sananmuang, T., Tunlayadechanont, P., Tighe, P. J., Mancuso, A., & Forghani, R. (2023). Applications of artificial intelligence in the radiology roundtrip: Process streamlining, workflow optimization, and beyond. *Seminars in Roentgenology*, *58*(2), 158–169. DOI: 10.1053/j.ro.2023.02.003 PMID: 37087136

Plummer, D. (2024). Ethical AI and the Future of Healthcare: Combining Academic Theory and Industry Practice to Ensure Patient-Centered Care. *European Journal of Technology*, *8*(1), 1–13. Advance online publication. DOI: 10.47672/ejt.1727

Polevikov, S. (2023). Advancing AI in healthcare: A comprehensive review of best practices. *Clinica Chimica Acta*, *548*, 117519. https://doi.org/https://doi.org/10.1016/j.cca.2023.117519. DOI: 10.1016/j.cca.2023.117519 PMID: 37595864

Poloju, N., & Rajaram, A. (2024). Transformation with yolo tiny network architecture for multimodal fusion in lung disease classification. *Cybernetics and Systems*, ●●●, 1–22. DOI: 10.1080/01969722.2024.2343992

Pourzolfaghar, Z., Alfano, M., & Helfert, M. (2023). Application of ethical AI requirements to an AI solution use-case in healthcare domain. *American Journal of Business*, *38*(3), 112–128. Advance online publication. DOI: 10.1108/AJB-12-2022-0201

Pradhan, B., Bhattacharyya, S., & Pal, K. (2021). IoT-based applications in healthcare devices. *Journal of Healthcare Engineering*, *2021*(1), 6632599. PMID: 33791084

Pradhan, B., Bhattacharyya, S., & Pal, K. (2021). IoT-Based Applications in Healthcare Devices. *Journal of Healthcare Engineering*, *2021*, 1–18. Advance online publication. DOI: 10.1155/2021/6632599 PMID: 33791084

Preum, S. M., Munir, S., Ma, M., Yasar, M. S., Stone, D. J., Williams, R., Alemzadeh, H., & Stankovic, J. A. (2021). A Review of Cognitive Assistants for Healthcare: Trends, Prospects, and Future Directions. *ACM Computing Surveys*, *53*(6), 1–37. Advance online publication. DOI: 10.1145/3419368

Priya, B., Rajendran, S., Bala, R., & Gobbi, R. (2009, July). Remote wireless health monitoring systems. In 2009 Innovative Technologies in Intelligent Systems and Industrial Applications (pp. 383-388). IEEE

Prorok, M., & Takacs, I. (2023). Legal and Moral Issues Related to Artificial Intelligence Technology in Business. *SISY 2023 - IEEE 21st International Symposium on Intelligent Systems and Informatics, Proceedings*. DOI: 10.1109/SISY60376.2023.10417881

Qamar, S., Amaan, M., Rahman, M. I., Aqeel, I., Shuaib, M., Khormi, I., & Alam, S. (2023). Cloud data transmission based on security and improved routing through hybrid machine learning techniques. *Soft Computing*. Advance online publication. DOI: 10.1007/s00500-023-08417-0

Qi, J., Yang, P., Min, G., Amft, O., Dong, F., & Xu, L. (2017). Advanced internet of things for personalised healthcare systems: A survey. *Pervasive and Mobile Computing*, *41*, 132–149. DOI: 10.1016/j.pmcj.2017.06.018

Qin, W. F., Xue, Y., Peng, H., Li, G., Chen, W., Zhao, X., Pang, J., & Zhou, B. (2024). Wearable real-time multi-health parameter monitoring system. *International Journal of Clothing Science and Technology*, *36*(1), 17–33. Advance online publication. DOI: 10.1108/IJCST-04-2023-0054

Qureshi, H. N., Manalastas, M., Zaidi, S. M. A., Imran, A., & Al Kalaa, M. O. (2020). Service level agreements for 5G and beyond: Overview, challenges and enablers of 5G-healthcare systems. *IEEE Access : Practical Innovations, Open Solutions*, *9*, 1044–1061. DOI: 10.1109/ACCESS.2020.3046927 PMID: 35211361

Rahim, M. J., Afroz, A., & Akinola, O. (2025). Predictive Analytics in Healthcare: Big Data, Better Decisions. *International Journal of Scientific Research and Modern Technology*, *4*(1), 1–21.

Rahman, S. M., Ibtisum, S., Podder, P., & Hossain, S. M. (2023). Progression and challenges of IoT in healthcare: A short review. *ArXiv Preprint ArXiv:2311.12869*.

Rahman, A., Debnath, T., Kundu, D., Khan, M. S. I., Aishi, A. A., Sazzad, S., Sayduzzaman, M., & Band, S. S. (2024). Machine learning and deep learning-based approach in smart healthcare: Recent advances, applications, challenges and opportunities. *AIMS Public Health*, *11*(1), 58–109. DOI: 10.3934/publichealth.2024004 PMID: 38617415

Rajagopal, A., Ahmad, S., Jha, S., Alagarsamy, R., Alharbi, A., & Alouffi, B. (2023). A Robust Automated Framework for Classification of CT Covid-19 Images Using MSI-ResNet. *Computer Systems Science and Engineering*, *45*(3), 3215–3229. DOI: 10.32604/csse.2023.025705

Rajesh, R., Hemalatha, S., Nagarajan, S. M., Devarajan, G. G., Omar, M., & Bashir, A. K. (2024). Threat detection and mitigation for tactile internet driven consumer IoT-healthcare system. *IEEE Transactions on Consumer Electronics*.

Rajkomar, A., Dean, J., & Kohane, I. (2019). Machine Learning in Medicine. *The New England Journal of Medicine*, *380*(14), 1347–1358. DOI: 10.1056/NEJMra1814259 PMID: 30943338

Ramalingam, S., Dharani, S. P., Priya, R., Devi, E. P., & Pavithra, S. (2024). Machine Learning Based Remote Health Care Data Monitoring and Prediction System Using IoMT. *2024 10th International Conference on Advanced Computing and Communication Systems (ICACCS)*, *1*, 2113–2118.

Ramanathan, A., Vijaya Rani, K. R., Bhupathyraaj, M., Chacko, L., & Alharbi, H. F. (2023). An Ethical Outlook on the Applications of Artificial Intelligence in Medicine and Pharmacy. In *Artificial Intelligence in Pharmaceutical Sciences*. DOI: 10.1201/9781003343981-10

Ramanayake, R., Wicke, P., & Nallur, V. (2023). Immune moral models? Pro-social rule breaking as a moral enhancement approach for ethical AI. *AI & Society*, *38*(2), 801–813. Advance online publication. DOI: 10.1007/s00146-022-01478-z PMID: 35645466

Rasid, M. F., Musa, W. M., Kadir, N. A., Noor, A. M., Touati, F., Mehmood, W., Khriji, L., Al-Busaidi, A., & Mnaouer, A. B. (2014, May 28–30). *Embedded gateway services for Internet of Things applications in ubiquitous healthcare*. In 2014 2nd International Conference on Information and Communication Technology (ICoICT) (pp. 145–148). IEEE. DOI: 10.1109/ICoICT.2014.6914055

Rasouli, J. J., Shao, J., Neifert, S., Gibbs, W. N., Habboub, G., Steinmetz, M. P., Benzel, E., & Mroz, T. E. (2021). Artificial Intelligence and Robotics in Spine Surgery. *Global Spine Journal*, *11*(4), 556–564. DOI: 10.1177/2192568220915718 PMID: 32875928

Rattanawiboomsom, V., Korejo, M. S., Ali, J., & Thatsaringkharnsakun, U. (2023). Blockchain-Enabled Internet of Things (IoT) Applications in Healthcare: A Systematic Review of Current Trends and Future Opportunities. *International Journal of Online & Biomedical Engineering*, *19*(10), 99–117. DOI: 10.3991/ijoe.v19i10.41399

Ravindranathan, P.. (2024). Illuminating the dark: Gaining insights and managing risks with dark analytics. In *2024 International Conference on Intelligent and Innovative Technologies in Computing, Electrical and Electronics (IITCEE)* (pp. 1–6). IEEE. DOI: 10.1109/IITCEE59897.2024.10467380

Rawas, S., Tafran, C., AlSaeed, D., & Al-Ghreimil, N. (2024). Transforming Healthcare: AI-NLP Fusion Framework for Precision Decision-Making and Personalized Care Optimization in the Era of IoMT. *Computers, Materials & Continua*, *81*(3), 4575–4601. DOI: 10.32604/cmc.2024.055307

Reddy, C. K. K., & Satvika, P. (2023). An Efficient Early Diagnosis and Healthcare Monitoring System for Mental Disorder using Machine learning Approach.

Reddy, C. K. K., Pujala, N., & Doss, S. (2024). From Industry 4.0 to 5.0: Navigating the human-tech symbiosis in the era of COVID-19. In Ethical artificial intelligence in power electronics. CRC Press Taylor and Francis. https://doi.org/DOI: 10.1201/9781032648323

Reddy, C. K. K. (2023). An Efficient Early Diagnosis and Healthcare Monitoring System for Mental Disorders Using Machine Learning. In *Sustainable Science and Intelligent Technologies for Societal Development* (pp. 22–43). IGI Global.

Reddy, C. K. K., Rangarajan, A., Rangarajan, D., Shuaib, M., Jeribi, F., & Alam, S. (2024). A Transfer Learning Approach: Early Prediction of Alzheimer's Disease on US Healthy Aging Dataset. *Mathematics*, *12*(14), 2204. DOI: 10.3390/math12142204

Reddy, C. K. K., Reddy, P. A., Janapati, H., Assiri, B., Shuaib, M., Alam, S., & Sheneamer, A. (2024). A fine-tuned vision transformer based enhanced multi-class brain tumor classification using MRI scan imagery. *Frontiers in Oncology*, *14*, 1400341. DOI: 10.3389/fonc.2024.1400341 PMID: 39091923

Reddy, K. K., Badam, R., Alam, S., & Shuaib, M. (2024). IoT Driven Accessibility:A Refreshable OCR-Braille Solution for Visually Impaired and Deaf-Blind Users through WSN. *JETECH Elsevier*, *2*(April), 128–137. Advance online publication. DOI: 10.1016/j.ject.2024.04.007

Reegu, F., Daud, S. M., & Alam, S. (n.d.). BLOCKCHAIN AND INTEROPERABLE STANDARDS FOR EHR-A COMPREHENSIVE REVIEW. *Turkish Journal of Physiotherapy and Rehabilitation, 32*(2).

Reegu, F. A., Daud, S. M., Alam, S., & Shuaib, M. (2021). *Blockchain-based Electronic Health Record System for efficient Covid-19 Pandemic Management*. DOI: 10.20944/preprints202104.0771.v1

Rehman, M. U., Shafique, A., Khan, M. S., Driss, M., Boulila, W., Ghadi, Y. Y., Changalasetty, S. B., Alhaisoni, M., & Ahmad, J. (2024). A Novel Medical Image Data Protection Scheme for Smart Healthcare System. *CAAI Transactions on Intelligence Technology*, *9*(4), 821–836. DOI: 10.1049/cit2.12292

Rehman, S. U., Usman, M., Toor, M. H. Y., & Hussaini, Q. A. (2024). Advancing structural health monitoring: A vibration-based IoT approach for remote real-time systems. *Sensors and Actuators. A, Physical*, *365*, 114863. DOI: 10.1016/j.sna.2023.114863

Rohokale, V. M., Prasad, N. R., & Prasad, R. (2011, February 28–March 3). *A cooperative Internet of Things (IoT) for rural healthcare monitoring and control.* In 2011 2nd International Conference on Wireless Communication, Vehicular Technology, Information Theory and Aerospace & Electronic Systems Technology (Wireless VITAE) (pp. 1–6). IEEE. DOI: 10.1109/WIRELESSVITAE.2011.5940920

Rojas, J. C., Rohweder, G., Guptill, J., Arora, V. M., & Umscheid, C. A. (2022). Predictive analytics programs at large healthcare systems in the USA: A national survey. *Journal of General Internal Medicine, 37*(15), 4015–4017. DOI: 10.1007/s11606-022-07517-1 PMID: 35396657

Rosa, B. M. G., Anastasova, S., & Yang, G. Z. (2023). NFC-Powered Implantable Device for On-Body Parameters Monitoring With Secure Data Exchange Link to a Medical Blockchain Type of Network. *IEEE Transactions on Cybernetics, 53*(1), 31–43. DOI: 10.1109/TCYB.2021.3088711 PMID: 34197334

Roy, C., Saha, R., Misra, S., & Niyato, D. (2021). Soft-health: Software-defined fog architecture for IoT applications in healthcare. *IEEE Internet of Things Journal, 9*(3), 2455–2462. DOI: 10.1109/JIOT.2021.3097554

Sabry, F., Eltaras, T., Labda, W., Alzoubi, K., & Malluhi, Q. (2022). Machine learning for healthcare wearable devices: The big picture. *Journal of Healthcare Engineering, 2022*(1), 4653923. DOI: 10.1155/2022/4653923 PMID: 35480146

Safavi, K. C., Driscoll, W., & Wiener-Kronish, J. P. (2019). Remote surveillance technologies: Realizing the aim of right patient, right data, right time. *Anesthesia and Analgesia, 129*(3), 726–734. DOI: 10.1213/ANE.0000000000003948 PMID: 31425213

Saha, E., & Ray, P. K. (2019). Modelling and analysis of inventory management systems in healthcare: A review and reflections. *Computers & Industrial Engineering, 137*, 106051. DOI: 10.1016/j.cie.2019.106051

Saif, S., Das, P., Biswas, S., Khan, S., Haq, M. A., & Kovtun, V. (2024). A Secure Data Transmission Framework for IoT Enabled Healthcare. *Heliyon, 10*(16), e36269. DOI: 10.1016/j.heliyon.2024.e36269 PMID: 39224301

Sakhare, N. N., Limkar, S., Mahadik, R. V., Phursule, R., Godbole, A., Shirkande, S. T., & Patange, A. (2023). Ethical considerations of AI applications in medicine: A policy framework for responsible deployment. In *Journal of Krishna Institute of Medical Sciences University* (Vol. 12, Issue 4).

Salah, W. A., & Zneid, B. A. (2019). Evolution of microcontroller-based remote monitoring system applications. *International Journal of Electrical and Computer Engineering, 9*(4), 2354. DOI: 10.11591/ijece.v9i4.pp2354-2364

Sanchez, P., Voisey, J. P., Xia, T., Watson, H. I., O'Neil, A. Q., & Tsaftaris, S. A. (2022). Causal machine learning for healthcare and precision medicine. *Royal Society Open Science, 9*(8), 220638. DOI: 10.1098/rsos.220638 PMID: 35950198

Saraswat, D., Bhattacharya, P., Verma, A., Prasad, V. K., Tanwar, S., Sharma, G., Bokoro, P. N., & Sharma, R. (2022). Explainable AI for Healthcare 5.0: Opportunities and Challenges. *IEEE Access : Practical Innovations, Open Solutions, 10*(July), 84486–84517. DOI: 10.1109/ACCESS.2022.3197671

Saripalle, R., Runyan, C., & Russell, M. (2019). Using HL7 FHIR to achieve interoperability in patient health record. *Journal of Biomedical Informatics, 94*, 103188. https://doi.org/https://doi.org/10.1016/j.jbi.2019.103188. DOI: 10.1016/j.jbi.2019.103188 PMID: 31063828

Sarker, S., Jamal, L., Ahmed, S. F., & Irtisam, N. (2021). Robotics and artificial intelligence in healthcare during the COVID-19 pandemic: A systematic review. *Robotics and Autonomous Systems*, *146*, 103902. DOI: 10.1016/j.robot.2021.103902 PMID: 34629751

Sathya, D., & Ganesh Kumar, P. (2017). Secured remote health monitoring system. *Healthcare Technology Letters*, *4*(6), 228–232. DOI: 10.1049/htl.2017.0033 PMID: 29383257

Satti, F. A., Ali, T., Hussain, J., Khan, W. A., Khattak, A. M., & Lee, S. (2020). Ubiquitous Health Profile (UHPr): A big data curation platform for supporting health data interoperability. *Computing*, *102*(11), 2409–2444. DOI: 10.1007/s00607-020-00837-2

Saxena, Y.. (2024). Cloud renaissance: Thriving in the post-pandemic digital landscape. In *2024 Fourth International Conference on Advances in Electrical, Computing, Communication and Sustainable Technologies (ICAECT)* (pp. 1–6). IEEE. DOI: 10.1109/ICAECT60202.2024.10469149

Sayeed, R., Gottlieb, D., & Mandl, K. D. (2020). SMART Markers: Collecting patient-generated health data as a standardized property of health information technology. *NPJ Digital Medicine*, *3*(1), 9. DOI: 10.1038/s41746-020-0218-6 PMID: 31993507

Schaeffer, C., Haque, A., Booton, L., Halleck, J., & Coustasse, A. (2016). Big data management in United States hospitals: Benefits and barriers.

Schaich, F., Hamon, M. H., Hunukumbure, M., Lorca, J., Pedersen, K., Schubert, M., Kosmatos, E., Wunder, G., & Reaz, K. (2018, June 3–6). *The ONE5G approach towards the challenges of multi-service operation in 5G systems.* In 2018 IEEE 87th Vehicular Technology Conference (VTC Spring) (pp. 1–6). IEEE. https://doi.org/DOI: 10.1109/VTCSpring.2018.8417832

Schütz, N., Knobel, S. E. J., Botros, A., Single, M., Pais, B., Santschi, V., Gatica-Perez, D., Buluschek, P., Urwyler, P., Gerber, S. M., Müri, R. M., Mosimann, U. P., Saner, H., & Nef, T. (2022). A systems approach towards remote health-monitoring in older adults: Introducing a zero-interaction digital exhaust. *NPJ Digital Medicine*, *5*(1), 116. DOI: 10.1038/s41746-022-00657-y PMID: 35974156

Selvam, P., Karthikeyan, P., Manochitra, S., Sujith, A., Ganesan, T., Ayyasamy, R., Shuaib, M., Alam, S., & Rajendran, A. (2025). Federated learning-based hybrid convolutional recurrent neural network for multi-class intrusion detection in IoT networks. *Discover Internet of Things*, *5*(1), 39. DOI: 10.1007/s43926-025-00130-8

Serrano, M., Dang, H. N., & Hoan, M. Q. N. 2018. "Recent Advances on Artificial Intelligence and Internet of Things Convergence for Human-Centric Applications." *ACM International Conference Proceeding Series*. DOI: 10.1145/3277593.3277638

Shafik, W. (2023). Wearable Medical Electronics in Artificial Intelligence of Medical Things. In *Handbook of Security and Privacy of AI-Enabled Healthcare Systems and Internet of Medical Things*. https://doi.org/DOI: 10.1201/9781003370321-2

Shafik, W. (2024a). 2 Deep Field of Learning Artificial Impacts Intelligence in the. *Deep Learning Concepts in Operations Research*, 9.

Shafik, W. (2024c). Artificial Intelligence-Enabled Internet of Medical Things (AIoMT) in Modern Healthcare Practices. In *Clinical Practice and Unmet Challenges in AI-Enhanced Healthcare Systems* (pp. 42–69). IGI Global. DOI: 10.4018/979-8-3693-2703-6.ch003

Shafik, W. (2024f). Community and Artificial Intelligence-Enabled Disaster Management and Preparedness. In *Navigating Natural Hazards in Mountainous Topographies: Exploring the Challenges and Opportunities of Living* (pp. 243–266). Springer. DOI: 10.1007/978-3-031-65862-4_13

Shafik, W. (2024k). Generative AI for Social Good and Sustainable Development. In *Generative AI: Current Trends and Applications* (pp. 185–217). Springer. DOI: 10.1007/978-981-97-8460-8_10

Shafik, W. (2024l). IoMT Future Trends and Challenges: Emerging Technologies, Policy Implications, and Research Questions. *Lightweight Digital Trust Architectures in the Internet of Medical Things (IoMT)*, 348–370.

Shafik, W. (2024o). Smart Health Revolution: Exploring Artificial Intelligence of Internet of Medical Things. In *Healthcare Industry Assessment: Analyzing Risks, Security, and Reliability* (pp. 201–229). Springer. DOI: 10.1007/978-3-031-65434-3_9

Shafik, W. (2025a). Artificial Intelligence Assisted Internet of Medical Things (AIoMTs) in Sustainable Healthcare Ecosystem. *Wellness Management Powered by AI Technologies*, 75–101.

Shafik, W. (2025d). Generative Adversarial Networks: Security, Privacy, and Ethical Considerations. In *Generative Artificial Intelligence (AI) Approaches for Industrial Applications* (pp. 93–117). Springer.

Shafik, W. (2025e). Human-Artificial Intelligence Collaborations in Polycystic Ovary Syndrome (PCOS) Clinical Trials and Research. In *AI-Based Nutritional Intervention in Polycystic Ovary Syndrome (PCOS)* (pp. 307–330). Springer Nature Singapore. DOI: 10.1007/978-981-96-2120-0_13

Shafik, W. (2025g). Investigating Generative Artificial Intelligence Readiness in the Internet of Medical Things: Are We Progressing Technologically? In *Convergence of Internet of Medical Things (IoMT) and Generative AI* (pp. 31–58). IGI Global Scientific Publishing.

Shafik, W. (2025h). Quantum Computing and Generative Adversarial Networks (GANs): Ethics, Privacy, and Security. In *Quantum AI and its Applications in Blockchain Technology* (pp. 111–156). IGI Global Scientific Publishing.

Shafik, W. (2025i). Revolutionizing Skin Cancer Diagnosis With Artificial Intelligence: Insights Into Machine Learning Techniques. In *Impact of Digital Solutions for Improved Healthcare Delivery* (pp. 167–194). IGI Global.

Shafik, W. (2025j). Revolutionizing Skin Cancer Diagnosis With Artificial Intelligence: Insights Into Machine Learning Techniques. In *Impact of Digital Solutions for Improved Healthcare Delivery* (pp. 167–194). IGI Global.

Shafik, W. (2025m). Sustainable Agriculture and Diet in the Metaverse Era: Sustainable Farming and Nutritious Eating in the Metaverse. In *Food in the Metaverse and Web 3.0 Era: Intersecting Food, Technology, and Culture* (pp. 159–184). IGI Global Scientific Publishing.

Shafik, W., & Kalinaki, K. (2024). Societal and Ethical Implications of Technology-Enhanced Agriculture and Healthcare: An African Context. *2024 IST-Africa Conference (IST-Africa)*, 1–11. DOI: 10.23919/IST-Africa63983.2024.10569306

Shafik, W., Tufail, A., Liyanage, C. D. S., & Apong, R. A. A. H. M. (2024). Medical Robotics and AI-Assisted Diagnostics Challenges for Smart Sustainable Healthcare. In *AI-Driven Innovations in Digital Healthcare: Emerging Trends, Challenges, and Applications* (pp. 304–323). IGI Global. DOI: 10.4018/979-8-3693-3218-4.ch016

Shafik, W. (2024b). Artificial Intelligence and the Medical Tourism. In *Examining Tourist Behaviors and Community Involvement in Destination Rejuvenation* (pp. 207–233). IGI Global. DOI: 10.4018/979-8-3693-6819-0.ch016

Shafik, W. (2024d). Artificial Intelligence-Enabled Internet of Medical Things for Enhanced Healthcare Systems. In *Smart Healthcare Systems* (pp. 119–134). CRC Press., DOI: 10.1201/9781032698519-9

Shafik, W. (2024e). Blockchain's impetus for secure IoT-enabled applications in smart city. In *Big Data and Blockchain Technology for Secure IoT Applications* (pp. 48–71). CRC Press., DOI: 10.1201/9781032663005-4

Shafik, W. (2024g). Connected healthcare—the impact of Internet of Things on medical services. In *Artificial Intelligence and Internet of Things based Augmented Trends for Data Driven Systems* (pp. 181–217). CRC Press., DOI: 10.1201/9781003497318-10

Shafik, W. (2024h). Consumer. *Advances in Marketing, Customer Relationship Management, and E-Services*, •••, 75–108. DOI: 10.4018/979-8-3693-9122-8.ch004

Shafik, W. (2024i). Digital healthcare systems in a federated learning perspective. In *Federated Learning for Digital Healthcare Systems* (pp. 1–35). Elsevier., DOI: 10.1016/B978-0-443-13897-3.00001-1

Shafik, W. (2024m). IoT-Enabled Secure and Intelligent Smart Healthcare. In *Secure and Intelligent IoT-Enabled Smart Cities* (pp. 308–333). IGI Global., DOI: 10.4018/979-8-3693-2373-1.ch015

Shafik, W. (2024n). Science of Emotional Intelligence. In *Enhancing and Predicting Digital Consumer Behavior with AI* (pp. 284–310). IGI Global. DOI: 10.4018/979-8-3693-4453-8.ch015

Shafik, W. (2024p). The Future of Healthcare: AIoMT—Redefining Healthcare with Advanced Artificial Intelligence and Machine Learning Techniques. In *Artificial Intelligence and Machine Learning in Drug Design and Development* (pp. 605–634). Wiley., DOI: 10.1002/9781394234196.ch19

Shafik, W. (2024q). Toward a More Ethical Future of Artificial Intelligence and Data Science. In *The Ethical Frontier of AI and Data Analysis* (pp. 362–388). IGI Global., DOI: 10.4018/979-8-3693-2964-1.ch022

Shafik, W. (2025b). Artificial Intelligence-Enabled Cybersecurity and Internet of Things Applications in Smart Cities. In *Building Tomorrow's Smart Cities With 6G Infrastructure Technology* (pp. 301–334). IGI Global Scientific Publishing.

Shafik, W. (2025c). Digital twins tools and technologies. In *Digital Twins for Smart Cities and Villages* (pp. 55–80). Elsevier., https://doi.org/https://doi.org/10.1016/B978-0-443-28884-5.00003-8 DOI: 10.1016/B978-0-443-28884-5.00003-8

Shafik, W. (2025f). Introduction to Machine Learning and Its Applications to Neuroscience. In *Machine Learning for Neurodegenerative Disorders* (pp. 1–32). CRC Press., DOI: 10.1201/9781032661025-1

Shafik, W. (2025k). Smart biomedical devices for smart healthcare. In *Machine Learning Models and Architectures for Biomedical Signal Processing* (pp. 421–448). Elsevier. DOI: 10.1016/B978-0-443-22158-3.00017-X

Shafik, W. (2025l). Sustainable Agriculture and Diet for Urban Development. In *Sustainable Smart Cities and the Future of Urban Development* (pp. 165–192). IGI Global Scientific Publishing.

Shafik, W., Kalinaki, K., Fahim, K. E., & Adam, M. (2024). Safeguarding Data Privacy and Security in Federated Learning Systems. In *Federated Deep Learning for Healthcare* (pp. 170–190). CRC Press., DOI: 10.1201/9781032694870-13

Shameer, K., Johnson, K. W., Glicksberg, B. S., Dudley, J. T., & Sengupta, P. P. (2018). Machine Learning in Cardiovascular Medicine: Are We There Yet? *Heart (British Cardiac Society)*, *104*(14), 1156–1164. DOI: 10.1136/heartjnl-2017-311198 PMID: 29352006

Sharma, S. K., Rao, R. S., Singh, P., & Khan, S. A. (2022). Evaluation of VANETs routing protocols for data-based smart health monitoring in intelligent transportation systems. *International Journal of Mathematical. Engineering and Management Sciences*, *7*(2), 211.

Sharma, V., Mishra, N., Kukreja, V., Alkhayyat, A., & Elngar, A. A. (2023). Framework for Evaluating Ethics in AI. *International Conference on Innovative Data Communication Technologies and Application, ICIDCA 2023 - Proceedings*. DOI: 10.1109/ICIDCA56705.2023.10099747

Shastry, K. A., & Shastry, A. (2023). An Integrated Deep Learning and Natural Language Processing Approach for Continuous Remote Monitoring in Digital Health. *Decision Analytics Journal*, *8*(August), 100301. DOI: 10.1016/j.dajour.2023.100301

Shehab, M., Abualigah, L., Shambour, Q., Abu-Hashem, M. A., Shambour, M. K. Y., Alsalibi, A. I., & Gandomi, A. H. (2022). Machine learning in medical applications: A review of state-of-the-art methods. *Computers in Biology and Medicine*, *145*, 105458. DOI: 10.1016/j.compbiomed.2022.105458 PMID: 35364311

Shen, Y., Yu, J., Zhou, J., & Hu, G. (2025). Twenty-Five Years of Evolution and Hurdles in Electronic Health Records and Interoperability in Medical Research: Comprehensive Review. *Journal of Medical Internet Research*, *27*, e59024. https://doi.org/https://doi.org/10.2196/59024. DOI: 10.2196/59024 PMID: 39787599

Shuaib, M., Hassan, N. H., Usman, S., Alam, S., Sam, S. M., & Samy, G. A.-L. N. (2022). Effect of Quantum computing on Blockchain-based Electronic Health Record Systems. *2022 4th International Conference on Smart Sensors and Application (ICSSA)*, 179–184. DOI: 10.1109/ICSSA54161.2022.9870964

Shuaib, M., Alam, S., & Reegu, F. A. (2023). Blockchain-based self-sovereign identity for COVID-19 medical passports and immunity certificates. *AIP Conference Proceedings, 2587*(1), 070003. DOI: 10.1063/5.0150394

Siddiqui, S. T. (2023). Integrating IoT and blockchain-enabled device-to-device communication to improve privacy in intelligent quarantine environments. *2023 7th International Conference on Computation System and Information Technology for Sustainable Solutions (CSITSS)*, 1–7.

Siddiqui, S. T., Shuaib, M., Gupta, A. K., & Alam, S. (2020). Implementing Blockchain Technology: Way to Avoid Evasive Threats to Information Security on Cloud. In *2020 International Conference on Computing and Information Technology, ICCIT 2020*. DOI: 10.1109/ICCIT-144147971.2020.9213798

Silvestri, S., Islam, S., Papastergiou, S., Tzagkarakis, C., & Ciampi, M. (2023). A Machine Learning Approach for the NLP-Based Analysis of Cyber Threats and Vulnerabilities of the Healthcare Ecosystem †. *Sensors (Basel), 23*(2), 1–26. DOI: 10.3390/s23020651 PMID: 36679446

Singh, L. (2022). Automated Kantian Ethics: A Faithful Implementation. *Lecture Notes in Computer Science (Including Subseries Lecture Notes in Artificial Intelligence and Lecture Notes in Bioinformatics), 13404 LNAI*. DOI: 10.1007/978-3-031-15791-2_16

Singh, A., Joshi, K., Alam, S., Bharany, S., Shuaib, M., & Ahmad, S. (2022). Internet of Things-Based Integrated Remote Electronic Health Surveillance and Alert System: A Review. *2022 IEEE International Conference on Current Development in Engineering and Technology (CCET)*, 1–6. DOI: 10.1109/CCET56606.2022.10080629

Singh, A., Nagabhooshanam, N., Kumar, R., Verma, R., Mohanasundaram, S., Manjith, R., & Rajaram, A. (2025). Deep learning based coronary artery disease detection and segmentation using ultrasound imaging with adaptive gated SCNN models. *Biomedical Signal Processing and Control, 105*, 107637. DOI: 10.1016/j.bspc.2025.107637

Singh, B., & Kaunert, C. (2024). Integration of cutting-edge technologies such as internet of things (IoT) and 5G in health monitoring systems: A comprehensive legal analysis and futuristic outcomes. *GLS Law Journal, 6*(1), 13–20. DOI: 10.69974/glslawjournal.v6i1.123

Singh, G., Schulthess, D., Hughes, N., Vannieuwenhuyse, B., & Kalra, D. (2018). Real World Big Data for Clinical Research and Drug Development. *Drug Discovery Today, 23*(3), 652–660. DOI: 10.1016/j.drudis.2017.12.002 PMID: 29294362

Singh, R., Shafik, W., Crowther, D., & Kumar, V. (Eds.). (2024). *Transforming Healthcare Sector Through Artificial Intelligence and Environmental Sustainability* (1st ed., Vol. 1). Springer Nature Singapore., DOI: 10.1007/978-981-97-9555-0

Singh, T. M., & Lippert, K. (2024). Digital Twins in Human Activity Prediction on Gait Using Extreme Gradient Boosting Local Binary Pattern: Healthcare 6.0. In Dubey, A., Kumar Reddy, C., Doss, S., & Hanafiah, M. (Eds.), *Exploring the Advancements and Future Directions of Digital Twins in Healthcare 6.0* (pp. 240–261). IGI Global., DOI: 10.4018/979-8-3693-5893-1.ch012

Singh, T. M., Reddy, C. K. K., & Lippert, K. (2024). Advancing human-centric solutions: The future trajectory of soft computing in modern society. In Kumar, N., Pal, S., Agarwal, P., Rosak-Szyrocka, J., & Jain, V. (Eds.), *Human-machine collaboration and emotional intelligence in Industry 5.0* (pp. 1–18). IGI Global., DOI: 10.4018/979-8-3693-6806-0.ch001

Singh, V. K., Bangari, N., Ali, Z., Vyas, A., Verma, R. K., & Saxena, A. (2023). Parachute shape ultra-wideband wearable antenna for remote health care monitoring. *International Journal of Communication Systems*, *36*(10), e5488. DOI: 10.1002/dac.5488

Sinha, S., & Vohora, D. (2017). *Drug Discovery and Development: An Overview*. Elsevier Inc.

Sisodiya, M., ... (2024). The transformative power of robotic process automation: Redefining business in Industry 4.0. In *2024 14th International Conference on Cloud Computing, Data Science & Engineering (Confluence)* (pp. 498–503). IEEE. DOI: 10.1109/Confluence60223.2024.10463415

Sivani, T., & Mishra, S. (2022). Wearable devices: evolution and usage in remote patient monitoring system. In *Connected e-Health: Integrated IoT and Cloud Computing* (pp. 311–332). Springer International Publishing. DOI: 10.1007/978-3-030-97929-4_14

Smith, H. (2021). Clinical AI: Opacity, accountability, responsibility and liability. *AI & Society*, *36*(2), 535–545. DOI: 10.1007/s00146-020-01019-6

Solanki, P., Grundy, J., & Hussain, W. (2023). Operationalising ethics in artificial intelligence for healthcare: A framework for AI developers. *AI and Ethics*, *3*(1), 223–240. Advance online publication. DOI: 10.1007/s43681-022-00195-z

Steinberg, D. (2009). CART: classification and regression trees. In *The top ten algorithms in data mining* (pp. 193–216). Chapman and Hall/CRC. DOI: 10.1201/9781420089653.ch10

Stellmach, C., Muzoora, M. R., & Thun, S. (2022). Digitalization of Health Data: Interoperability of the Proposed European Health Data Space. In *Studies in health technology and informatics* (Vol. 298, pp. 132–136). DOI: 10.3233/SHTI220922

Stylianides, C., Alexandropoulou, C. A., Sulaiman, W., Panagiotopoulos, I., Kleanthous, S., Dimitrakopoulos, G., Constantinou, I., Vassiliou, S., Garcia, F., Politi, E., Ntalaperas, D., Papageorgiou, X., Ioannides, N., Palazis, L., Pattichis, C. S., & Panayides, A. S. (2023). AI-based solutions for predicting sepsis in ICUs. *2023 IEEE EMBS Special Topic Conference on Data Science and Engineering in Healthcare, Medicine and Biology, IEEECONF 2023*. DOI: 10.1109/IEEECONF58974.2023.10404309

Su, B., Wang, B., Cao, Y., Dou, H., Zhang, T., & He, X. (2024). A multi-functional flexible piezoresistive sensor based on sericin-functionalized CNTs decorated carbon foams for wearable thermal-therapy devices. *Ceramics International*, *50*(7), 10305–10313. Advance online publication. DOI: 10.1016/j.ceramint.2023.12.342

Subasi, A., Ozaltin, O., Mitra, A., Subasi, M. E., & Sarirete, A. (2023). Trustworthy artificial intelligence in healthcare. In *Accelerating Strategic Changes for Digital Transformation in the Healthcare Industry: Volume 2* (Vol. 2). DOI: 10.1016/B978-0-443-15299-3.00015-4

Subasi, A. (2021, August). 2024. "Artificial Intelligence in Drug Discovery and Development.". *Applications of Artificial Intelligence in Healthcare and Biomedicine*, *23*, 417–454. DOI: 10.1016/B978-0-443-22308-2.00018-4

Suboyin, A., Sreedeth, D., Rahman, M. M., Diaz, S., Kannan, J., Sreedeth, H. S., Rehman, A., Valiyapalathingal, M., Noor, Y., & Somra, B. (2024). Transforming Strategy with AI-Augmented Personas for Sustainability, Data Management, Regulatory Frameworks, Healthcare and Compliance. *Abu Dhabi International Petroleum Exhibition and Conference*, D011S016R005.

Swain, S., Oyekola, P. O., & Muduli, K. (2022). Intelligent technologies for excellency in sustainable operational performance in the healthcare sector. [IJSESD]. *International Journal of Social Ecology and Sustainable Development*, *13*(5), 1–16. DOI: 10.4018/IJSESD.313963

Swaroop, K. N., Chandu, K., Gorrepotu, R., & Deb, S. (2019). A health monitoring system for vital signs using IoT. *Internet of Things : Engineering Cyber Physical Human Systems*, *5*, 116–129. DOI: 10.1016/j.iot.2019.01.004

Swathi, G. (2024, August 29). Navigating the Integration of Machine Learning in Healthcare: Challenges, Strategies, and Ethical Considerations. *Journal of Computational and Cognitive Engineering*. Advance online publication. DOI: 10.47852/bonviewJCCE42023600

Syamala, M., Chandrasekaran, R., Balamurali, R., Rani, R., Hashmi, A., Kiran, A., & Rajaram, A. (2024). Evaluating generative adversarial networks for virtual contrast-enhanced kidney segmentation using Res-UNet in non-contrast CT images. *Multimedia Tools and Applications*, •••, 1–24. DOI: 10.1007/s11042-024-19626-6

Taliento, M. (2023). AI in Healthcare Management and Accounting: Novelties and Trends from a Literature Review and Illustrative Cases. *Proceedings of the 42nd International Business Information Management Association Conference*, 1685–1696. DOI: 10.5171/2023.4252023

Terkelsen, C., Nørgaard, B., Lassen, J., Gerdes, J., Ankersen, J., Rømer, F., Nielsen, T., & Andersen, H. (2002). Telemedicine used for remote prehospital diagnosing in patients suspected of acute myocardial infarction. *Journal of Internal Medicine*, *252*(5), 412–420. DOI: 10.1046/j.1365-2796.2002.01051.x PMID: 12528759

Thakur, G. K., Thakur, A., Khan, N., & Anush, H. (2024). The role of natural language processing in medical data analysis and healthcare automation. *2024 International Conference on Knowledge Engineering and Communication Systems (ICKECS)*, Chikkaballapur, India, 1–5. https://doi.org/DOI: 10.1109/ICKECS61492.2024.10616749

Thantharate, P., & Thantharate, A. (2023). ZeroTrustBlock: Enhancing Security, Privacy, and Interoperability of Sensitive Data through ZeroTrust Permissioned Blockchain. In *Big Data and Cognitive Computing* (Vol. 7, Issue 4). DOI: 10.3390/bdcc7040165

Thorat, V., Rao, P., Joshi, N., Talreja, P., & Shetty, A. R. (2024, May 7). Role of Artificial Intelligence (AI) in Patient Education and Communication in Dentistry. *Cureus*, *16*(5), e59799. DOI: 10.7759/cureus.59799 PMID: 38846249

Thuemmler, C., & Bai, C. (2017). *Health 4.0: How virtualization and big data are revolutionizing healthcare*. Springer. DOI: 10.1007/978-3-319-47617-9

Tidjon, L. N., & Khomh, F. (2023). The Different Faces of AI Ethics Across the World: A Principle-to-Practice Gap Analysis. *IEEE Transactions on Artificial Intelligence*, *4*(4), 820–839. Advance online publication. DOI: 10.1109/TAI.2022.3225132

Timme, R. E., Wolfgang, W. J., Balkey, M., Venkata, S. L. G., Randolph, R., Allard, M., & Strain, E. (2020). Optimizing open data to support one health: Best practices to ensure interoperability of genomic data from bacterial pathogens. *One Health Outlook*, *2*(1), 20. DOI: 10.1186/s42522-020-00026-3 PMID: 33103064

Topol, E. (2019). High-performance medicine: The convergence of human and artificial intelligence. *Nature Medicine*, *25*(1), 44–56. DOI: 10.1038/s41591-018-0300-7 PMID: 30617339

Treacy, S. (2023). Mechanisms and Constraints Underpinning Ethically Aligned Artificial Intelligence Systems: An Exploration of Key Performance Areas. *Human-Centric Intelligent Systems*, *3*(3), 189–196. Advance online publication. DOI: 10.1007/s44230-023-00036-0

Truong, H. T. T., Almeida, M., Karame, G., & Soriente, C. 2019. "Towards Secure and Decentralized Sharing of IoT Data." *Proceedings - 2019 2nd IEEE International Conference on Blockchain, Blockchain 2019* 176–83. DOI: 10.1109/Blockchain.2019.00031

Tsantikidou, K., & Sklavos, N. (2022). Hardware limitations of lightweight cryptographic designs for IoT in healthcare. *Cryptography*, *6*(3), 45. DOI: 10.3390/cryptography6030045

Tudora, E., Tîrziu, E., Nicolau, N.-D., & Gheorghe-Moisii, M. (2021). Fog and cloud computing-based IoT in healthcare monitoring system for healthy ageing. *2021 23rd International Conference on Control Systems and Computer Science (CSCS)*, 489–494.

Tuli, S., Tuli, S., Wander, G., Wander, P., Gill, S. S., Dustdar, S., Sakellariou, R., & Rana, O. (2020). Next Generation Technologies for Smart Healthcare: Challenges, Vision, Model, Trends and Future Directions. *Internet Technology Letters*, *3*(2), 1–6. DOI: 10.1002/itl2.145

Udo, B. (2023). Robotic Process Automation (RPA) in Healthcare. *International Research Journal on Advanced Science Hub*, *5*(05S), 229–235. DOI: 10.47392/irjash.2023.S030

Vaiyapuri, T., Mahalingam, J., Ahmad, S., Abdeljaber, H. A. M., Yang, E., & Jeong, S.-Y. (2023). Ensemble Learning Driven Computer-Aided Diagnosis Model for Brain Tumor Classification on Magnetic Resonance Imaging. *IEEE Access : Practical Innovations, Open Solutions*, *11*, 91398–91406. DOI: 10.1109/ACCESS.2023.3306961

Valaboju, P. K. (2024). *Transformative Impact of AI and Cloud Technologies: A Comparative Analysis across Healthcare*. Retail, and Mobile Financial Services.

Vankadara, Y.. (2024). 6G revolution: Redefining communication systems. In *2024 International Conference on Smart Systems for Applications in Electrical Sciences (ICSSES)* (pp. 1–6). IEEE. DOI: 10.1109/ICSSES62373.2024.10561292

Varshney, K. (2021)... *Application of IoT in Healthcare*, (6), 192–196.

Vayena, E., & Blasimme, A. (2018). Challenges in the ethics of AI in healthcare. *Nature Medicine*, *24*(9), 1303–1305.

Veeraiah, V., Kumar, G. K. R., Singh, D. P., Chaudhary, A., Elkady, G., & Ross, D. S. (2022). A Descriptive Research on Internet of Things Implementation in Healthcare Sector. *2022 5th International Conference on Contemporary Computing and Informatics (IC3I)*, 308–312.

Venkatesh, R. (2024). A Lightweight Quantum Blockchain-Based Framework to Protect Patients Private Medical Information. *IEEE Transactions on Network Science and Engineering*, *11*(4), 3577–3584. DOI: 10.1109/TNSE.2024.3378922

Verma, N., Singh, S., & Prasad, D. (2022). A review on existing IoT architecture and communication protocols used in healthcare monitoring system. Journal of The Institution of Engineers (India): Series B, 103(1), 245-257.

Vidhya, S., Siva Raja, P. M., & Sumithra, R. P. (2024). Blockchain-Enabled Decentralized Healthcare Data Exchange: Leveraging Novel Encryption Scheme, Smart Contracts, and Ring Signatures for Enhanced Data Security and Patient Privacy. *International Journal of Network Management*, *34*(5), e2289. https://doi.org/https://doi.org/10.1002/nem.2289. DOI: 10.1002/nem.2289

Vijayan, V., Connolly, J. P., Condell, J., McKelvey, N., & Gardiner, P. (2021). Review of wearable devices and data collection considerations for connected health. *Sensors (Basel)*, *21*(16), 5589. DOI: 10.3390/s21165589 PMID: 34451032

Vijayasarveswari, V., & Lim Jia Chyin, N. M. (1962). Wafi, and I. Iszaidy. 2021. "Development of E-Healthcare Management System Using PHP, Javascript and Cascading Style Sheets.". *Journal of Physics: Conference Series*, (1). Advance online publication. DOI: 10.1088/1742-6596/1962/1/012030

Waheed, N., Rehman, A. U., Nehra, A., Farooq, M., Tariq, N., Jan, M. A., Khan, F., Alalmaie, A. Z., & Nanda, P. (2023). Fedblockhealth: A synergistic approach to privacy and security in iot-enabled healthcare through federated learning and blockchain. *GLOBECOM 2023-2023 IEEE Global Communications Conference*, 3855–3860.

Walsh, G., Stogiannos, N., van de Venter, R., Rainey, C., Tam, W., McFadden, S., McNulty, J. P., Mekis, N., Lewis, S., O'Regan, T., Kumar, A., Huisman, M., Bisdas, S., Kotter, E., Pinto dos Santos, D., Sá dos Reis, C., van Ooijen, P., Brady, A. P., & Malamateniou, C. (2023). Responsible AI practice and AI education are central to AI implementation: a rapid review for all medical imaging professionals in Europe. *BJR|Open, 5*(1). DOI: 10.1259/bjro.20230033

Wang, B., Hu, X., Zhang, J., Xu, C., & Gao, Z. (2022). Intelligent Internet of Things in mammography screening using multicenter transformation between unified capsules. *IEEE Internet of Things Journal*, *10*(2), 1536–1545. DOI: 10.1109/JIOT.2022.3209895

Wang, C., Wang, Z., Guan, W., Wang, W., Xu, L., Li, L., Huang, S., & Wang, W. (2024). Trustworthy Health Monitoring Based on Distributed Wearable Electronics With Edge Intelligence. *IEEE Transactions on Consumer Electronics*, *70*(1), 2333–2341. Advance online publication. DOI: 10.1109/TCE.2024.3358803

Wang, F., & Preininger, A. (2019). AI in healthcare: Applications, challenges, and future directions. *Computers in Biology and Medicine*, *112*, 103–119.

Wang, K., Chen, C.-M., Tie, Z., Shojafar, M., Kumar, S., & Kumari, S. (2021). Forward privacy preservation in IoT-enabled healthcare systems. *IEEE Transactions on Industrial Informatics, 18*(3), 1991–1999. DOI: 10.1109/TII.2021.3064691

Wasswa Shafik. (2024). Challenges and Future Prospectives of Ultrasound-Assisted Extraction. In Bancha Yingngam, M. S. A. (Ed.), *Ultrasound Assisted Extraction: Methods and Applications* (1st ed., Vol. 1). Nova, Science and Technology.

Wasswa, S. (2025). The Role of Emotional Intelligence in Career Development and Career Success. In K. D. Pushan, G. Sachin, K. Shafali, G. Anita, Rita Karmakar, & Pronaya Bhattacharya (Eds.), *Emotional Intelligence in the Digital Era: Concepts, Frameworks, and Applications* (1st ed., Vol. 1, pp. 108–128). Taylor & Francis Group. DOI: 10.1201/9781032715377-7

Watson, A., & Wozniak-O'Connor, V. (2025). The promise of artificial intelligence in health: Portrayals of emerging healthcare technologies. *Sociology of Health & Illness, 47*(1), e13840. DOI: 10.1111/1467-9566.13840 PMID: 39311476

Wazid, M., Singh, J., Das, A. K., & Rodrigues, J. J. P. C. (2023). An ensemble-based machine learning-envisioned intrusion detection in industry 5.0-driven healthcare applications. *IEEE Transactions on Consumer Electronics, 70*(1), 1903–1912. DOI: 10.1109/TCE.2023.3318850

Wen, A., Fu, S., Moon, S., El Wazir, M., Rosenbaum, A., Kaggal, V. C., Liu, S., Sohn, S., Liu, H., & Fan, J. (2019). Desiderata for delivering NLP to accelerate healthcare AI advancement and a Mayo Clinic NLP-as-a-service implementation. npj. *Digital Medicine, 2*(1), 130. DOI: 10.1038/s41746-019-0208-8 PMID: 31872069

Whig, V., Othman, B., Gehlot, A., Haque, M. A., Qamar, S., & Singh, J. 2022. "An Empirical Analysis of Artificial Intelligence (AI) as a Growth Engine for the Healthcare Sector." Pp. 2454–57 in *2022 2nd International Conference on Advance Computing and Innovative Technologies in Engineering (ICACITE)*. IEEE. DOI: 10.1109/ICACITE53722.2022.9823607

Wu, H., Lu, X., & Wang, H. (2023). The application of artificial intelligence in health care resource allocation before and during the COVID-19 pandemic: Scoping review. *JMIR AI, 2*, e38397. DOI: 10.2196/38397

Xia, Q., Gao, J., & Amofa, S. (2021). Blockchain Medical Data Sharing. In *Wireless Blockchain* (pp. 245–268). https://doi.org/https://doi.org/10.1002/9781119790839.ch11

Xu, J., & Yang, P. (2020). Real-time monitoring in healthcare with machine learning techniques. *Journal of Artificial Intelligence in Medicine, 106*, 101865. Topol, E. J. (2019). *Deep Medicine: How Artificial Intelligence Can Make Healthcare Human Again.* Basic Books.

Xu, B., Xu, L., Cai, H., Jiang, L., Luo, Y., & Gu, Y. (2017). The design of an m-Health monitoring system based on a cloud computing platform. *Enterprise Information Systems, 11*(1), 17–36. DOI: 10.1080/17517575.2015.1053416

Xu, X., Ge, Z., Chow, E. P., Yu, Z., Lee, D., Wu, J., & Zhang, L. (2022). A machine-learning-based risk-prediction tool for HIV and sexually transmitted infections acquisition over the next 12 months. *Journal of Clinical Medicine, 11*(7), 1818.

Yadav, G., Bokhari, M. U., Alzahrani, S. I., Alam, S., & Shuaib, M. (2025). Emotion-Aware Ensemble Learning (EAEL): Revolutionizing Mental Health Diagnosis of Corporate Professionals via Intelligent Integration of Multi-Modal Data Sources and Ensemble Techniques. *IEEE Access : Practical Innovations, Open Solutions*, *13*, 11494–11516. DOI: 10.1109/ACCESS.2025.3529032

Yang, G., Urke, A. R., & Øvsthus, K. (2018, March 22–23). *Mobility support of IoT solution in home care wireless sensor network*. In 2018 Ubiquitous Positioning, Indoor Navigation and Location-Based Services (UPINLBS) (pp. 475–480). IEEE. https://doi.org/DOI: 10.1109/UPINLBS.2018.8559724

Yin, Y., Zeng, Y., Chen, X., & Fan, Y. (2016). The Internet of Things in Healthcare: An Overview. *Journal of Industrial Information Integration*, *1*, 3–13. DOI: 10.1016/j.jii.2016.03.004

Yogeshappa, V. G. (2024). AI-driven precision medicine: Revolutionizing personalized treatment plans. [IJCET]. *International Journal of Computer Engineering and Technology*, *15*(5), 455–474. DOI: 10.5281/zenodo.13843057

Yu, K. H., Beam, A. L., & Kohane, I. S. (2018). Artificial Intelligence in Healthcare. *Nature Biomedical Engineering*, *2*(10), 719–731. DOI: 10.1038/s41551-018-0305-z PMID: 31015651

Zadeh, L. A. (1996). Fuzzy logic, neural networks, and soft computing. In Fuzzy sets, fuzzy logic, and fuzzy systems: selected papers by Lotfi A Zadeh (pp. 775-782).

Zahid, N., Sodhro, A. H., Kamboh, U. R., Alkhayyat, A., & Wang, L. (2022). AI-Driven Adaptive Reliable and Sustainable Approach for Internet of Things Enabled Healthcare System. *Mathematical Biosciences and Engineering*, *19*(4), 3953–3971. DOI: 10.3934/mbe.2022182 PMID: 35341282

Zeb, S., Fnu, N., Abbasi, N., & Fahad, M. (2024). AI in Healthcare: Revolutionizing Diagnosis and Therapy. *International Journal of Multidisciplinary Sciences and Arts*, *3*(3), 118–128. DOI: 10.47709/ijmdsa.v3i3.4546

Zhang, P., & Kamel Boulos, M. N. (2023). Generative AI in Medicine and Healthcare: Promises, Opportunities and Challenges. In *Future Internet* (Vol. 15, Issue 9). DOI: 10.3390/fi15090286

Zhang, J., Yang, M., Ge, Y., Ivers, R., Webster, R., & Tian, M. (2022). The role of digital health for post-surgery care of older patients with hip fracture: A scoping review. *International Journal of Medical Informatics*, *160*, 104709. DOI: 10.1016/j.ijmedinf.2022.104709 PMID: 35144101

Zhang, L., Xu, J., Vijayakumar, P., Sharma, P. K., & Ghosh, U. (2022). Homomorphic encryption-based privacy-preserving federated learning in IoT-enabled healthcare system. *IEEE Transactions on Network Science and Engineering*, *10*(5), 2864–2880. DOI: 10.1109/TNSE.2022.3185327

Zhang, W., Thurow, K., & Stoll, R. (2014). A knowledge-based telemonitoring platform for application in remote healthcare. *International Journal of Computers, Communications & Control*, *9*(5), 644–654. DOI: 10.15837/ijccc.2014.5.661

Zhang, Y., Zheng, X. T., Zhang, X., Pan, J., & Thean, A. V. Y. (2024). Hybrid integration of wearable devices for physiological monitoring. *Chemical Reviews*, *124*(18), 10386–10434. DOI: 10.1021/acs.chemrev.3c00471 PMID: 39189683

Zizheng, H. (2024, February). Computer vision-aided mmWave communications for indoor medical healthcare. *Computers in Biology and Medicine*, *169*, 107869. Advance online publication. DOI: 10.1016/j.compbiomed.2023.107869

About The Contributors

Mohammed Shuaib is an Assistant Professor at Jazan University, Saudi Arabia, with over 11 years of academic experience. . His international experience includes a visiting research position at INTI International University, Malaysia. Dr. Shuaib's research achievements include 65 peer-reviewed publications in high-impact journals like Elsevier, Springer, and IEEE Access, four patents, and an H-index of 26 with over 1860 citations. He was recognized among the World's Top 2% Scientists by Stanford University in 2024. In addition to research, Dr. Shuaib currently serves as an Associate Editor for Sustainable Computing: Informatics and Systems (Elsevier) and the International Journal of Electrical and Computer Engineering (IAES). He also serves as an Academic Editor for PLOS ONE and the International Journal of RF and Microwave Computer-Aided Engineering (Wiley). Moreover, he is on the editorial boards of Mobile Information Systems (Wiley), Discover Internet of Things (Springer), Journal of Economy and Technology (Elsevier), and International Journal of Information Technology and Web Engineering (IGI Global). These journals are indexed in top databases such as ISI, Web of Science, and Scopus. Currently, he holds editorial roles as follows: 1. Associate Editor, Sustainable Computing: Informatics and Systems, Elsevier. 2. Editor Board member, "Journal of Economy and Technology " Elsevier. 3. Academic Editor in Hindawi, International Journal of RF and Microwave Computer-Aided 4. Academic Editor in PLOS ONE Journal 5. Academic Editor in PLOS COMPLEX SYSTEMS Journal

Shadab Alam, currently an Associate Professor at Jazan University, KSA, is an accomplished computer science researcher focusing on information security, blockchain, IoT, and smart healthcare. He completed his PhD in Computer Science from Aligarh Muslim University, India, where he also earned his master's and bachelor's degrees. Dr. Shadab Alam has made substantial contributions to the field of computer science, as evidenced by his publication of over 80 research papers in high-impact journals and prominent international conference proceedings. His innovative work has also led to the acquisition of 05 international patents, including those in the US and Australia, and 03 national patents.He was recognized among the World's Top 2% Scientists by Stanford University in 2024. Beyond his research, Dr. Alam is actively involved in the professional community as a senior member of IEEE (SMIEEE), and holds memberships in several esteemed organizations, including CSI, CRSI, ACM, IAENG, CSTA, IACSIT, and ICSE, reflecting his wide-ranging influence and commitment to the field. Dr. Shadab Alam's editorial achievements include serving as an Academic Editor for several renowned journals: PLOS ONE, Computational and Mathematical Methods in Medicine, Computational and Mathematical Methods, Security and Communication Networks, and Journal of Computational and Cognitive Engineering. These roles are facilitated through collaborations with publishers like Hindawi, John Wiley & Sons, Inc., and BON VIEW PUBLISHING PTE. LTD, Singapore, signify his expertise and influence in the field.

Kishor Kumar Reddy C. is currently working as Associate Professor, Dept. of Computer Science and Engineering, Stanley College of Engineering and Technology for Women, Hyderabad, India. He has research and teaching experience of more than 13 years. He has published more than 90 research papers in National and International Conferences, Book Chapters, and Journals indexed by Scopus and others. He is an author for 2 text books and 15 edited books. He is the member of ISTE, CSI, IAENG, UACEE, IACSIT.

A. Rajaram He received the B.E. degree in Electronics and Communication Engineering from the Government College of Technology, Coimbatore, Anna University, Chennai. He received the M.E. degree in Electronics and Communication Engineering (Applied Electronics) from the Government College of Technology, Anna University, Chennai. He received the Full Time Ph.D. degree in Electronics and Communication Engineering from the Anna University of Technology, Coimbatore. He is currently working as a Professor, ECE Department in E.G.S. Pillay Engineering College, Nagapattinam, India. His research interests include Mobile Ad Hoc networks, wireless communication networks (WiFi, WiMax HighSlot GSM), novel VLSI NOC Design approaches to address issues such as low-power, cross-talk, hardware acceleration,Design issues includes OFDM MIMO and noise Suppression in MAI Systems, ASIC design, Control systems, Fuzzy logic and Networks, AI, Sensor Networks. He has published more SCIE indexed journals

***

Sultan Ahmad has been associated with the Department of Computer Science, College of Computer Engineering and Sciences, Prince Sattam Bin Abdulaziz University, Alkharj, Saudi Arabia. He is also an Adjunct Professor with Chandigarh University, Gharuan, Punjab, India. He received his Master of computer science and applications from Aligarh Muslim University, India, in 2006, and the Ph.D. degree in CSE from Glocal University. He has more than 18 years of teaching and research experience. He has around 130 accepted and published research papers and book chapters in reputed SCI, SCIE, ESCI, and SCOPUS-indexed journals and conferences. He also serves as Guest Editor for SCIE/ESCI/SCOPUS indexed journals. He has an Australian, a Chinese, an Indian and two UK design patent in his name. He has authored and edited 5 books on cutting-edge topics. His research has also secured funding from national and international projects. He also took up the roles of resource person and technical panel member and headed several international conferences. He has presented his research papers at many national and international conferences. He has been an integral part of accreditation processes in the university such as ABET and NCAAA. His research interests include Intelligent computing, data Science, machine learning, and the Internet of Things. He is a member of IEEE, IACSIT and the Computer Society of India

Harishchander Anandaram completed a PhD in bioengineering, an M.Tech., and a B.Tech. in bioinformatics from the Sathyabama Institute of Science and Technology, Chennai, in 2020, 2011, and 2009. In his bachelor's and master's theses, he worked on analysing resistance in HIV protease inhibitors based on molecular mechanics and machine learning studies, a collaborative project with IIT Madras. In his PhD thesis, he worked on pharmacogenomics and miRNA-regulated networks in psoriasis, a collaborative project with Georgetown University, USA; JIPMER, India; CIBA, India; and ILS, India. His thesis illustrated a multi-disciplinary approach by combining computational biophysics and molecular biology machine learning. While doing a PhD, he had the opportunity to collaborate with international researchers and have publications in reputed international journals in bioinformatics and systems biology. He has received the prestigious "Young Scientist Award" from "The Melinda Gates Foundation" for his research abstract on "The Implications of miRNA Dynamics in Infectious Diseases.". To date, he has reviewed more than 200 manuscripts in systems biology.

B. Arunsundar, Assistant Professor Department of Data Science and Business Systems, School of Computing, Faculty of Engineering and Technology, SRM Institute of Science and Technology, Kattankulathur, Chennai-603203

T.R.Chenthil, was born in Nagercoil on 31st May 1985. He received his Bachelor Degree in Electronics and communication Engineering, from St.Xavier's Catholic College of Engineering, Chunkankadai, Kanyakumari District,Tamilnadu. India in the year 2006. He received his Masters Degree in APPLIED ELECTRONICS from St.Joseph's College of Engineering, Chennai, Tamilnadu, India in the year 2008, and Ph.D degrees in Electronics Engineering from Sathyabama University, Chennai, Tamilnadu, India in the year 2023. He is working as Associate Professor and Head in Department of Artificial Intelligence & Data Science in Jeppiaar Engineering College, Chennai. His interested areas of research are wireless communication, wireless sensor network, Underwater wireless sensor Networks, Low Power VLSI Design and Mixed Signal circuits. He has Research publications in SCI, WEB OF SCIENCE and SCOPUS National / International Journals / Conferences.

Vishal Eswaran is an accomplished Senior Big Data Engineer with an impressive career spanning over 6 years. His fervor for constructing robust data pipelines, unearthing insights from intricate datasets, identifying trends, and predicting future trajectories has fueled his journey. Throughout his tenure, Vishal has lent his expertise to empower numerous prominent US healthcare clients, including CVS Health, Aetna, and Blue Cross and Blue Shield of North Carolina, with informed business decisions drawn from expansive datasets. Vishal's ability to distill intricate data into comprehensive documents and reports stands as a testament to his proficiency in managing multifaceted internal and external data analysis responsibilities. His aptitude for synthesizing complex information ensures that insights are both accessible and impactful for strategic decision-making. Moreover, Vishal's distinction extends to his role as a co-author of the book "Internet of Things - Future Connected Devices." This book not only underscores his prowess in the field but also showcases his visionary leadership in the realm of Internet of Things (IoT). His insights resonate with a forward-looking perspective, emphasizing the convergence of technology and human life. As the author of "Secure Connections: Safeguarding the Internet of Things (IoT) with Cybersecurity," Vishal Eswaran's reputation as a thought leader is further solidified. His work is a manifestation of his commitment to ensuring the security of interconnected devices within the IoT landscape, a vital consideration in our digitally driven world. Vishal's dedication to enhancing the safety and integrity of IoT ecosystems shines through in his work.

Vivek Eswaran, With 8 years of experience as a Senior Software Engineer specializing in front-end development, Vivek Eswaran brings a vital perspective to securing the Internet of Things (IoT). At Medallia, Vivek played an instrumental role in crafting engaging user interfaces and optimized digital experiences. This profound expertise in front-end engineering equips them to illuminate the crucial synergy between usability and cybersecurity as IoT adoption accelerates. In the new book "Secure Connections: Safeguarding the Internet of Things with Cybersecurity," Vivek combines their real-world experiences building intuitive and secure software systems with cutting-edge insights into strengthening IoT ecosystems. Drawing parallels between front-end best practices and security imperatives, they offer readers an invaluable guide for fortifying IoT without compromising usability. As businesses and consumers continue rapidly connecting people, processes, and devices, Vivek's contribution provides timely insights. Blending user empathy with security proficiency, Vivek empowers audiences to realize the potential of IoT through resilient and human-centered systems designed for safety without friction.

Ushaa Eswaran is the Principal and Professor at Mahalakshmi Tech Campus in Chennai, Tamil Nadu, India. With over 34 years of experience in academia, she is a distinguished author, researcher, and educator. Dr. Eswaran is also a proud recipient of the REX Karmaveer Global Fellowship and the Karmaveer Chakra PLATINUM MEDAL Award. Her academic foundation is in Electronics Engineering, and she has made significant contributions to the field of biosensors, pioneering work that led to her earning a Doctorate. She has published more than 80 papers in reputed journals, authored 44 chapters in various books, and has 26 Scopus-indexed publications. Dr. Eswaran is the co-author of several acclaimed books, including "The Internet of Things: The Future of Connected Devices," published by Euphoria Publishers in 2023, and "Secure Connections: Safeguarding the Internet of Things (IoT) with Cyber Security," published by Sarvad Publication in the same year. In 2024, she co-authored "Converging Technologies: The Intersection of IoTs, AI, ML, DL, Cloud Computing, Blockchain, Data Science, AR, VR, and 3D Printing," along with "AI-Integrated Biosensors and Technologies for Automated Disease Detection and Drug Delivery," which is currently under process with Taylor & Francis Group. She is also working on an upcoming title, "AI-Driven Revolution: Transforming the Skies and Roads." Dr. Eswaran is passionate about equipping the younger generation with knowledge grounded in ethical principles. Her work serves as a beacon of practical wisdom in the evolving IoT landscape, shedding light on its future societal impacts. Her scholarly contributions are further evidenced by her ORCID identifier (0000-0002-5116-3403), highlighting her prolific research journey. Through her dedication to academic excellence and holistic student development, Dr. Ushaa Eswaran continues to explore the dynamic interface between technology and human values, ensuring her contributions significantly impact the field.

Shugufta Fatima is an Assistant Professor in the Department of Computer Science and Engineering at Stanley College of Engineering and Technology for Women in Hyderabad, India. With eight years of teaching experience, she brings a unique perspective to the academic community. She earned her Bachelor's and Master's degrees in Computer Science and Engineering from Osmania University. Her academic journey has been marked by excellence, as evidenced by her receipt of Academic Excellence awards throughout her studies. Her dedication to advancing knowledge in her areas of interest, which include Machine Learning, Deep Learning, and Artificial Intelligence, is reflected in her research and teaching, and she is committed to further exploration in these fields. Through her research, teaching, and community engagement efforts, she is making valuable contributions to both the academic community and society at large. She has published book chapters, research papers in reputable academic journals that have received significant citations, serves as a book chapter reviewer with IGI Global, and has guided students in their projects. She also holds a patent in her name. She has conducted numerous national-level workshops, organized events, and participated in conferences and faculty development programs on a large scale. As an educator, she is dedicated to fostering critical thinking and intellectual curiosity in her students. She believes in creating an inclusive learning environment where students feel empowered to engage with complex ideas and develop their analytical skills through mentoring sessions. By employing innovative teaching methods and real-world examples, she strives to inspire a passion for learning among her students.

Gaurav Gupta is an esteemed Associate Professor at the Yogananda School of Artificial Intelligence, Computers, and Data Science, within the Faculty of Engineering & Technology at Shoolini University, Solan, Himachal Pradesh, India . In his role, Dr. Gupta is dedicated to both teaching and conducting pioneering research in the field of machine learning, with a particular focus on its applications in healthcare and agriculture. Dr. Gupta commenced his academic journey with a Bachelor of Engineering degree in 2006 from Dr. B.R. Ambedkar University, Agra, Uttar Pradesh, followed by a Postgraduate degree in 2011, and a Ph.D. in Computer Science Engineering in 2019 from KSOU-VIT, Karnataka, and Shoolini University, respectively. With over 18+ years of rich teaching/research experience, Dr. Gupta has made significant academic contributions that span across international scientific papers, reviews, book chapters, and both edited and authored books, with publications recognized by prestigious entities such as IEEE, Elsevier, Springer Nature, Taylor & Francis, and Wiley. Furthermore, Dr. Gupta has published over 15+ books with renowned national and international publishers.

Md. Alimul Haque is currently working as Assistant Professor in the Department of Computer Science, Veer Kunwar Singh University, Ara, India. He received his Bachelor and Master degree in Computer Application in 2004 and 2008 respectively and the Ph.D. Degree on "Security and Privacy aspects on Wireless Communication Networks" from V. K. S. University, Ara, India in 2017. His research interests include cyber security, wireless communication networks, IoT and Artificial Intelligence. He has served as a reviewer in many international journals such as the International Journal of Web-Based Learning and Teaching Technologies (IJWLTT) - IGI Global, Elsevier and IEEE Sensors Journals. He has published multi-focused research articles, and his research has led to numerous papers in peer-reviewed journals (Elsevier, Springer, IEEE and IGI) of the world. He has authored book on Blockchain that are available on Amazon. He has been a Life member of ISCA, Kolkata, India and the International Association of Engineers (IAENG), Hong Kong.

Madiha Munawar, a second-year Computer Science and Engineering (CSE) student with a keen interest in software engineering and research. I have contributed to book chapters on emerging technologies and have also participated as a reviewer, critically reviewing book chapters, and am looking forward to conducting more research and publishing chapters, conference papers and journal articles. With a deep passion for coding, I actively explore diverse programming languages and innovative problem-solving techniques. I have participated in International conference and presented my paper in that, also in coding competitions and contributed to book chapters on emerging technologies. Driven by an insatiable thirst for knowledge, I aspire to create impactful software solutions that address real-world challenges with efficiency and creativity.

Keerthna Murali, With over 5 years of experience as a Site Reliability Engineer at Dell, Keerthna Murali has honed an intricate expertise in maintaining and optimizing robust digital infrastructures. On the frontlines of ensuring seamless online experiences, Keerthna specialized in troubleshooting complex issues and proactively enhancing system performance and availability. These capabilities uniquely position them to tackle the critical challenge of security for rapidly emerging IoT ecosystems. In their new book "Secure Connections," Keerthna channels their real-world experiences maintaining enterprise-scale platforms into a compelling vision for building security into the foundation of IoT systems. Blending software engineering best practices with cybersecurity insights, they offer a prescient guide for developers, IT leaders, and security experts seeking to realize IoT's potential while mitigating its risks.

Keerthy N, Assistant Professor, Department of Electronics & Communication Engineering Global Academy of Technology, Aditya Layout, Rajarajeshwari Nagar, Bengaluru, Karnataka 560098.

Jagadeshwari Puttanapura is a dedicated Computer Science and Engineering student at Stanley College of Engineering and Technology for Women, India. With a keen interest in software development, machine learning, and data science, she have consistently demonstrated strong academic performance and a passion for technology. She has actively participated in several coding competitions, securing top positions in contests.

D Prabakar, Assistant Professor, Department of Data Science and Business Systems, School of Computing, Faculty of Engineering and Technology, SRM Institute of Science and Technology, Kattankulathur, Chennai-603203, India.

Nirmalkumar S. Benni, Associate Professor, Department of Information Science & Engineering, RNS Institute of Technology, R R Nagar Post, Channasandra, Bengaluru - 560 098, Karnataka, India.

Satyajeet Sahoo, Department of ECE, Vignan's Foundation for Science, Technology and Research, Vadlamudi, Guntur, AP-522213, India.

Wasswa Shafik (Member, IEEE) received a Bachelor of Science degree in information technology from Ndejje University, Uganda, a Master of Engineering degree in Information Technology (Computer and Communication Networks) from Yazd University, Iran, and a PhD in Computer Science with the School of Digital Science, Universiti Brunei Darussalam, Brunei Darussalam. He is also the Founder and Research Director of the Dig Connectivity Research Laboratory (DCRLab) after serving as a Research Associate at the Network Interconnectivity Research Laboratory at Yazd University. Prior to this, he worked as a Community Data Analyst at Population Services International (PSI-Uganda), a Community Data Officer at the Programme for Accessible Health Communication (PACE-Uganda), a Research Assistant at the Socio-Economic Data Centre (SEDC-Uganda), Uganda, an Assistant Data Officer at TechnoServe, Kampala, Uganda, and Asmaah Charity Organization as Cheif Executive Officer. He has hundreds of publications with renowned publishers. His research interests include Artificial Intelligence, Smart Agriculture, Digital Health, Green Computing, Security and Privacy.

T. Monika Singh holds an M.Tech in Computer Science and Engineering from Osmania University and is currently pursuing a Ph.D. in the same field at KL University. Since 2017, she has been a faculty member in the Computer Science and Engineering Department at Stanley College of Engineering and Technology for Women. With a rich background in teaching and research, she is also a certified project-based learning mentor by Wipro and holds a TalentNext certification in Java Full Stack development. Her research interests focus on Machine Learning, and she has published several papers in national and international journals. Additionally, she holds a patent to her name.

K. Suganthi, Department of Electronics & Communication Engineering, Faculty of Engineering and Technology, SRM Institute of Science and Technology, Kattangulathur, Chengalpattu District, Tamil, Nadu - 603 203, India.

Index

I

M

N

O

P

R

S

T

W

www.ingramcontent.com/pod-product-compliance
Lightning Source LLC
LaVergne TN
LVHW080534300926
849162LV00007B/1607
* 9 7 9 8 3 3 7 3 1 0 2 2 0 *